MELANOMA IN THE CLINIC – DIAGNOSIS, MANAGEMENT AND COMPLICATIONS OF MALIGNANCY

Edited by **Mandi Murph**

Melanoma in the Clinic – Diagnosis, Management and Complications of Malignancy
Edited by Mandi Murph

Published by InTech
Janeza Trdine 9, 51000 Rijeka, Croatia

Technical Editor Sonja Mujacic

Cover Designer InTech Design Team

Additional hard copies can be obtained from orders@intechopen.com

Melanoma in the Clinic – Diagnosis, Management and Complications of Malignancy,
Edited by Mandi Murph
p. cm.
ISBN 978-953-307-571-6

For EU product safety concerns:
IN TECH d.o.o., Prolaz Marije Krucifikse Kozulić 3, 51000 Rijeka, Croatia,
info@intechopen.com or visit our website at intechopen.com.

Meet the editor

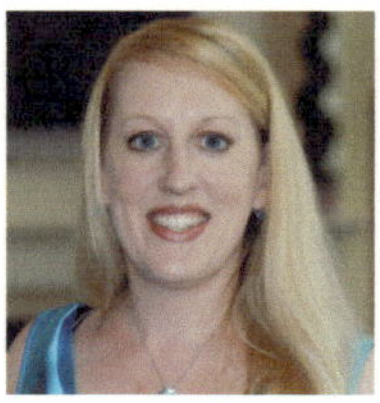

Mandi Murph is a Georgia Cancer Coalition Scholar and an Assistant Professor in the College of Pharmacy at the University of Georgia in Athens, Georgia. Before coming to Georgia, Murph was a postdoctoral fellow in Systems Biology at the University of Texas M.D. Anderson Cancer Center in Houston. She won a young investigator award from the Biochemical Journal. She is an author on publications in Cancer Cell, Molecular Cancer, Journal of the National Cancer Institute, Molecular Cancer Research, PLoS ONE, Clinical Cancer Research and the Journal of Biological Chemistry. She has received grant funding from the Georgia Cancer Coalition and the National Cancer Institute, which is part of the National Institutes of Health.

Contents

Preface

Melanoma Oncologists who have in the past struggled with resolving how best to treat their patients given the few effective therapeutics available are now beginning to confront the disease directly. These new tools are likely to change clinical practice surrounding melanoma.

In the first section of this book, several manuscripts discuss imaging techniques for diagnosis – currently the best way to cure melanoma early before it develops into a late - stage, metastatic disease. Further, this book discusses the clinical aspects of melanoma treatment in surgery and long-term management. Acral, cutaneous and mucosal melanomas are represented in this book, along with some rather unusual clinical observations. As such, it provides insight into rare case studies only observed by a few clinicians. When most people consider melanoma, it is likely to be regarded as cutaneous melanoma derived by overexposure to a lifetime of UV radiation. In contrast, manuscripts presented here discuss melanoma in the gastrointestinal tract, genito-urinary tract, female genital tract, pulmonary metastases, familial mutations leading to melanoma, canine melanoma and melanoma in pregnancy. It is a fascinating representation of the diversity of clinical cases that exist globally.

Again, I have to thank several outstanding people, without whom this would not have otherwise been possible – Ana Pantar, Petra Nenadic, Juliet Eneh and Molly Altman. These people helped me throughout this process. In addition, I would also like to thank my loving spouse, Gary Rollie, who is always a supportive champion of my career. This past year he listened to me say that, "This will only take a few more minutes," knowing that it wasn't true, but understanding that at some point I would finish. And I did.

I hope you enjoy reading this book as much as I did.

Sincerely,

Mandi Murph, Ph.D.
Assistant Professor
Department of Pharmaceutical and Biomedical Sciences
University of Georgia
College of Pharmacy
Athens, GA, USA

Part 1

Melanoma Models and Diagnostic Techniques

1

Acral Melanoma: Clinical, Biologic and Molecular Genetic Characteristics

Minoru Takata
Department of Dermatology, Okayama University Postgraduate School of Medical, Dentistry, and Pharmaceutical Sciences Japan

1. Introduction

Acral melanomas (AM) is a distinct subtype of melanoma affecting the palms, soles and nail apparatuses. It is mostly identical to acral lentiginous melanoma according to Clark's classification (Clark et al., 1986), but it may also include nodular melanoma and superficial spreading melanoma that developed on glabrous skin and nail apparatus (Curtin et al., 2005). While AM is the least frequent subtype of cutaneous melanoma overall in Caucasians, it is the most prevalent type of melanoma in people of color. Prognosis of AM is generally poor, which may be in part due to delay in diagnosis (Bradford et al., 2009).

The distinct histological and phenotypic characteristics suggest that AM might differ biologically from other types of cutaneous melanomas. Recent molecular genetic studies characterized AM as a unique type of melanoma showing higher frequency of chromosomal aberrations, especially focused amplifications of particular chromosome regions (Bastian et al., 2000; Curtin et al., 2005). Furthermore, recent discovery of frequent mutation or amplification of *KIT* gene in AM and mucosal melanoma has led to the molecular targeted therapy by approved drugs targeting KIT, such as imatinib, for advanced cases (Curtin et al., 2006). This would represent a first decisive step toward the individualized treatment of melanoma (Garrido &Bastian, 2010)

2. Epidemiology

Although AM accounts for 5% of all melanomas in the United States (Markovic et al., 2007)(Table 1), it is a predominant form of melanoma in individuals with darker skin (ie, Blacks, Asians and Hispanics) (Cormier et al., 2006). The proportion of AM among all melanoma subtypes is greatest in blacks followed by Asians/Pacific islanders and Hispanic whites (Bradford et al., 2009). The nation-wide survey in Japan shows that AM accounts for 41% of all melanomas (Ishihara et al., 2008)(Table 1), the rate being almost the same in Chinese (Chi et al., 2011). However, the absolute incidence of AM in darker-skinned individuals is similar to that in whites (Stevens et al., 1990; Bradford et al., 2009), who have a much higher incidence of melanoma overall due to the strong susceptibility to sunlight (Cormier et al., 2006). Thus, carcinogens other than ultraviolet light (UVL) equally affecting all ethnic groups or endogenous mutagenesis may play a role in the development of AM. Trauma may have a role in AM development, since 13% to 25% of patients with AM reported prelesional trauma, such as puncture wounds, friction blisters and stone bruises (Coleman et al., 1980; Phan et al.,

2006). The mean age at diagnosis of AM is 62.8 years, compared with 58.5 years for cutaneous melanoma overall. Incidence of AM significantly increases with each year of advancing age, which is seen across the different racial groups (Bradford et al., 2009).

Type of Melanoma[1)]	United States (Markovic et al., 2007)	Japan (Ishihara et al., 2008)
SSM	70%	17%
NM	5%	20%
LMM	4~15%	7%
ALM	5%	41%
Unknown	5~11%	13%

[1)]SSM, superficial spreading melanoma; NM, nodular melanoma; LMM, lentigo maligna melanoma; ALM, acral lentiginous melanoma

Table 1. Comparison of melanoma types between the United States and Japan.

Although acral volar skin and nail beds constitutes only a few % of skin surface, the fact that nearly half of cutaneous melanomas arise on these anatomical sites in darker-skinned individuals indicates that these are predilection sites of melanomas not causally related to UVL exposure. The melanocyte density in palmoplantar skin is five times lower than that found in nonpalmoplantar sites. Furthermore, the growth and differentiation of palmoplantar melanocytes are suppressed by dickkopf 1 (DKK1) secreted from dermal fibroblasts through the down-regulation of microphthalmia-associated transcription factor (MITF) and beta-catenin (Yamaguchi et al., 2004). The reason why such growth-suppressed melanocytes in palmoplantar skin are more susceptible to melanoma development is currently unknown.

3. Clinical features

Clinically, AMs on palms and soles begin with irregularly pigmented macular lesions. The soles of the feet are most commonly involved. Morphological characteristics of early AM lesions include variable shades of brown from tan to black color, irregular and asymmetric shape often accompanied by notching at the periphery, and over 7mm in diameter (Saida, 1989) (Fig. 1a).

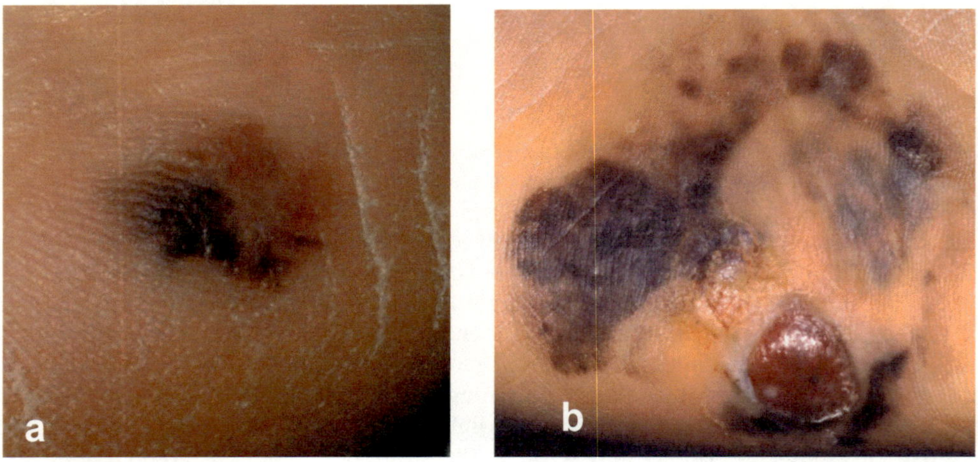

Fig. 1. Clinical pictures of radial growth phase (a) and tumorgenic vertical growth phase (b) of AM.

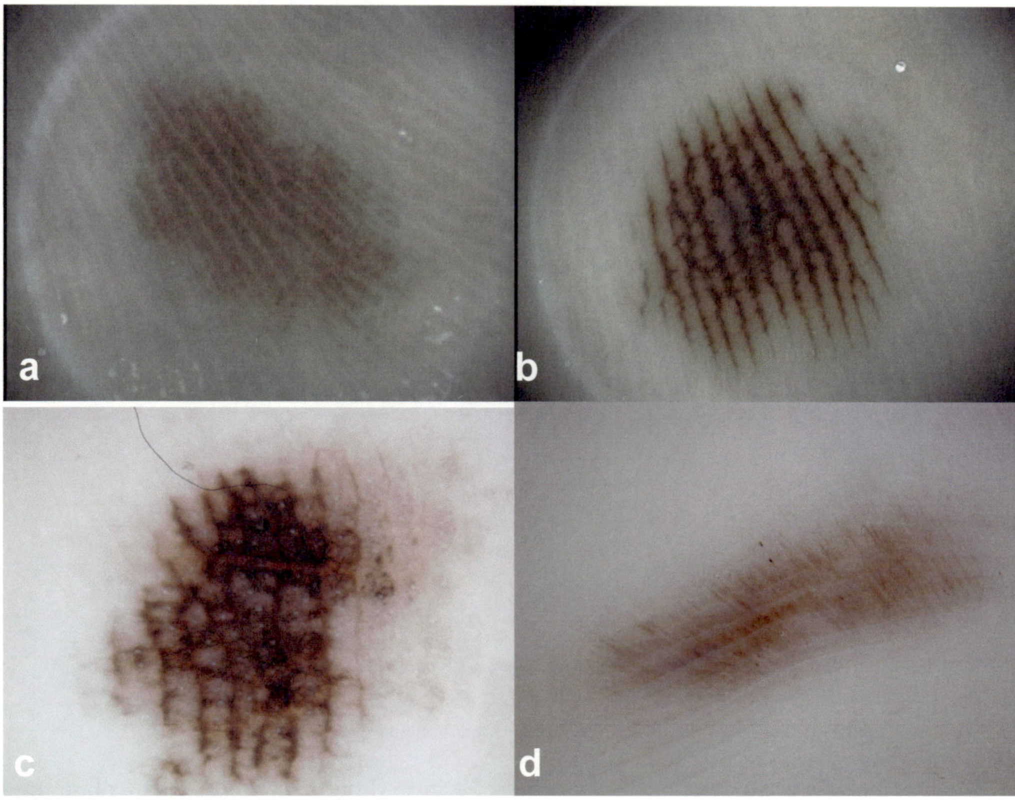

Fig. 2. Dermoscopy of early AM (a) and melanocytic nevus on acral volar skin (b, c, and d). a, palarelle ridge pattern; b, pararelle furrow pattern; c, lattice-like pattern; d, fibrillar pattern.

Dermoscopic observations of these early lesions show band-like pigmentation on ridges of the skin markings, designated as a "parallel ridge pattern"(Fig. 2a). This is in sharp contrast to the dermoscopic patterns in acral melanocytic nevi, which show parallel linear pigmentation along the sulci of the skin markings, designated as a "parallel furrow pattern"(Fig. 2b) and its variants "lattice-like pattern" (Fig. 2c) and "fibrillar pattern"(Fig. 2d) (Oguchi et al., 1998; Miyazaki et al., 2005). The sensitivity and specificity of the parallel ridge pattern in diagnosing early AM is 86% and 99%, respectively (Saida et al., 2004). A simple three-step algorism effectively discriminating early AM from acral melanocytic nevi has been proposed (Fig. 3) (Saida et al., 2011). This algorism classifies acquired pigmented lesions on acral volar skin by the dermoscopic findings and the maximal diameter, and recommends three management options including "no need to follow-up", "periodic follow-up", and "excision of the lesion for histopathological evaluation".

In contrast to the palmoplantar melanoma, nail apparatus melanoma more often affects fingers than the toes. The digits most commonly affected are the thumb followed by the great toe. If the AM is situated in the nail matrix, a longitudinal pigmented band of the nail plate is the earliest sign (Fig. 4a). As melanocytic nevi of the nail matrix also typically accompany longitudinal melanonychia, identifying early nail matrix melanoma is challenging. Dermoscopy again provides useful information for this differentiation. The suspicious dermoscopic features of early nail matrix melanoma are irregular lines on a brown background, pigmentation of the cuticle (micro-Hutchingson's sign), a wide pigmented band, and triangular pigmentation on the nail plate (Fig. 4b) (Koga et al., 2011).

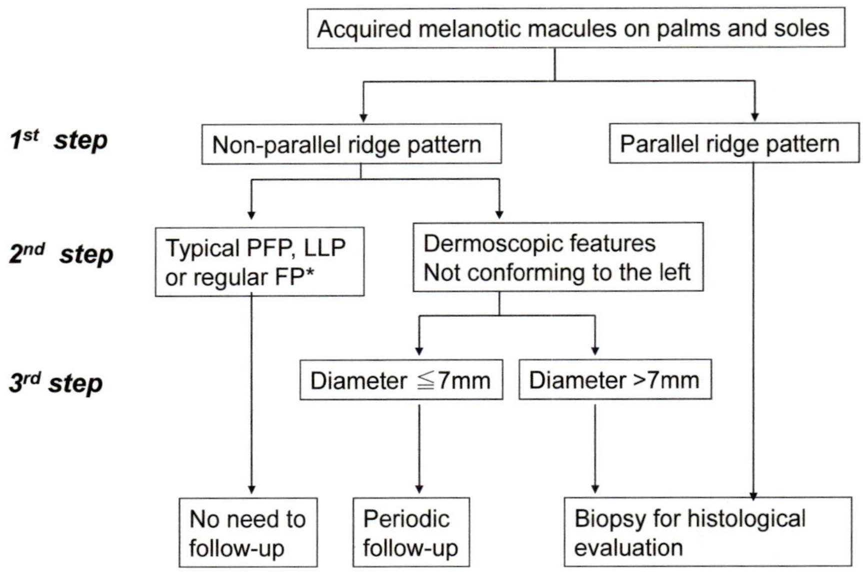

*PFP: parallel furrow pattern, LLP: lattice-like pattern, FP: fibrillar pattern

Fig. 3. Three-step algorism for the management of acquired pigmented lesions on plams and soles (Adapted from Saida et al., 2011, with permision).

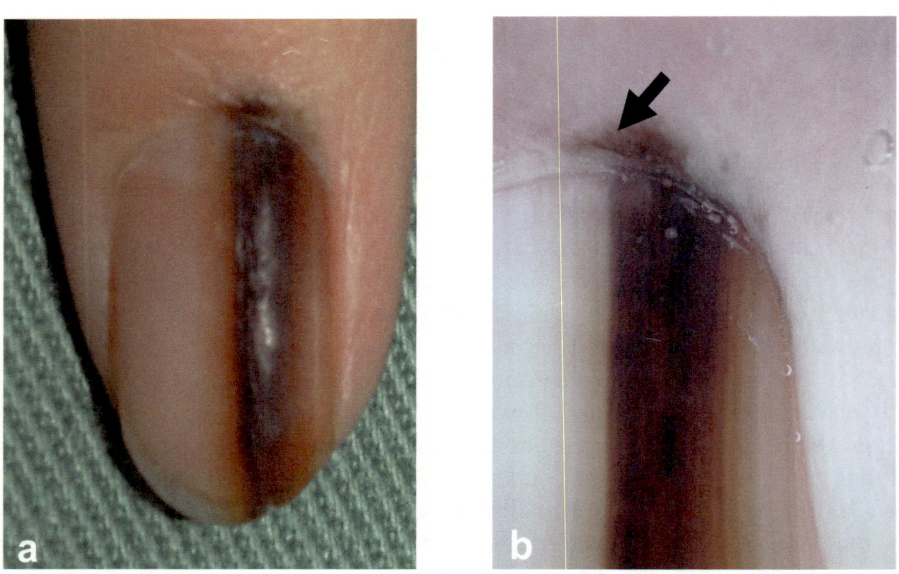

Fig. 4. Clinical (a) and dermoscopic (b) photographs of early nail matrix melanoma. The arrow indicates micro-Hutchingson's sign.

The tumorigenic vertical growth phase of palmoplantar melanoma is characterized by the development of a nodule often associated with ulceration (Fig. 1b). The development of a subungal tumor and the destruction of the nail plate are observed in the vertical growth phase of nail apparatus melanoma.

4. Histopathology

Histopathology of the earliest lesions of palmoplantar melanoma shows proliferation of solitary arranged slightly atypical melanocytes mainly detected in the crista profunda intermedia, the epidermal rete ridge underlying the ridges of the skin markings (Ishihara et al., 2006). In early nail apparatus melanoma, slightly atypical melanocytes proliferate in the epidermis of nail matrix. Eventually, large atypical melanocytes, frequently with prominent pigmented dendrites, proliferate as single cells in the basal layer of the hyperplastic epidermis while some tumor cells can be found in the upper layer of the epidermis. Nesting of melanocytes is not prominent, and tends to occur at the tips of the rete ridges. Brisk lichenoid lymphocytic infiltrate that may obscure the dermal-epidermal junction is common. In the vertical growth phase, atypical tumor cells are often spindle-shaped. Desmoplastic change is not uncommon (Clark et al., 1986).

5. Molecular genetics

There exists clinical heterogeneity in cutaneous melanoma with different susceptibility to UVL, which may be explained by differences in somatic genetic changes. Recent molecular genetic investigations have revealed that melanomas from intermittently sun-exposed skin, most of which are located on trunk and extremities, show frequent mutations in either *BRAF* or *NRAS* gene. In contrast, *BRAF* or *NRAS* mutations are rather infrequent in melanomas arising from sun-protected areas, such as acral skin, nail apparatus and mucosa (Table 2). Instead, these types of melanomas show a higher degree of chromosomal aberrations; specifically, genomic amplifications involving small portions of chromosome arms (Curtin et al., 2005). In AM, the most frequently amplified region is chromosome 11q13 which contains the *cyclin D1* gene. Narrow amplifications of other chromosome regions, including 4q12, 5p15, 11q14 and 22q11-13, are also found (Bastian et al., 2000). Target genes of 4q12 and 11q14 amplifications appear to be *KIT* and *GAB2*, respectively (Curtin et al., 2006; Chernoff et al., 2009).

	Acral melanomas	Melanomas from intermittently sun-exposed skin	Reference
BRAF	23% mutated	59% mutated	(Curtin et al., 2005)
NRAS	10% mutated	22% mutated	(Curtin et al., 2005)
KIT	14% mutated 24% amplified	0% mutated 0% amplified	(Curtin et al., 2006)
Cyclin D1	44% amplified	5% amplified	(Sauter et al., 2002)
GAB2	19% amplified	3% amplified[a]	(Chernoff et al., 2009)

[a] including one melanoma on face

Table 2. Comparison of somatic genetic changes between acral melanomas and melanomas from intermittently sun-exposed skin.

Cyclin D1 positively regulates the activity of cyclin dependent kinases, leading to phosphorylation of retinoblastoma protein promoting entry into mitosis, and acts as an oncogene (reviewed in (Tashiro et al., 2007)). Interestingly, while gene amplifications are usually found in association with disease progression in other cancers, *cyclin D1* gene amplifications in AM are detected early in the radial growth phase (Bastian et al., 2000). Furthermore, copy number increase of *cyclin D1* gene was observed even in normal-looking melanocytes in the epidermis beyond the histopathologically recognizable margin of melanoma (Bastian et al., 2000; North et al., 2008), as well as in very early acral melanoma *in situ* lesions, which shows slight increase of non-atypical melanocytes in the basal cell layer of the epidermis (Yamaura et al., 2005). These genetically aberrant cells with normal morphology are " field cells" (Bastian, 2003), which represent a latent progression phase that precedes the stage of atypical melanocyte proliferation in the epidermis. These observations suggest that amplification of the *cyclin D1* gene might be one of the earliest events in AM development. The presence of amplifications, however, indicates that other aberrations likely cause genomic instability (North et al., 2008). Investigations in a radial growth phase AM cell line SMYM-PRGP harboring *cyclin D1* amplification (Fig. 5) suggest that overly expressed cyclin D1 protein may act as a survival factor (Murata et al., 2007). While the progressive increase of the *cyclin D1* copy number from normal-looking melanocytes to the *in situ* portion to the invasive melanoma was observed, suggesting that the increased *cyclin D1* gene dosage confers a growth advantage during later stages of tumor progression (North et al., 2008), this may simply reflect the increase of genomic instability associated with melanoma progression (Takata et al., 2010).

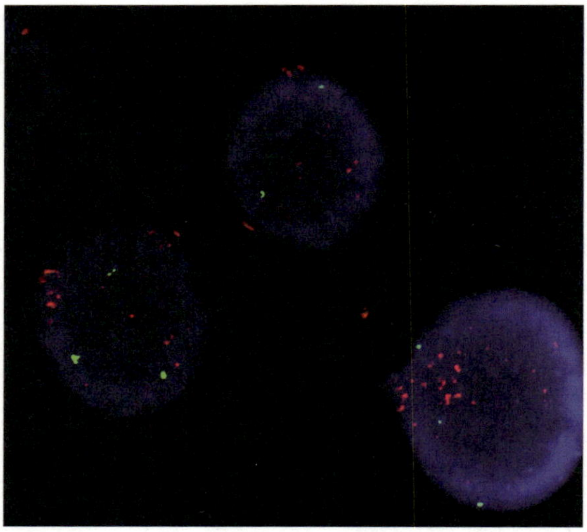

Fig. 5. Amplification of the *cyclin D1* gene in radial growth phase acral melanoma cell line SMYM-PRGP (Murata et al., 2007). Green signals, chromosome 11 centromere; red signals, *cyclin D1*.

While mutations of the *BRAF* and *NRAS* genes are infrequent in AM, a substantial number of AM harbor mutations or amplifications of the *KIT* gene encoding a receptor tyrosine kinase (Curtin et al., 2006). Recent studies have revealed *KIT* mutations and amplification in 14% and 24% of AMs, respectively (Table 2) (Woodman &Davies, 2010). About 30% of the tumors with *KIT* mutations also show increased copy number/amplification of *KIT*. The *KIT* mutations identified in AM differ from those found in gastrointestinal stromal tumors (GIST). The majority of *KIT* mutations in GIST are deletions or insertions, whereas those found in melanoma are substitution mutations. In addition, *KIT* mutations are not present in exon 9, which is the location of 15% of *KIT* mutations in GIST. More than half of *KIT* mutations in melanoma are found in exon 11, which encodes juxtamembrane domain of KIT receptor, whereas mutations are also found in exons 13, 17 and 18 encoding kinase domains (Woodman &Davies, 2010).

GAB2 is a scaffolding protein that mediates interactions with various signaling pathways including RAS-RAF-ERK and PI3K-AKT signaling, and is a critical molecule for melanoma progression (Horst et al., 2009). A recent study found *GAB2* amplification in 5 of 23 (19%) AMs, while amplifications were rare in other types of cutaneous melanomas (Table 2). The majority of *GAB2* amplification occurred independent from genetic alterations in *BRAF, NRAS, KIT* and *cyclin D1*, suggesting a critical role of *GAB2* in a subset of AM (Chernoff et al., 2009).

6. Molecular targeted therapy

Since *KIT* mutations are detected in ~15% of AM, KIT is a promising molecular target of metastatic AM. Several *in vitro* experiments using melanoma cell lines harboring *KIT* mutations have actually shown significant growth suppressive effects of small molecular KIT inhibitors, such as imatinib, which are already approved for other cancers. Imatinib dramatically decreased proliferation, and was cytotoxic to a mucosal melanoma cell line demonstrating a highly amplified *KIT* exon 11 V559D mutation (Jiang et al., 2008). In contrast, cell viability of another melanoma cell line with *KIT* exon 11 L576P mutation, the most common *KIT* mutation in melanoma (34%) (Woodman &Davies, 2010), was not reduced by imatinib. However, dasatinib reduced cell viability of this cell line at concentrations as low as 10nM. Molecular modeling studies found that the L576P mutation induces structural changes in KIT that reduce the affinity for imatinib but not for dasatinib (Woodman et al., 2009). An acral melanoma cell line with non-amplified *KIT* exon 17 D820Y was also resistant to imatinib treatment. The *KIT* D820Y mutation usually arises as a secondary mutation in the setting of imatinib treatment in GIST, which was shown to be sensitive to sunitinib. As expected, treatment of the *KIT* D820Y cell line with 1 μM of sunitinib showed modest reduction in cell proliferation. (Ashida et al., 2009).

Clinically, dramatic response to imatinib therapy has been observed in several sporadic cases with metastatic acral and mucosal melanomas with *KIT* mutations, such as exon 13 K642E, 7-codon duplication in exon 11, and exon 11 V599A (Hodi et al., 2008; Lutzky et al., 2008; Terheyden et al., 2010). However, gene amplification and overexpression of wild-type *KIT*, which is frequently present in acral and mucosal melanomas (Woodman &Davies, 2010), did not translate into clinical efficacy of imatinib (Hofmann et al., 2009). Consistent with an *in vitro* study, metastatic melanoma patients with the *KIT* L576P mutation showed marked reduction (>50%) and elimination of tumor F18-fluorodeoxyglucose (FDG)-avidity by positron emission tomography(PET) imaging after dasatinib treatment (Woodman &Davies, 2010). Partial response by dasatinib was also observed in a patient with the *KIT* exon 13 K642E mutation (Kluger et al., 2010).

Three phase-II trials of imatinib in unselected metastatic melanomas were mostly disappointing, and highlighted the importance of proper patient selection (Ugurel et al., 2005; Wyman et al., 2006; Kim et al., 2008). There are currently three ongoing clinical trials prospectively testing imatinib in selected patients with melanoma showing *KIT* mutations or amplifications (mostly acral and mucosal melanomas)(Table 3). The NCT00470470 trial selected stage III or IV patients with somatic mutations in *KIT*. Of the 12 evaluable patients, 2 demonstrated a complete response. Of note, these two patients had both amplification and mutation of *KIT*. A partial response was observed in two patients. All but two, who had mutations known to be resistant to imatinib in GIST, of the remaining patients had stable disease (Carvajal et al., 2009). In another phase-II trial of imatinib in patients with advanced melanoma from acral skin, mucosa or chronically sun-damaged skin (NCT00424515), five of ten patients with *KIT* mutations demonstrated a partial response. In contrast, none of the ten patients who had wild-type/amplified *KIT* showed a clinical response (Fisher et al., 2010). In the NCT00881049 trial which recruited Chinese patients with metastatic melanoma harboring *KIT* aberrations, a rate of 20% partial response and 40% stable disease was achieved, with 60% overall disease control rate (Guo et al., 2010). These results show clinical benefit of imatinib in a proportion of molecularly selected patients.

	Phase	NCT number	*KIT* aberrations required for eligibility
Imatinib	2	00470470	Mutation or amplification
Imatinib	2	00424515	Mutation or amplification
Imatinib	2	00881049	Mutation or amplification
Imatinib and temozolomide	1/2	00667953	Mutation
Nilotinib	2	00788775	Mutation or amplification
Nilotinib and dacarbazine	3	01028222	Mutation
Sunitinib	2	00631618	Mutation or amplification
Sunitinib	2	00577382	None
Dasatinib	2	00700882	None
Dasatinib and dacarbazine	1/2	00597038	None

Table 3. Clinical trials of KIT inhibitors for melanoma (Modified from Romano et al., 2011).

Nilotinib is a second-generation tyrosine kinase inhibitor of KIT, PDGFR and BCR-ABL. Nilotinib is potent as imatinib against mutant *KIT*, and is significantly more potent than imatinib against wild-type *KIT*. A phase-II trial of nilotinib in patients with melanoma characterized by a *KIT* mutation or amplification is ongoing, and a randomized phase-III, open-label study to compare the efficacy of nilotinib versus dacarbazine for treatment of patients with metastatic melanoma harboring a *KIT* mutation has been initiated. Phase-II trials testing other tyrosine kinase inhibitors targeting KIT, such as sunitinib and dasatinib, for melanoma are also ongoing (Table 3).

7. Conclusions

It is now clear that melanoma arises from multiple pathways, with initiating and promoting factors differing for each. Melanomas on intermittently sun-exposed skin preferentially affect Caucasians who have an inherently high propensity for melanocyte proliferation characterized by high nevus counts (Whiteman et al., 2003). Exposure to intense bursts of UVL radiation, especially in childhood, is the major risk factor. This type of melanomas may arise from pre-existing melanocytic nevus, and the mutation of the *BRAF* gene may be a key initiating somatic genetic event (Michaloglou et al., 2008). By contrast, AM arises *de novo*, and equally affects all ethnic groups. The first genetic aberration affecting normal melanocytes in acral volar skin would be one that disrupts the maintenance of genomic integrity. This would lead to the amplification of *cyclin D1* and the selection for clonal expansion of affected melanocytes. Then, acquiring activating mutations in oncogenes, such as *KIT* (Curtin et al., 2006), may be a crucial step inducing proliferation of transformed melanocytes (Takata et al., 2010). Understanding molecular pathogenesis in different types of melanomas will lead to the development of effective prevention and treatment strategies for individual patients.

8. Acknowledgments

The author's works were supported by the Grants-in-Aid for Cancer Research from the Ministry of Health, Labor, and Welfare of Japan (15–10 and 21S-7), Grants-in-Aid for Scientific Research from the Japan Society for the Promotion of Science (17659336 and 20591318), and a Management Expenses Grant from the Japanease Government to the National Cancer Center (21S-7(6)). I thank many colleagues who worked with me at the Department of Dermatology, Shinshu University, Japan, for their contributions to the studies of acral melanoma.

9. References

Ashida, A., Takata, M., Murata, H., Kido, K. & Saida, T. (2009). Pathological activation of KIT in metastatic tumors of acral and mucosal melanomas. *Int J Cancer,* Vol. 124, No. 4, pp. 862-868, ISSN 1097-0215

Bastian, B. C. (2003). Understanding the progression of melanocytic neoplasia using genomic analysis: from fields to cancer. *Oncogene,* Vol. 22, No. 20, pp. 3081-3086, ISSN 0950-9232

Bastian, B. C., Kashani-Sabet, M., Hamm, H., Godfrey, T., Moore, D. H., 2nd, Brocker, E. B., LeBoit, P. E. & Pinkel, D. (2000). Gene amplifications characterize acral melanoma and permit the detection of occult tumor cells in the surrounding skin. *Cancer Res,* Vol. 60, No. 7, pp. 1968-1973, ISSN 0008-5472

Bradford, P. T., Goldstein, A. M., McMaster, M. L. & Tucker, M. A. (2009). Acral lentiginous melanoma: incidence and survival patterns in the United States, 1986-2005. *Arch Dermatol,* Vol. 145, No. 4, pp. 427-434, ISSN 1538-3652

Carvajal, R. D., Chapman, P. B., Wolchok, J. D., Cane, L., Teitcher, J. B. & Lutzky, J. (2009). A phase II study of imatinib mesylate (IM) for patients with advanced melanoma harboring somatic alterations of KIT. *Proceedings of the American Society of Clinical Oncology*, Orlando, May-June, 2009.

Chernoff, K. A., Bordone, L., Horst, B., Simon, K., Twadell, W., Lee, K., Cohen, J. A., Wang, S., Silvers, D. N., Brunner, G. & Celebi, J. T. (2009). GAB2 amplifications refine molecular classification of melanoma. *Clin Cancer Res,* Vol. 15, No. 13, pp. 4288-4291, ISSN 1078-0432

Chi, Z., Li, S., Sheng, X., Si, L., Cui, C., Han, M., & Guo, J. (2011). Clinical presentation, histology, and prognosis of malignent melanoma in ethnic Chinese: A study of 522 consecutive cases. *BMC Cancer*, Vol. 11, pp. 85-94, ISSN 1471-2407

Clark, W. H., Jr., Elder, D. E. & Van Horn, M. (1986). The biologic forms of malignant melanoma. *Hum Pathol,* Vol. 17, No. 5, pp. 443-450, ISSN 0046-8177

Coleman, W. P., 3rd, Loria, P. R., Reed, R. J. & Krementz, E. T. (1980). Acral lentiginous melanoma. *Arch Dermatol,* Vol. 116, No. 7, pp. 773-776, ISSN 0003-987X

Cormier, J. N., Xing, Y., Ding, M., Lee, J. E., Mansfield, P. F., Gershenwald, J. E., Ross, M. I. & Du, X. L. (2006). Ethnic differences among patients with cutaneous melanoma. *Arch Intern Med,* Vol. 166, No. 17, pp. 1907-1914, ISSN 0003-9926

Curtin, J. A., Busam, K., Pinkel, D. & Bastian, B. C. (2006). Somatic activation of KIT in distinct subtypes of melanoma. *J Clin Oncol,* Vol. 24, No. 26, pp. 4340-4346, ISSN 1527-7755

Curtin, J. A., Fridlyand, J., Kageshita, T., Patel, H. N., Busam, K. J., Kutzner, H., Cho, K. H., Aiba, S., Brocker, E. B., LeBoit, P. E., Pinkel, D. & Bastian, B. C. (2005). Distinct sets of genetic alterations in melanoma. *N Engl J Med,* Vol. 353, No. 20, pp. 2135-2147, ISSN 1533-4406

Fisher, D. E., Barnhill, R., Hodi, F. S., Herlyn, M., Merlino, G., Medrano, E., Bastian, B., Landi, M. T. & Sosman, J. (2010). Melanoma from bench to bedside: meeting report from the 6th international melanoma congress. *Pigment Cell Melanoma Res,* Vol. 23, No. 1, pp. 14-26, ISSN 1755-148X

Garrido, M. C. & Bastian, B. C. (2010). KIT as a therapeutic target in melanoma. *J Invest Dermatol,* Vol. 130, No. 1, pp. 20-27, ISSN 1523-1747

Guo, J., Si, L., Kong, Y., Xu, X. w., Flaherty, K. T., Corless, C. L., Zhu, Y. Y., Li, L. & Li, H. F. (2010). A phase II study of imatinib for advanced melanoma patients with KIT aberrations. *Proceedings of the American Society of Clinical Oncology,* Chicago, June, 2010.

Hodi, F. S., Friedlander, P., Corless, C. L., Heinrich, M. C., Mac Rae, S., Kruse, A., Jagannathan, J., Van den Abbeele, A. D., Velazquez, E. F., Demetri, G. D. & Fisher, D. E. (2008). Major response to imatinib mesylate in KIT-mutated melanoma. *J Clin Oncol,* Vol. 26, No. 12, pp. 2046-2051, ISSN 1527-7755

Hofmann, U. B., Kauczok-Vetter, C. S., Houben, R. & Becker, J. C. (2009). Overexpression of the KIT/SCF in uveal melanoma does not translate into clinical efficacy of imatinib mesylate. *Clin Cancer Res,* Vol. 15, No. 1, pp. 324-329, ISSN 1078-0432

Horst, B., Gruvberger-Saal, S. K., Hopkins, B. D., Bordone, L., Yang, Y., Chernoff, K. A., Uzoma, I., Schwipper, V., Liebau, J., Nowak, N. J., Brunner, G., Owens, D., Rimm, D. L., Parsons, R. & Celebi, J. T. (2009). Gab2-mediated signaling promotes melanoma metastasis. *Am J Pathol,* Vol. 174, No. 4, pp. 1524-1533, ISSN 1525-2191

Ishihara, K., Saida, T., Otsuka, F. & Yamazaki, N. (2008). Statistical profiles of malignant melanoma and other skin cancers in Japan: 2007 update. *Int J Clin Oncol,* Vol. 13, No. 1, pp. 33-41, ISSN 1341-9625

Ishihara, Y., Saida, T., Miyazaki, A., Koga, H., Taniguchi, A., Tsuchida, T., Toyama, M. & Ohara, K. (2006). Early acral melanoma in situ: correlation between the parallel ridge pattern on dermoscopy and microscopic features. *Am J Dermatopathol,* Vol. 28, No. 1, pp. 21-27, ISSN 0193-1091

Jiang, X., Zhou, J., Yuen, N. K., Corless, C. L., Heinrich, M. C., Fletcher, J. A., Demetri, G. D., Widlund, H. R., Fisher, D. E. & Hodi, F. S. (2008). Imatinib targeting of KIT-mutant oncoprotein in melanoma. *Clin Cancer Res,* Vol. 14, No. 23, pp. 7726-7732, ISSN 1078-0432

Kim, K. B., Eton, O., Davis, D. W., Frazier, M. L., McConkey, D. J., Diwan, A. H., Papadopoulos, N. E., Bedikian, A. Y., Camacho, L. H., Ross, M. I., Cormier, J. N., Gershenwald, J. E., Lee, J. E., Mansfield, P. F., Billings, L. A., Ng, C. S.,

Charnsangavej, C., Bar-Eli, M., Johnson, M. M., Murgo, A. J. & Prieto, V. G. (2008). Phase II trial of imatinib mesylate in patients with metastatic melanoma. *Br J Cancer,* Vol. 99, No. 5, pp. 734-740, ISSN 1532-1827

Kluger, H. M., Dudek, A. Z., McCann, C., Ritacco, J., Southard, N., Jilaveanu, L. B., Molinaro, A. & Sznol, M. (2010). A phase 2 trial of dasatinib in advanced melanoma. *Cancer,* Vol. 117, No. 10, pp. 2202-2208 ISSN 0008-543X

Koga, H., Saida, T. & Uhara, H. (2011). Key point in dermoscopic differentiation between early nail apparatus melanoma and benign longitudinal melanonychia. *J Dermatol,* Vol. 38, No. 1, pp. 45-52, ISSN 1346-8138

Lutzky, J., Bauer, J. & Bastian, B. C. (2008). Dose-dependent, complete response to imatinib of a metastatic mucosal melanoma with a K642E KIT mutation. *Pigment Cell Melanoma Res,* Vol. 21, No. 4, pp. 492-493, ISSN 1755-1471

Markovic, S. N., Erickson, L. A., Rao, R. D., Weenig, R. H., Pockaj, B. A., Bardia, A., Vachon, C. M., Schild, S. E., McWilliams, R. R., Hand, J. L., Laman, S. D., Kottschade, L. A., Maples, W. J., Pittelkow, M. R., Pulido, J. S., Cameron, J. D. & Creagan, E. T. (2007). Malignant melanoma in the 21st century, part 1: epidemiology, risk factors, screening, prevention, and diagnosis. *Mayo Clin Proc,* Vol. 82, No. 3, pp. 364-380, ISSN 0025-6196

Michaloglou, C., Vredeveld, L. C., Mooi, W. J. & Peeper, D. S. (2008). BRAF(E600) in benign and malignant human tumours. *Oncogene,* Vol. 27, No. 7, pp. 877-895, ISSN 1476-5594

Miyazaki, A., Saida, T., Koga, H., Oguchi, S., Suzuki, T. & Tsuchida, T. (2005). Anatomical and histopathological correlates of the dermoscopic patterns seen in melanocytic nevi on the sole: a retrospective study. *J Am Acad Dermatol,* Vol. 53, No. 2, pp. 230-236, ISSN 1097-6787

Murata, H., Ashida, A., Takata, M., Yamaura, M., Bastian, B. C. & Saida, T. (2007). Establishment of a novel melanoma cell line SMYM-PRGP showing cytogenetic and biological characteristics of the radial growth phase of acral melanomas. *Cancer Sci,* Vol. 98, No. 7, pp. 958-963, ISSN 1347-9032

North, J. P., Kageshita, T., Pinkel, D., Leboit, P. E. & Bastian, B. C. (2008). Distribution and Significance of Occult Intraepidermal Tumor Cells Surrounding Primary Melanoma. *J Invest Dermatol,* Vol.128 No.8 pp.2024-2030, ISSN 1523-1747

Oguchi, S., Saida, T., Koganehira, Y., Ohkubo, S., Ishihara, Y. & Kawachi, S. (1998). Characteristic epiluminescent microscopic features of early malignant melanoma on glabrous skin. A videomicroscopic analysis. *Arch Dermatol,* Vol. 134, No. 5, pp. 563-568, ISSN 0003-987X

Phan, A., Touzet, S., Dalle, S., Ronger-Savle, S., Balme, B. & Thomas, L. (2006). Acral lentiginous melanoma: a clinicoprognostic study of 126 cases. *Br J Dermatol,* Vol. 155, No. 3, pp. 561-569, ISSN 0007-0963

Romano, E., Schwartz, G. K., Chapman, P. B., Wolchock, J. D. & Carvajal, R. D. (2011). Treatment implications of the emerging molecular classification system for melanoma. *Lancet Oncol,* Vol. No. pp. ISSN 1474-5488

Saida, T. (1989). Malignant melanoma in situ on the sole of the foot. Its clinical and histopathologic characteristics. *Am J Dermatopathol,* Vol. 11, No. 2, pp. 124-130, ISSN 0193-1091

Saida, T., Koga, H. & Uhara, H. (2011). Key points in dermoscopic differentiation between early acral melanoma and acral nevus. *J Dermatol,* Vol. 38, No. 1, pp. 25-34, ISSN 1346-8138

Saida, T., Miyazaki, A., Oguchi, S., Ishihara, Y., Yamazaki, Y., Murase, S., Yoshikawa, S., Tsuchida, T., Kawabata, Y. & Tamaki, K. (2004). Significance of dermoscopic patterns in detecting malignant melanoma on acral volar skin: results of a multicenter study in Japan. *Arch Dermatol,* Vol. 140, No. 10, pp. 1233-1238, ISSN 0003-987X

Sauter, E. R., Yeo, U. C., von Stemm, A., Zhu, W., Litwin, S., Tichansky, D. S., Pistritto, G., Nesbit, M., Pinkel, D., Herlyn, M. & Bastian, B. C. (2002). Cyclin D1 is a candidate oncogene in cutaneous melanoma. *Cancer Res,* Vol. 62, No. 11, pp. 3200-3206, ISSN 0008-5472

Stevens, N. G., Liff, J. M. & Weiss, N. S. (1990). Plantar melanoma: is the incidence of melanoma of the sole of the foot really higher in blacks than whites? *Int J Cancer,* Vol. 45, No. 4, pp. 691-693, ISSN 0020-7136

Takata, M., Murata, H. & Saida, T. (2010). Molecular pathogenesis of malignant melanoma: a different perspective from the studies of melanocytic nevus and acral melanoma. *Pigment Cell Melanoma Res,* Vol. 23, No. 1, pp. 64-71, ISSN 1755-148X

Tashiro, E., Tsuchiya, A. & Imoto, M. (2007). Functions of cyclin D1 as an oncogene and regulation of cyclin D1 expression. *Cancer Sci,* Vol. 98, No. 5, pp. 629-635. ISSN

Terheyden, P., Houben, R., Pajouh, P., Thorns, C., Zillikens, D. & Becker, J. C. (2010). Response to imatinib mesylate depends on the presence of the V559A-mutated KIT oncogene. *J Invest Dermatol,* Vol. 130, No. 1, pp. 314-316, ISSN 1523-1747

Ugurel, S., Hildenbrand, R., Zimpfer, A., La Rosee, P., Paschka, P., Sucker, A., Keikavoussi, P., Becker, J. C., Rittgen, W., Hochhaus, A. & Schadendorf, D. (2005). Lack of clinical efficacy of imatinib in metastatic melanoma. *Br J Cancer,* Vol. 92, No. 8, pp. 1398-1405, ISSN 0007-0920

Whiteman, D. C., Watt, P., Purdie, D. M., Hughes, M. C., Hayward, N. K. & Green, A. C. (2003). Melanocytic nevi, solar keratoses, and divergent pathways to cutaneous melanoma. *J Natl Cancer Inst,* Vol. 95, No. 11, pp. 806-812, ISSN 1460-2105

Woodman, S. E. & Davies, M. A. (2010). Targeting KIT in melanoma: a paradigm of molecular medicine and targeted therapeutics. *Biochem Pharmacol,* Vol. 80, No. 5, pp. 568-574, ISSN 1873-2968

Woodman, S. E., Trent, J. C., Stemke-Hale, K., Lazar, A. J., Pricl, S., Pavan, G. M., Fermeglia, M., Gopal, Y. N., Yang, D., Podoloff, D. A., Ivan, D., Kim, K. B., Papadopoulos, N., Hwu, P., Mills, G. B. & Davies, M. A. (2009). Activity of dasatinib against L576P KIT mutant melanoma: molecular, cellular, and clinical correlates. *Mol Cancer Ther,* Vol. 8, No. 8, pp. 2079-2085, ISSN 1538-8514

Wyman, K., Atkins, M. B., Prieto, V., Eton, O., McDermott, D. F., Hubbard, F., Byrnes, C., Sanders, K. & Sosman, J. A. (2006). Multicenter Phase II trial of high-dose imatinib mesylate in metastatic melanoma: significant toxicity with no clinical efficacy. *Cancer,* Vol. 106, No. 9, pp. 2005-2011, ISSN 0008-543X

Yamaguchi, Y., Itami, S., Watabe, H., Yasumoto, K., Abdel-Malek, Z. A., Kubo, T., Rouzaud, F., Tanemura, A., Yoshikawa, K. & Hearing, V. J. (2004). Mesenchymal-epithelial interactions in the skin: increased expression of dickkopf1 by palmoplantar fibroblasts inhibits melanocyte growth and differentiation. *J Cell Biol,* Vol. 165, No. 2, pp. 275-285, ISSN 0021-9525

Yamaura, M., Takata, M., Miyazaki, A. & Saida, T. (2005). Specific dermoscopy patterns and amplifications of the cyclin D1 gene to define histopathologically unrecognizable early lesions of acral melanoma in situ. *Arch Dermatol,* Vol. 141, No. 11, pp. 1413-1418, ISSN 0003-987X

2

Histopathological Diagnosis of Early Stage of Malignant Melanoma

Eiichi Arai, Lin Jin, Koji Nagata and Michio Shimizu
Department of Pathology, Saitama Medical University International Medical Center Saitama, Japan

1. Introduction

Macroscopically, malignant melanoma (MM) is diagnosed by the so-called ABCDE rule(asymmetry, border irregularity, color variation, diameter generally greater than 6 mm, and elevation)[1]. Nowadays, D may stand for dark color. In addition to this, the dermoscope has been an indispensable tool to diagnose MM, allowing MMs of less than 4 mm in diameter to be found. Therefore, D may also stand for dermoscopic structure[2].

There are variations in approaches for the histopathological diagnosis of MM. By putting them in order according to the clinical ABCDE rules, they are as follows: Asymmetry (including asymmetrical silhouette and color imbalance), Buckshot scatter (= pagetoid spread), Cytological atypia, Deep mitosis, Enclosing (= surrounding) lymphocytes, Fibrosis, and Gainsaying (= no) maturation. Moreover, the diagnosis will be made by adding the specific findings related to the site of the body such as palms, soles, subungual region, genital area, oral cavity and conjunctiva[2].

In general, the pathological diagnostic clues of MM in situ are as follows:

1. single melanocytes predominance and irregular distribution of nests,
2. cytological atypia (larger than the normal melanocytes, abundant cytoplasm, distinct nucleoli), and
3. pagetoid spread of melanocytes.[3]

We chose three important conditions in early stage lesions of MM, which are difficult to be applicable to the above clues of MM in situ. They are (1) early stage of lentigo maligna pattern of maligna melanoma in situ, (2) early stage of melanoma in situ on volar skin, and (3) Spitzoid or nevoid melanoma without invasion beyond the mid-dermis.

Here, in this session, we describe these three conditions. In particular, we describe No (2) item, which is common in the Japanese, in detail. Moreover, although immunostainigs are not useful for the differential diagnosis between MM and benign lesion, we selected some useful immunohistochemical findings which serve to differentiate them.

2. Lehtigo maligna (early stage of lentigo maligna pattern of maligna melanoma *in situ*)

Lentigo maligna (LM=early stage of lentigo maligna pattern of maligna melanoma in situ) is clinically only found on chronically sun-exposed areas of elderly people. Macroscopically, changes of asymmetry, border irregularity, color variation in the ABCDE rule and dermoscopically irregular reticular pigment network are important findings for their diagnosis. Histologically, in typical LMs, three of the diagnostic clues of MM in situ described above are used for the diagnosis of LM. In the early lesions of LM, melanocytes do not show buckshot scatter (pagetoid spread) and alignment along the basal layer. Their nuclei are hyperchromatic, and show slight cytological atypia and few mitoses. Single melanocytic proliferation is present broadly[4], continuously[3], or generally (almost diffusely)[5], and is lentiginous along the basal layer.

However, in earlier stages of LM the distribution is not lentiginous but sparse. The diagnostic clues for the early stage of LM are follows: 1) melanocytes are irregularly distributed (Fig. 1); 2) melanocytes lose their polarity of nuclei against the basement membrane (Fig. 2); and 3) melanocytes show a rather large shape, hyperchromatic nuclei and clear halo with moth-eaten appearance of nuclei (Fig. 3). Although these large melanocytes in LM are needed for differentiating them from activated melanocytes in benign lesions (lentigo senilis, lichen planus-like keratosis, lichenoid actinic keratosis and so on), benign lesions have neither loss of polarity nor a moth-eaten appearance. In addition, benign lesions usually show vacuolar degeneration and pigment incontinence.

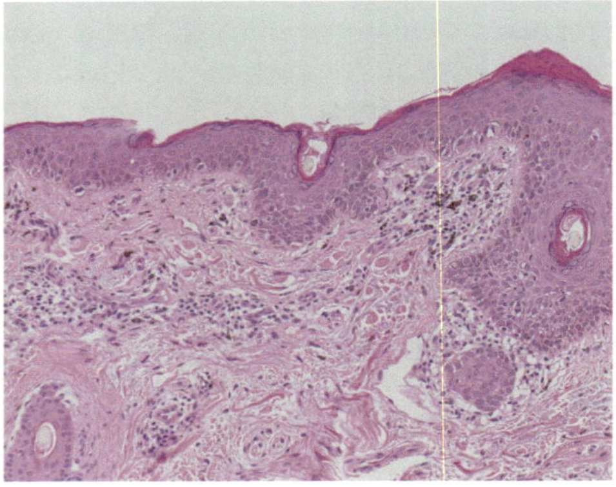

Fig. 1. Early stage of lentigo maligna (low power view): The distribution of melanocytes is irregular.

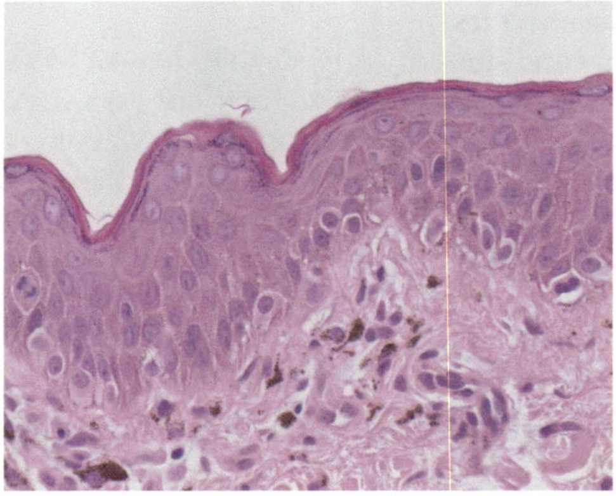

Fig. 2. Early stage of lentigo maligna melanoma (middle power view): Melanocytes lose their polarity of nuclei against the basement membrane.

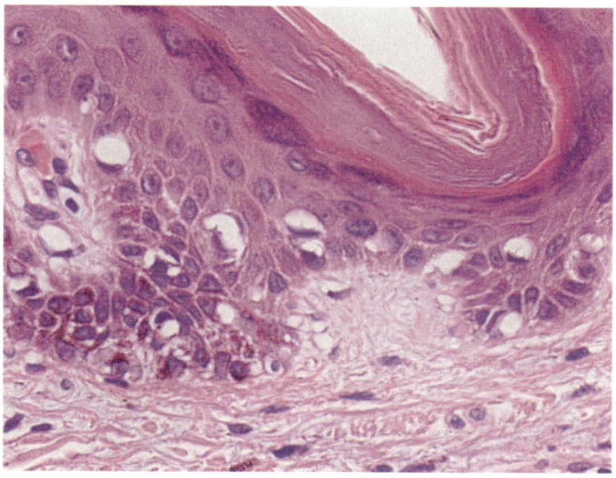

Fig. 3. Early stage of lentigo maligna melanoma (high power view): Melanocytes show a rather large shape, hyperchromatic nuclei and clear halo with moth-eaten appearance of nuclei. They also show hyperchromatic nuclei and loss of polarity against the basement membrane.

3. Early stage of melanoma *in situ* on volar skin

Histopathological criteria of early stage of melanoma in situ on volar skin have been thought to be so far as follows:

1. melanocytes arranged as solitary units predominate over melanocytes in nests[6];
2. irregular distribution of nests are frequently seen[3]; nests of melanocytes vary in size and shape[6];
3. slight cytological atypia is seen[3];
4. single cells often extend irregularly far down to the eccrine duct epithelium[3,6]; and
5. pagetoid spread of melanocytes is seen, especially an ascent up to the granular layer[3,6].

Moreover, on the sole, benign melanocytic lesions are frequently observed to have melanocytes ascending up to the granular layer. As in the early volar MM in situ, when only a few melanocytes show slight nuclear enlargement and slight cytological atypia, such a lesion has been called atypical melanosis of the foot[7]. However, nowadays these lesions are thought to be an early stage of MM in situ. With the recent development of dermoscopy for the diagnosis of MM in situ on the sole, it is important to find the melanocytes present on the crista profunda intermedia[8]. We found 5 cases of MM in situ from the review of 145 cases of melanocytic nevi on the sole previously diagnosed[9]. Separately from these five cases of MM in situ, we chose 14 cases of MM in situ on the volar skin in our institution. Resected specimens of these cases were cut perpendicularly against for cutaneous secant (the direction of skin crista and furrow, Fig. 4). The diagnoses of these cases were confirmed after clinicopathological conference. By the detailed observation of melanocytes on the crista profunda intermedia as pointed out by Ishihara et al[8], we found important findings about the distribution pattern and cytological atypia. In the early lesion, the melanocytes on the slope of rete ridges on the crista profunda intermedia exist without a continuous pattern, showing irregular intervals of each melanocyte and loss of polarity of nuclei against the basement membrane (Fig. 5). The nuclei are larger than those of normal melanocytes, show hyperchromatic nuclei, and have large nucleoli (Fig. 6). These findings are reported in our report[9].

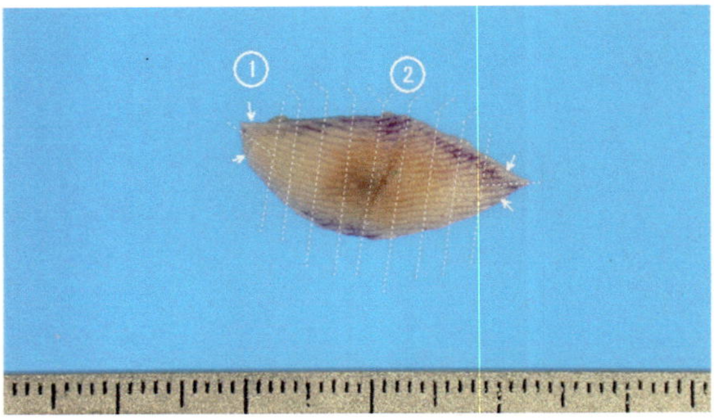

Fig. 4. How to cut the specimen of pigmented lesion on the volar skin. Lesions should be cut perpendicularly for cutaneous secant (the direction of skin crista and furrow).

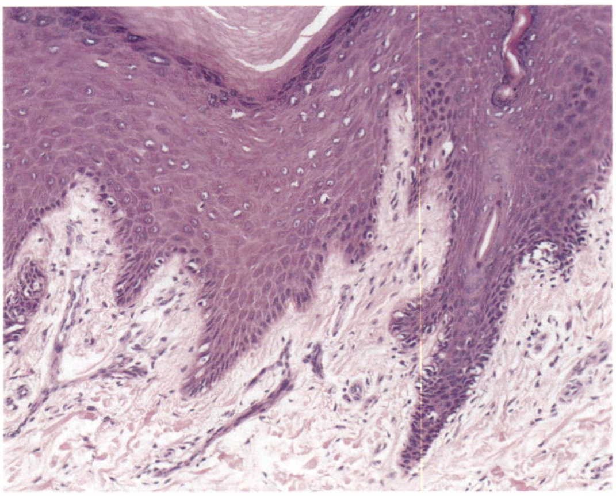

Fig. 5. Early lesion of MM in situ on the volar skin (low power view). Melanocytes on the slope of rete ridges on the crista profunda intermedia exist without continuous pattern, with irregular intervals of each melanocyte and loss of polarity of nuclei against the basement membrane.

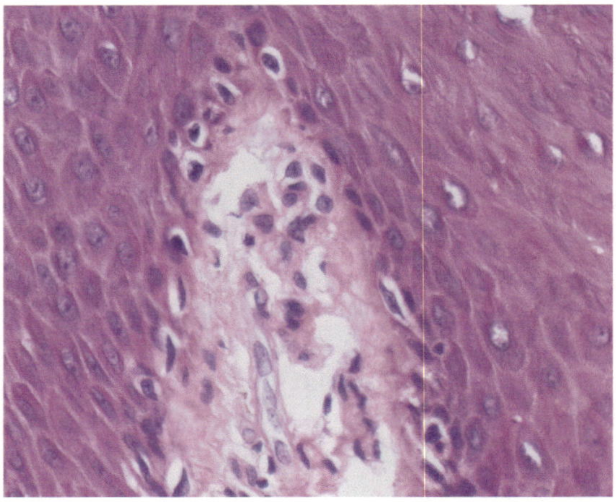

Fig. 6. Early lesion of MM in situ on the volar skin (high power view). The nuclei are larger than those of normal melanocytes, show hyperchromatiic nuclei, and have large nucleoli.

4. Spitzoid or nevoid melanoma without invasion beyond the mid-dermis

Melanocytic proliferative disorders include only melanocytic nevi and malignant melanomas. Therefore, the diagnosis of MM could be based on an exclusion of benign pigmented nevi. The differential points between Spitz nevi or compound nevi and early stage of MMs in this group are deep existence of high cellular density without maturation (Fig. 7), deep mitosis (Fig. 8) and jagged lesional base (Fig. 9). In addition, many well-formed large Kamino bodies favor a diagnosis of Spitz nevus [3].

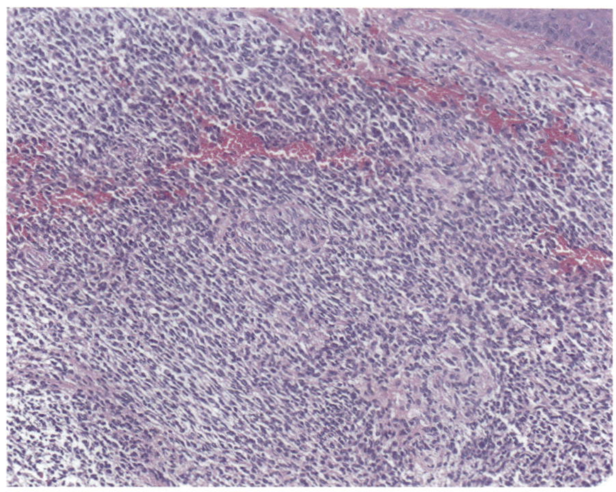

Fig. 7. Nevoid melanoma (middle power view). High cellular density without maturation is present.

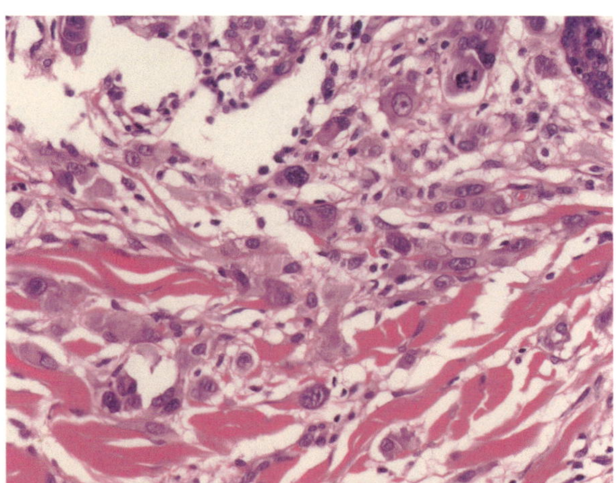

Fig. 8. Spitzoid melanoma (high power view). Deep mitosis is present.

5. Useful findings of immunostaining

Regarding the immunohistochemistry in the diagnosis of MM, combined immunohistochemical stains may be used to gain useful information in the diagnosis of early stage of MM. In Spitz nevus, nevoid nevus, blue nevus, melanocytic nevus and normal

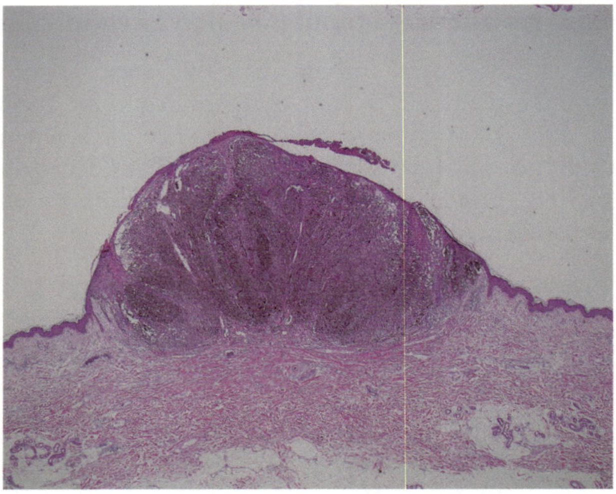

Fig. 9. Spitzoid melanoma (low power view): There is a jagged lesional base.

melanocyte, S-100 protein and Melan-A are diffusely positive. Furthermore, we must know that S-100 protein is positive for Langerhans cells, and melan-A is positive for melanophages. MM and blue nevus are diffusely positive for HMB-45 (Fig. 10, left), but normal melanocytes and benign melanocytic nevi are negative (Fig. 10. right). In Spitz nevus, nevoid nevus and activated melanocytic lesion are usually positive for HMB-45. Especially, the upper portion of these lesions is strongly positive for HMB-45, but the lower portion of these lesions is weakly positive or negative (Fig.11). This finding is indicative for maturation of melanocytes. Namely, melanocytes in the epidermis are positive but melanocytes in the dermis are negative. MIB-1 is also useful for seeking deep mitosis, which favor a diagnosis of MM (Fig.12).

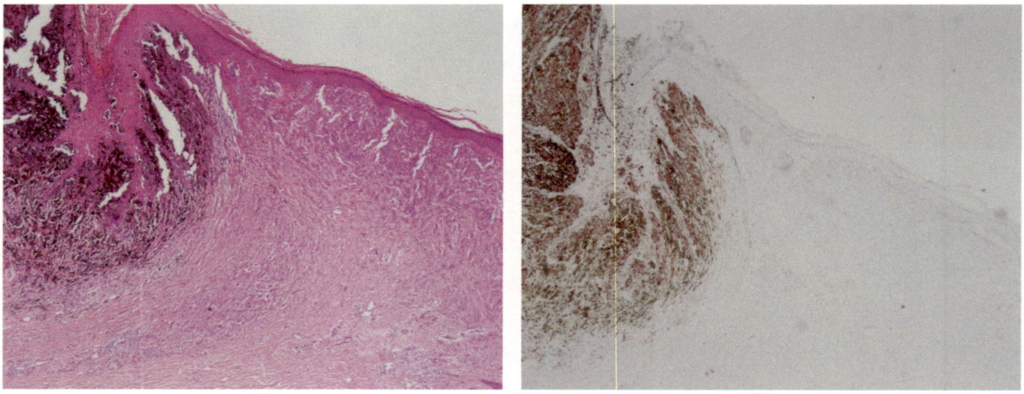

(a) (b)

Fig. 10. (a) Combined case with Spitzoid melanoma (left) and intradermal melanocytic nevus (right). (b) The Spitzoid melanoma is positive (left) but intradermal melanocytic nevus is negative for HMB-45 using alkaliphosphatase (right).

HMB-45 has been known to be positive for MM except for desmoplastic/spindle cell melanoma[2)]. However, early stage of MMs rarely shows this specific feature. In general, desmoplastic/spindle cell melanoma usually exists in the dermis and has little epidermal change. In differentiation between spindle cell melanoma and pigmented spindle cell nevus (Reed), it is useful to find maturation.

In immunohistochemical summary, combination of S-100 protein (high sensitivity for melanocytic lesions), melan-A (high specificity for melanocytic lesions), HMB-45 and MIB-1 is useful for making a diagnosis of early stage of MM.

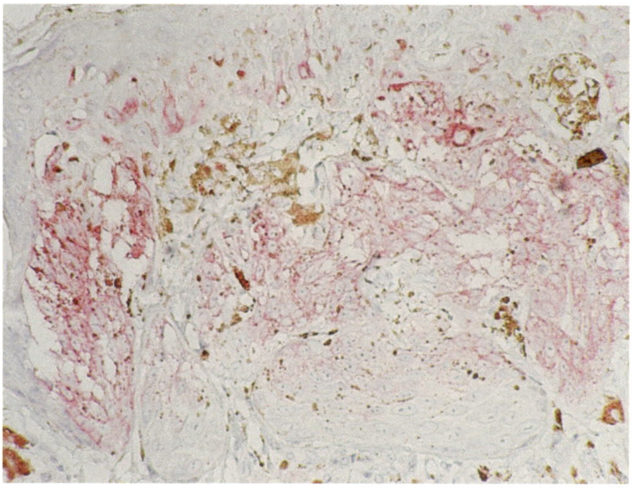

Fig. 11. Spitz nevus: The upper portion of these lesions is strongly positive, but the lower portion is weakly positive or negative (HMB-45 using alkaliphosphatase.

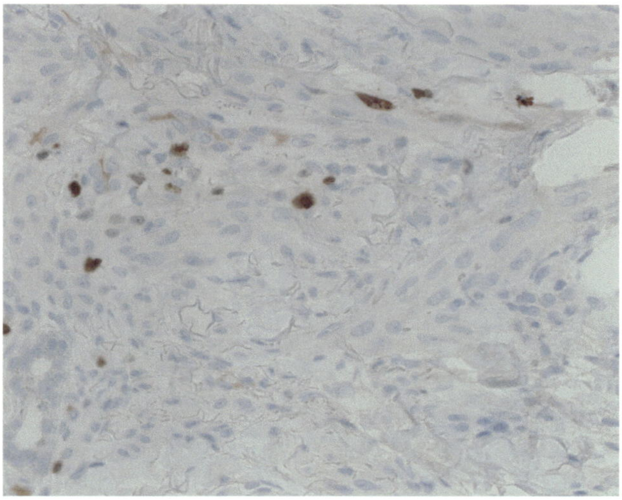

Fig. 12. Spitzoid melanoma: MIB-1 is positive for the lower part of the lesion.

6. References

[1] Elder DE and Murphy GF: Melanocytic Tumors of the Skin. AFIP Atlas of Tumor Pathology, 3rd series, Fascicle 2, Bethesda, Maryland, 2010.

[2] Weedon D: Weedon's Skin Pathology, 3rd ed, Churchill Livingstone Elsevier, 2010.
[3] Massi G and LeBiot PE: Histological Diagnosis of nevi and Melanoma, Steinkopff Darmstadt Springer, Germany, 2004
[4] King R et al: Lentiginous melanoma: a histologic pattern to melanoma to be distinguished form lentiginous nevus. Modern Pathology 2005;18:1397.
[5] Kwon IH, Lee JH, Cho KH: Acral lentiginous melanoma in situ: a study of nine cases. Am J Dermatopathol 2004;26:285-289.
[6] Ackerman AB, Cerroni L, Kerl H: Pitfalls in Histopathologic Diagnosis of Malignant Melanoma. Philadelphia: Lea & Fibiger, 1994.
[7] Nogita T, Wong TY, Ohara K et al: Atypical melanosis of the foot. A report of three cases in Japanese populations. Arch Dermatol 1994;130:1042.
[8] Ishihara Y, Saida T, Miyazaki A et al: Early acral melanoma in situ: Correlation between the parallel ridge pattern on dermoscopic features. Am J Dermatopathol 2006:28:21-7.
[9] Jin L, Arai E, Anzai S, Kimura T, Tsuchida T, Nagata K, Shimizu M: Reassessment of histopathology and dermoscopy findings in 145 Japanese cases of melanocytic nevus of the sole: toward a pathological diagnosis of early-stage malignant melanoma in situ. Pathol Int 60: 65-70, 2010.

3

Wnt/β-Catenin Signaling Pathway in Canine Skin Melanoma and a Possibility as a Cancer Model for Human Skin Melanoma

Jae-Ik Han and Ki-Jeong Na
College of Veterinary Medicine,
Chungbuk National University
Cheongju,
Korea

1. Introduction

Cutaneous melanoma is a relatively common skin tumor in the dog, accounting for 5 to 7% of canine skin tumors (Bostock, 1986; Rothwell et al., 1987). This tumor originates from the transformation of the melanocytes, which are present mainly in the epidermis and hair follicles. The transformed melanocytes lose their normal contact with surrounding keratinocytes and tend to proliferate to surrounding tissues (Smith et al., 2002). Breed has been reported to be prognostically significant; more than 75% of melanomas in Doberman pinschers and miniature schnauzers are behaviorally benign, whereas 85% of melanomas in miniature poodles are malignant (Bolon et al., 1990).

Cutaneous melanoma can be behaviorally benign or malignant, and can occur anywhere on the body. Some investigations into the molecular and genetic basis of melanoma were previously performed (Table 1), but the etiology of melanoma is largely unknown. These tumors usually can be diagnosed by simple fine-needle aspiration cytology; however, histologic examination is important to determine the potential for malignancy (Aronsohn & Carpenter 1990; Bolon et al., 1990).

The therapeutic treatment for local cutaneous melanoma in the dog is surgical excision. It shows an excellent prognosis after surgical excision of benign tumors, whereas the prognosis of tumors with malignant criteria is guarded or poor; metastatic rates of 30 to 75% have been reported after the surgery (Withrow & Vail 2007). Systemic chemotherapy for malignant melanoma has shown little promise. Some agents, including mitoxantrone (Ogilvie et al., 1991), doxorubicin (Moore, 1993), dacarbazine (Gillick & Spiegle, 1987), and carboplatin (Rassnick et al., 2001) have been used for treatment. However, in general, the effects of these drugs have been poor and the durations of the effects have been shortlived. A few researches have been conducted to develop effective therapeutic targets in the mechanism of melanoma progression and/or metastasis; however, there is no effective strategy until the present time (von Euler et al., 2008; Han et al., 2010; Thamm et al., 2010).

Factor	Normal function	Abnormality	Reference
p53 gene	: activate DNA repair protein : hold the cell cycle at the G1/S phase : initiate apoptosis if the DNA damage proves to be irreversible	: exclusion of p53 from the nucleus	Koenig et al., 2002
Metallothionein	: capture harmful oxidant radicals	: inactivates p53 functions	Dincer et al., 2001
RB-1 gene	: hold the cell cycle at the G1/S phase	: exclusion of RB-1 from the nucleus	Koenig et al., 2002
P16/P21/P27	: inhibits the activity of CDK2 and CDK4	: loss or reduction of ink-4a gene	Koenig et al., 2002
PTEN gene	: inhibits the AKT signaling pathway	: loss or reduction of PTEN expression	Koenig et al., 2002
N-RAS	: a member of the RAS signal transduction	: mutation of N-RAS gene	Mayr et al., 2003
VEGF	: important signaling protein in vasculogenesis and angiogenesis	: improves the angiogenesis in tumors	Rawlings et al., 2003

Table 1. Cutaneous melanoma-related molecular and genetic factors in dogs.

2. Wnt/β-catenin signaling pathway

2.1 Normal regulation of the Wnt/ β-catenin signaling pathway

2.1.1 Wnt signaling: ligands and receptors

The Wnt genes encode a group of 19 secreted cysteine rich glycoproteins that act as ligands to activate receptor-mediated signaling pathways that control cell differentiation, cell proliferation, and cell motility (Chlen & Moon, 2007). Wnt proteins are defined by sequence rather than by functional properties. Because it is difficult to solubilize active Wnt molecules, the purification of Wnts is complicated. Its insoluble nature is caused by the lipid modification causing hydrophobic state. For example, murine Wnt3a, the first identified Wnt protein, undergoes two kinds of lipid modification; first is the addition of palmitate to cysteine 77 causing diminishing the ability to activate β-catenin signaling and second is the addition of palmitoleoyl to serine 209 causing Wnt3a accumulation in the endoplasmic reticulum (Willert et al., 2003; Takada et al., 2006; Galli et al., 2007; Komekado et al., 2007). Until now, *Drosophila* Wingless (Wg) is the most investigated Wnt molecule *in vivo*. Those researches indicate that the hydrophobicity and membrane localization of Wg are lost when Porcupine (Porc) gene is eliminated (Zhai et al., 2004; Takeda et al., 2006; Hausmann et al., 2007). Porc encodes a transmembrane ER protein responsible for Wg lipid modification. Consequently, it suggests that Porc is a important mediator of both lipid modification and membrane targeting of Wg.

In Vertebrates, there are two kinds of Wnt signaling pathway; β-catenin-dependent (canonical) and β-catenin-independent (non-canonical) signaling pathways. Canonical or β-catenin-dependent signaling pathway is also called as the Wnt/β-catenin signaling pathway. Two distinct receptor families are important for the Wnt/β-catenin signaling pathway: the Frizzled (Fz) seven transmembrane receptors and the LDL receptor-related proteins 5 and 6 (LRP5 and LRP6) (He et al., 2004; Logan and Nusse, 2004). In Wnt/Fz interaction, Wnt proteins bind directly to the cysteine-rich domain of Fz receptor; however, without a cognate ligand, the complex of Wnt/Fz cannot activate Wnt signaling, indicating Fz activation is ligand dependent. For participating to Wnt signaling, LRPs need to transport to the cell surface by a specific molecule called Boca in *Drosophila* or Mesd in mice (Culi & Mann, 2003; Hsieh et al., 2003). Two LRPs act different functions at different developmental process; LRP6 is more important for embryogenesis while LRP5 is critical for adult bone homeostasis. In most data, Wnt induces the formation of Fz-LRP5/6 complex to activate Wnt signaling pathway.

2.1.2 Wnt signaling: off state

Cytoplasmic β-catenin phosphorylation and degradation is the characteristic feature (Fig. 1). The Axin protein coordinates sequential phosphorylation of β-catenin at serine 45 by CK 1α and then threonine 41, serine 37 and serine 33 by glycogen synthase kinase-3β (GSK-3β) through the interaction with separate domains of Axin (Kimelman & Xu, 2006). After then, the E3 ubiquitin ligase β-Trcp binds to serine 33 and 37 of β-catenin, and leads to β-catenin ubiquitination and degradation. GSK3 and CK1 also phosphorylate Axin and Adenomatous polyposis coli (APC), resulting in the enhancement of β-catenin phosphorylation and degradation through increased association between Axin/APC and β-catenin (Kimelman & Xu, 2006; Huang & He, 2008). Additional aspects on Axin complex deserve further discussion.

1. Serine/threonine phosphatases, PP1 and PP2A, counteract the role of GSK3 and/or CK1 in the Axin complex. PP1 promote the dissociation of the Axin complex through the dephosphorylation of Axin while PP2A dephosphorylates β-catenin. Both reactions result in reduced β-catenin degradation (Luo et al., 2007; Su et al., 2008).
2. Axin concentration is different among each component in *Xenopus*, indicating that Axin controls the rate of the complex assembly (Lee et al., 2003). However, it is not sure whether the different concentration of Axin in each component is universal to other organisms.

APC is a part of the Axin complex causing β-catenin phosphorylation. APC also inhibit the dephosphorylation of β-catenin, and thereby enhancing β-catenin degradation (Su et al., 2008). APC and Axin compete for same β-catenin, and APC also remove phosphorylated β-catenin from Axin for degradation and for making Axin available for another β-catenin phosphorylation (Xing et al., 2003; Kimelman & Xu, 2006). APC also promote to remove β-catenin from the nucleus and suppress β-catenin target genes.

Interestingly, APC can promote Wnt signaling through the acceleration of Axin degradation (Lee et al., 2003; Takacs et al., 2008). It depends on the APC amino acid terminal that is not involved in β-catenin degradation. Conversly, Axin can also promote APC degradation (Choi et al., 2004). However, the mechanisms of both APC and Axin degradation are not known.

2.1.3 Wnt signaling: on state

Wnt/β-catenin signaling pathway is important in many developmental processes including the formation of neural crest-derived melanocytes (Larue & Delmas 2006). In neural-crest

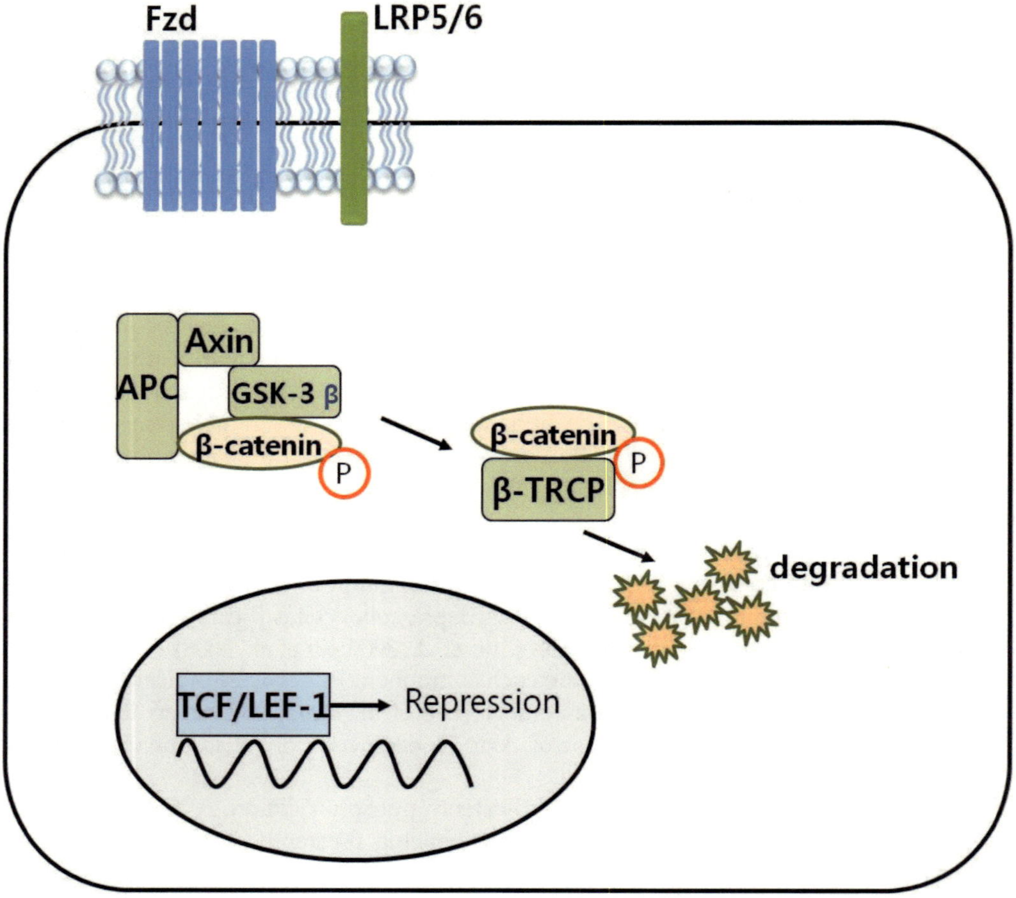

Fig. 1. Regulation of Wnt/β-catenin signaling pathway. In the absence of Wnt signals, the cellular concentration of free β-catenin is low, because a complex of the adenomatous polyposis coli (APC), glycogen synthase kinase 3β (GSK-3β) and axin protein is responsible for regulating the level of β-catenin, via GSK-3β-mediated phosphorylation of specific serin and threonine residues in β-catenin.

emigration and expansion during the embryogenesis, this pathway has been implicated in the migration and differentiation of the melanoblast by β-catenin dependent manner (Fig. 2) (Dunn *et al.* 2000; Ikeya *et al.* 1997). A hallmark of the activation of the pathway is the accumulation of β-catenin protein in the cytoplasm. Wnt signals influence the proteins that regulate β-catenin stability through several mechanisms and thereby induce the activation of Wnt target gene through the nuclear translocation of β-catenin as follows;

1. After the signaling of Wnt proteins, the receptor complex transduces a signal to several intracellular proteins that include Dishevelled (Dsh) through a direct binding between Dsh and Fz. Dsh is a ubiquitously expressed cytoplasmic protein and interacts with a C-terminal cytoplasmic Lys-Thr-X-X-X-Trp motif of Fz (Umbhauer et al., 2000). During the process, Dsh is also phosphorylated by several protein kinases such as Par1 (Yanagawa et al., 1995; Sun et al., 2001). Wnt-induced LRP phosphorylation is also important for the receptor activation. LRP5 and LRP6 have five repetitive Pro-Pro-Pro-(SerTrp)Pro [PPP(S/T)P] motifs, which are involved in constitutive β-catenin signaling (Tamai et al., 2004; MacDonald et al., 2008). GSK3 and CK1 are responsible for PPP(S/T)P phosphorylation after the stimulation of Wnt proteins (Davidson et al., 2005; Zeng et al., 2005). These dual phosphorylated motifs become a binding site for the Axin complex and recruit Axin to LRP6 under Wnt stimulation. Zeng et al. (2008) indicates that GSK3 is responsible for most PPP(S/T)P phosphorylation in GSK α/β null cell lines. Consequently, Axin/GSK3 interaction mediates LRP6 phosphorylation, resulting in the accumulation of β-catenin in the cytoplasm.
2. As described above, the receptors transduce a signal to several intracellular proteins that include Dishevelled (Dsh). Activated Dsh acts as a suppressor of the proteasome-mediated degradation, which is controlled by a complex of glycogen synthase kinase-3β (GSK-3β), Axin, Adenomatous polyposis coli (APC), and β-TrCP. In particular, Wnt signals promote to detach Axin from the complex and thereby, induce β-catenin stabilization (Cliffe et al., 2003; Tamai et al., 2004). Consequently, stabilized β-catenin accumulates in the cytoplasm.
3. In vertebrates, Caprin-2, a cytoplasmic protein, binds to LRP6 and promotes its phosphorylation by GSK3 (Ding et al., 2008). In addition, Caprin-2 promotes the formation of LRP6-Axin-GSK3 complex.
4. Microtubule actin cross-linking factor 1 (Macf1) is a member of the protein that links the cytoskeleton to junctional proteins. It seems that this protein is a transporter of Axin to LRP6. Its function may be vertebrate-specific (Chen et al., 2006).
5. Cytoplasmic β-catenin can enter and retain in the nucleus (Henderson & Fagotto, 2002; Stadeli et al., 2006). Though the mechanism of the movement is not well understand, Henderson and Fagotto (2002) suggests that nuclear pore protein interacts directly with β-catenin, resulting in the movement to the nucleus. A recent study indicates that JNK2 and Rac1 constitute a cytoplasmic complex with β-catenin and thereby promote its nuclear translocation (Wu et al., 2008).
6. In the nucleus, β-catenin interacts with transcription factors such as lymphoid enhancer-binding factor 1/T cell-specific transcription factor (LEF/TCF) DNA-binding proteins. In the absence of Wnt signal, TCF acts as a repressor of Wnt target genes, however, β-catenin convert the TCF repressor into a transcriptional activator complex and thereby activates the transcription of the target genes including c-myc and cyclin D1 that cause a cell proliferation and differentiation. The target genes of Wnt/β-catenin signaling pathway are summarized in Table 2.

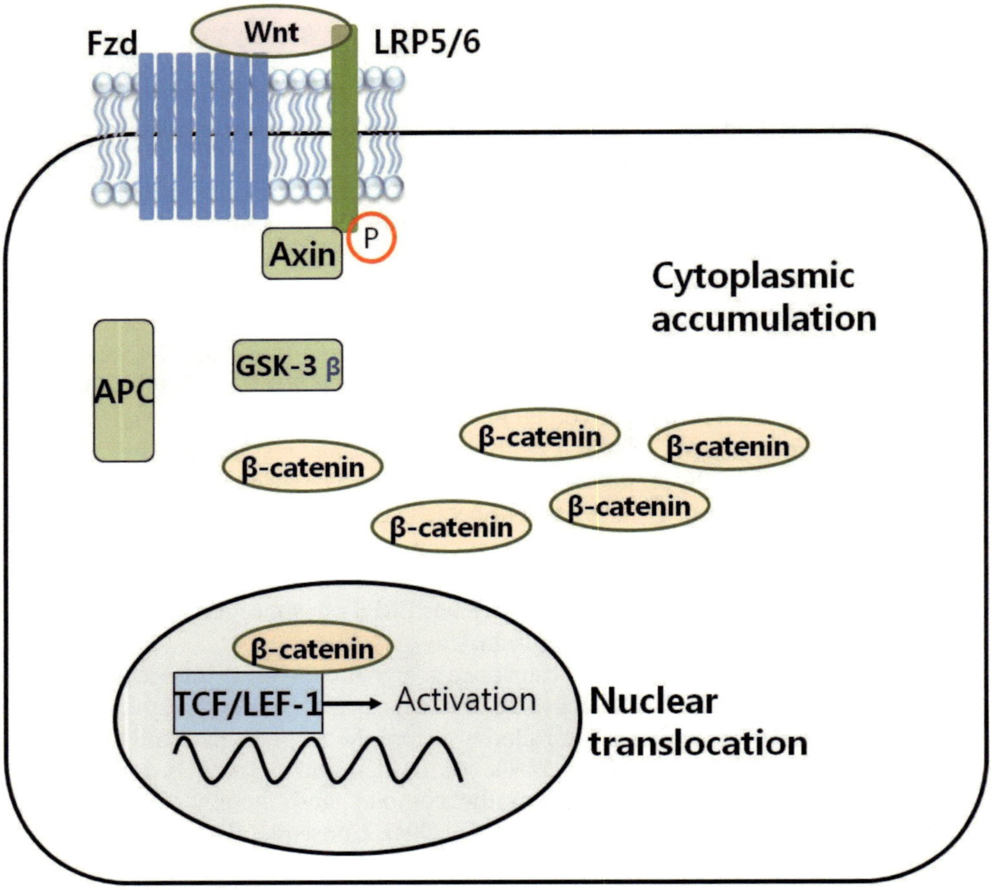

Fig. 2. Regulation of Wnt/β-catenin signaling pathway. Upon Wnt signaling, the activity of GSK-3β is inhibited by Dsh, hence β-catenin is accumulated in the cytoplasm. The accumulated β-catenin can enter the nucleus and activates the target genes such as *LEF-1*, c-myc and cyclin D1.

Target gene	Changes in target gene expression	Mediator	Reference
Fz	Suppress	Wnt	Muller et al., 1999
Dfz2	Suppress	Wnt	Cadigan et al., 1998
Dfz3	Activate	Wnt	Sato et al., 1999
Fz7	-	Wnt	Willert et al., 2002
LRP	Suppress	Wnt	Wehrli et al., 2000
Axin2	Suppress	β-catenin	Jho et al., 2002
β-TCRP	Suppress	β-catenin	Spiegelman et al., 2000
TCF1	Suppress	TCF	Roose et al., 2001
LEF1	Activate	β-catenin	Hovanes et al., 2001

Table 2. The target genes of Wnt/β-catenin signaling pathway.

2.2 Dysregulation of the Wnt/ β-catenin signaling pathway

2.2.1 Wnt signaling in human diseases

In human medicine, mutations of the Wnt/β-catenin signaling pathway have been introduced as a cause of many hereditary disorders, cancer, and other diseases (Table 3). These include mutations in several components of Wnt signaling pathway such as ligands and receptors. Also, the loss of E-cadherin or the abruption of cadherin-catenin complex by MET/RON receptor tyrosine kinases (RTKs) can cause the abnormal accumulation of β-catenin into the cells (Danikovitch-Miagkova *et al.* 2001; Nelson and Nusse 2004).

Gene	Function	Disease	References
Wnt3	Ligands	Tetra-amelia	Niemann et al., 2004
Wnt4		Mullerian-duct regression and viriliation	Biason-Lauber et al., 2004
Wnt7a		Fuhrmann syndrome	Woods et al., 2006
Wnt10a		Odonto-onchyo-dermal hypoplasia	Adaimy et al., 2007
LRP5	Receptor	Hyperparathyroid tumor High bone mass Osteoporosis-pseudoglioma FEVR eye vascular defects	Gong et al., 2001; Boyden et al., 2002; Little et al., 2002; Toomes et al., 2004; Bjorklund et al., 2007
LRP6		Early coronary disease and osteoporosis	Mani et al., 2007
Axin1	Facilitates β-catenin degradation	Caudal duplication, cancer	Satoh et al., 2000; Oates et al., 2006
Axin2		Tooth agenesis, cancer	Liu et al., 2000; Lammi et al., 2004
APC	Facilitates β-catenin degradation	Familial adenomatous polyposis, cancer	Kinzler et al., 1991; Nishisho et al., 1991
β-catenin	Signal transducer	Cancer	Korinek et al., 1997; Morin et al., 1997
TCF	Transcriptional partner of β-catenin	Type II diabetes (?)	Florez et al., 2006; Grant et al., 2006

Table 3. Human diseases caused by mutations of the Wnt/β-catenin signaling pathway

Association of dysregulated Wnt/β-catenin signaling pathway with human cancer has also been documented through constitutively activated β-catenin signaling. Dysfunction of APC/Axin/GSK3 complex or β-catenin mutation (especially in exon 3) blocks its degradation and consequently, accumulated β-catenin leads to excessive cell proliferation that predisposes cells to tumorigenesis. Particularly, in human skin melanoma, dysregulated Wnt/β-catenin signaling pathway is essential for metastasis. In this tumor, the transformation of normal melanocytes into melanoma cells is a multistep process (Albino et al., 1991; Haass et al., 2005; Meier et al., 2000; Shih & Herlyn 1993). The first step, considered as benign, is associated with the formation of a nevus and the radial growth phase (RGP). During RGP, melanocytes tend to proliferate superficially to the basement membrane of the epidermis. During the next stage, the vertical growth phase (VGP), the cells bypass senescence to proliferate actively in a vertical manner in the dermis, crossing the basement membrane. At this stage, the cells migrate and become clearly invasive (Fig. 3). In RGP and VGP, the alteration of Wnt/β-catenin signaling pathway has been considered to act fundamental roles (Sanders et al. 1999; Larue and Beermann 2007). However, in human, only infrequent mutation has been found in genes encoding the components, such as APC and β-catenin. Therefore, it is presumed that Wnt/β-catenin signaling is probably activated by changes in the expression of genes encoding the components directly involved in the signaling pathway or associated with the regulation of this pathway (Larue and Delmas 2006).

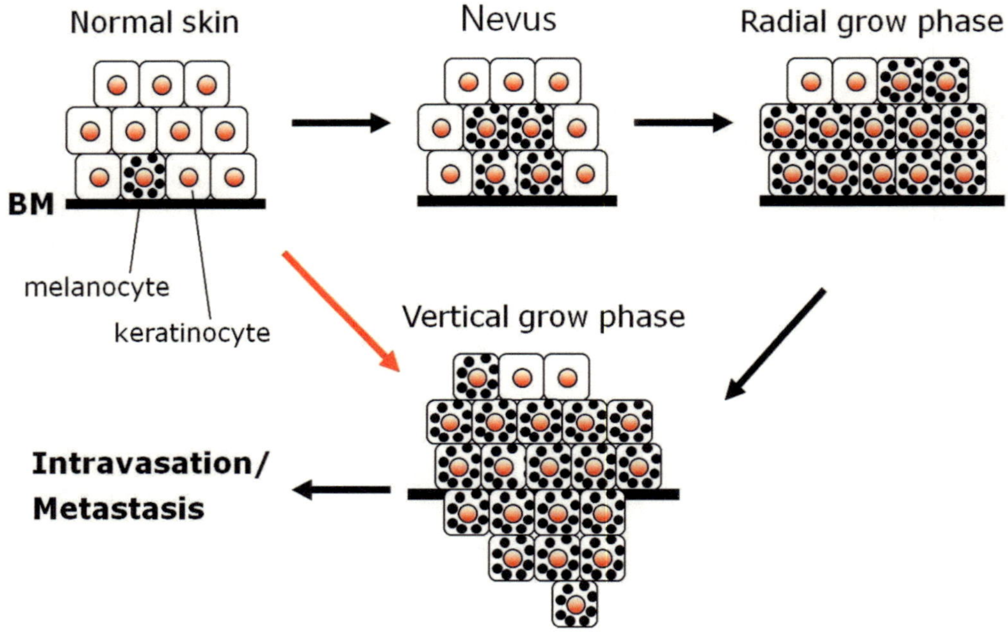

Fig. 3. Cutaneous melanomagenesis in human. After the formation of nervi, constitutively activated β-catenin results in the progress of RGP and VGP, inducing tumor cell metastasis. BM, basement membrane.

2.2.2 Wnt signaling in canine diseases

In dogs, abnormalities of the Wnt/β-catenin signaling pathway have been investigated in mammary tumor and skin melanoma (Gama et al., 2008; Han et al., 2010). In both studies, decreased membrane β-catenin expression was consistently observed, indicating the disruption of intercellular adhesion (Fig. 4). On plasma membrane level, β-catenin acts as a bridge that links cadherin to the cytoskeleton in the plasma membrane of the normal cell (Demunter et al. 2002; Sanders et al. 1999). Thus, the loss of cadherin molecule or the disruption of cadherin-catenin complex can induce the release of β-catenin into the cytoplasm. The loss of E-cadherin and the activated MET/RON receptor tyrosine kinases (RTKs) have been reported to cause the cytoplasmic release of β-catenin in human melanoma and normal canine kidney cells (Danilkovitch-Miagkova et al. 2001; Demunter et al. 2002; Sanders et al. 1999). In the study of canine skin melanoma, the authors observed significantly increased β-catenin expression in mRNA level (Han et al., 2010). It seems that the increased synthesis of β-catenin can also induce the cytoplasmic accumulation, besides the translocation of membrane β-catenin. Wnt factor has been considered to increase the synthesis of β-catenin in human (Danilkovitch-Miagkova et al. 2001; Larue and Delmas 2006). However, the expression level of β-catenin in protein level is needed to confirm our hypothesis as increased RNA synthesis does not always equate with increased protein synthesis. The authors also examined consistently decreased expression of membrane E-cadherin in all canine skin melanoma tissues, indicating the disruption of intercellular adhesion (Fig. 5, unpublished). However, the authors couldn't conclude the relationship between E-cadherin and β-catenin because of low sample number. In another study, the authors observed that only 28% of tumor tissues revealed overexpressed MET/RON RTKs indicating that those RTKs were not a major contributing factor for increased β-catenin expression in the cytoplasm (Han et al., 2009). As a next study, the authors are examining the mutation of β-catenin gene. GSK3/APC/Axin complex recognizes the amino acid sequence encoded by exon 3 of β-catenin gene and initiates phosphorylation, followed by degradation of β-catenin.

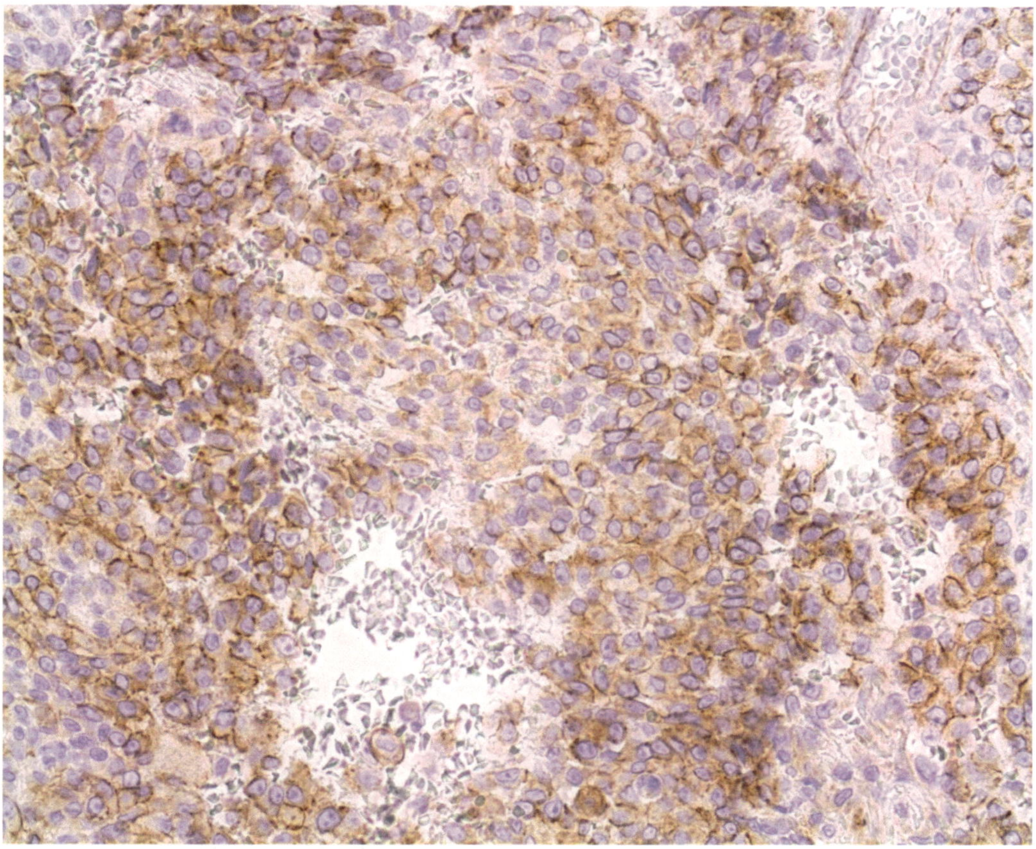

Fig. 4. Immunohistochemistry for β-catenin in canine skin melanoma showing variable membrane expression and cytoplasmic translocation of β-catenin (authors' study).

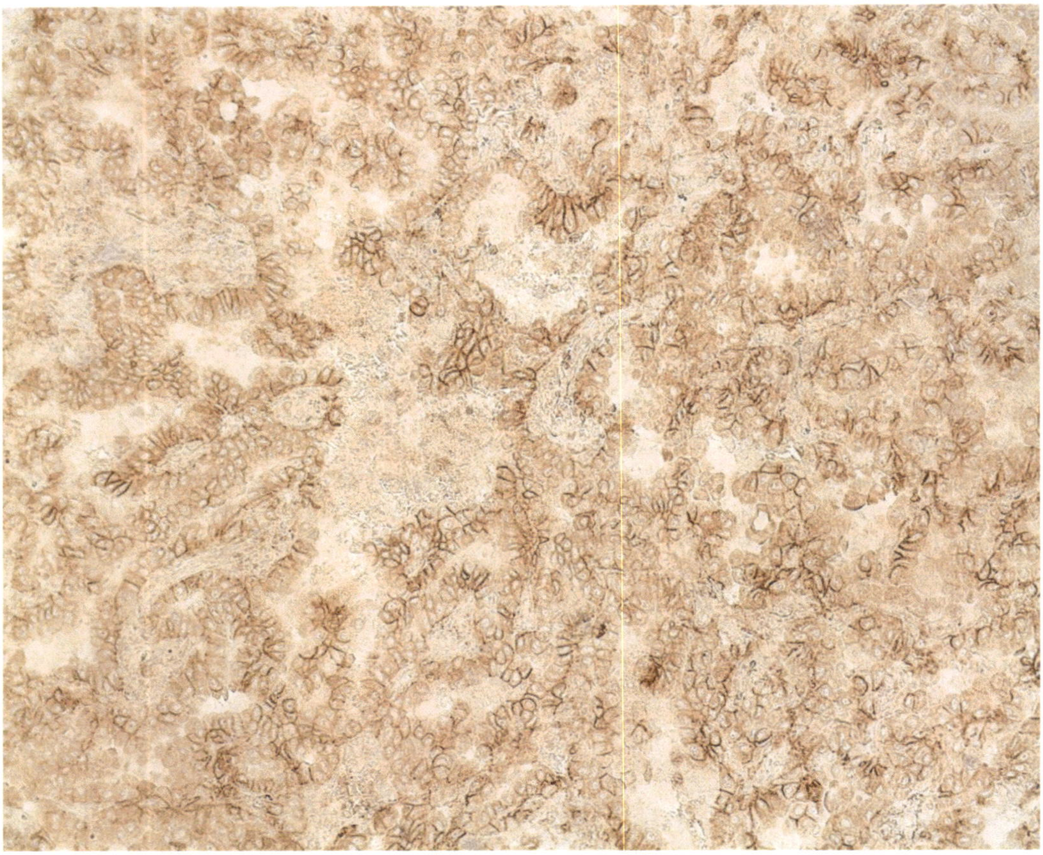

Fig. 5. Immunohistochemistry for E-cadherin in canine skin melanoma showing variable membrane expression of E-cadherin (authors' study).

3. Spontaneous canine skin melanoma as a model for human melanoma

Spontaneous tumors in companion animals are suitable models for human cancer. They share a similar lifestyle with human (their owner), and have a relatively high incidence of tumors, large body size and shorter life span (Vail & MacEwen, 2000). Their tumors are also spontaneously occurring and genetically heterogenous in contrast to the tumor of experimental animals induced by chemical or transplantation. In companion animals, tumors that have a potential to be a model for human are mammary carcinoma, osteosarcoma, melanoma, lymphoma and leukemia.

Although a lot of investigations and therapeutic trials have been conducted, the incidence and deaths by skin melanoma continue to increase in human, particularly Caucasian population (Longstreet, 1988; Woodhead et al., 1999). In human, melanoma classifies four subtypes; superficial spreading melanoma (SSM), nodular melanoma, lentigo maligna melanoma and acral lentiginous melanoma. SSM is the most common type of melanoma, accounting for about 70% of all diagnosed cases. The most aggressive type is, however, nodular melanoma. Nodular melanoma is the second common type, accounting for 15% of all diagnosed cases. Usually, it develops in people aged 60 and older. Because of high incidence of the alteration in Wnt/β-catenin signaling pathway, a genetically modified mouse model has been developed (Delmas et al. 2007). However, the location of melanocytes in mice differs from that in the human skin and a mouse model does not spontaneously develop melanoma (Larue and Beermann 2007). Whereas, in normal skin of the dog, the melanocyte is mainly present in the basal layer of the epidermis and hair follicle similar to that of the human. In addition, the age incidence, histopathology and biological behavior, which rapidly progression to vertical growth phase (VGP) without radial growth phase (RGP) in canine cutaneous melanoma are very similar to the feature of human cutaneous nodular melanoma (Chamberlain et al. 2003; Gross et al. 2005; Smith et al. 2002). It suggests that the canine cutaneous melanoma could be a suitable model for therapeutic trial by correcting the altered Wnt/β-catenin signaling pathway.

4. References

Adaimy, L., Chouery, E., Megarbane, H., Mroueh, S., Delague, V., Nicolas, E., Belguith, H., de Mazancourt, P. & Megarbane, A. (2007) Mutation in WNT10A is associated with an autosomal recessive ectodermal dysplasia: the odonto-onycho-dermal dysplasia. *American Journal of Human Genetics*: 81(4), 821-828.

Akiyama, T. (2000) Wnt/β-catenin signaling. *Cytokine & Growth Factor Review*: 11(4), 273-282.

Albino, A., Davis, B., & Nanus, D. (1991) Induction of growth factor RNA expression of activated N-rasQ61K on an INK4a-deficient background. *Cancer Research*: 65, 4005-4011.

Aronsohn, M. G., Carpenter, J. L. (1990) Distal extremity melanocytic nevi and malignant melanomas in dogs. *Journal of the American Animal Hospital Association*: 26(6), 605-612.

Behrens, J., von Kries, J. P., Kuhl, M., Bruhn, L., Wedlich, D., Grosschedl, R., and Birchmeier, W. (1996) Functional interaction of beta-catenin with the transcription factor LEF-1. *Nature*: 382(6592), 638-642.

Biason-Lauber, A., Konrad, D., Navratil, F. & Schoenle, E. J. (2004) A WNT4 mutation associated with Mullerian-duct regression and virilization in a 46, XX woman. *The New England Journal of Medicine*: 351(8), 792-798.

Bjorklund, P., Akerstrom, G. & Westin, G. (2007) An LRP5 receptor with internal deletion in hyperparathyroid tumors with implications for deregulated WNT/beta-catenin signaling. *PLoS medicine*: 4(11), e328.

Bolon, B., Calderwood Mays, M. B., & Hall, B. J. (1990) Characteristics of canine melanomas and comparison of histology and DNA ploidy to their biologic effect. *Veterinary Pathology*: 27(2), 96-102.

Bostock, D. E. (1986) Neoplasms of the skin and subcutaneous tissues in dogs and cats. *The British Veterinary Journal*: 142(1), 1-19.

Boyden, L. M., Mao, J., Belsky, J., Mitzner, L., Farhi, A., Mitnick, M. A., Wu, D., Insogna, K. & Lifton, R. P. (2002) High bone density due to a mutation in LDL-receptor-related protein 5. *The New England Journal of Medicine*: 346(20), 1513-1521.

Cadigan, K. M., Fish, M. P., Rulifson, E. J. & Nusse, R. (1998) Wingless repression of *Drosophila* frizzled 2 expression shapes the Wingless morphogen gradient in the wing. *Cell*: 93(5), 767-777.

Chamberlain, A. J., Fritschi, L. & Kelly, J. W. (2003) Nodular melanoma: patient's perceptions of presenting features and implications for earlier detection. *Journal of the American Academy of Dermatology*: 48(5), 694-701.

Chen, H. J., Lin, C. M., Lin, C. S., Perez-Olle, R., Leung, C. L. & Liem, R. K. (2006) The role of microtubule actin cross-linking factor 1 (MACF1) in the Wnt signaling pathway. *Genes & development*: 20(14), 1933-1945.

Chien, A. J. & Moon, R. T. (2007) WNTS and WNT receptors as therapeutic tools and targets in human disease processes. *Frontiers in Bioscience*: 12, 448-457.

Chin, L., Garraway, L. A., and Fisher, D. E. (2006) Malignant melanoma: genetics and therapeutics in the genomic era. *Genes & Development*: 20(16), 2149-2182.

Choi, J., Park, S. Y., Costantini, F., Jho, E. H. & Joo, C. K. (2004) Adenomatous polyposis coli is down-regulated by the ubiquitin-proteasome pathway in a process facilitated by Axin. *The Journal of Biological Chemistry*: 279(47), 49188-49198.

Clevers, H. (2006) Wnt/β-catenin signaling in development and disease. *Cell*: 127(3), 469-80.

Cliffe, A., Hamada, F. & Bienz, M. (2003) A role of Dishevelled in relocating Axin to the plasma membrane during wingless signaling. *Current Biology*: 13(11), 960-966.

Culi, J. & Mann, R. S. (2003) Boca, an endoplasmic reticulum protein required for wingless signaling and trafficking of LDL receptor family members in Drosophila. *Cell*: 112(3), 343-354.

Danilcovitch-Miagkova, A., Miagkov, A., Skeel, A., Nakaigawa, N., Zbar, B. & Leonard, E. J. (2001) Oncogenic mutants of RON and MET receptor tyrosine kinases causes activation of the beta-catenin pathway. *Molecular and Cellular Biology*: 21(17), 5857-5868.

Davidson, G., Wu, W., Shen, J., Bilic, J., Fenger, U., Stannek, P., Glinka, A. & Niehrs, C. (2005) Casein kinase 1 gamma couples Wnt receptor activation to cytoplasmic signal transduction. *Nature*: 438(7069), 867-872.

Delmas, V., Beermann, F., Martinozzi, S., Carreira, S., Ackermann, J., Kumasaka, M., Denat, L., Goodall, J., Luciani, F., Viros, A., Demirkan, N., Bastian, B. C., Goding, C. R. & Larue, L. (2007) β-catenin induces immortalization of melanocytes by suppressing p16INK4a expression and cooperates with N-Ras in melanoma development. *Genes & Development*: 21(22), 2923-2935.

Demunter, A., Libbrecht, L., Degreef, H., De Wolf-Peeters, C., a& van den Oord, J. J. (2002) Loss of membranous expression of β-catenin is associated with tumor progression in cutaneous melanoma and rarely caused by exon 3 mutations. *Modern Pathology*: 15(4), 454-461.

Dincer, Z., Jasani, B., & Haywood, S. (2001) Metallothionein expression in canine and feline mammary and melanocytic tumours. *Journal of Comparative Pathology*: 125(2-3), 130-136.

Ding, Y., Xi, Y., Chen, T., Wang, J. Y., Tao, D. L., Wu, Z. L., Li, Y. P., Li, C., Zeng, R. & Li, L. (2008) Caprin-2 enhances canonical Wnt signaling through regulating LRP5/6 phosphorylation. *The Journal of Cell Biology*: 182(5), 865-872.

Dunn, K. J., Williams, B. O., Li, Y., & Pavan, W. J. (2000) Neural crest-directed gene transfer demonstrates Wnt1 role in melanocyte expansion and differentiation during mouse development. *Proceedings of the National Academy of Sciences of the United States of America*: 97(18), 10050-10055.

Ikeya, M., Lee, S. M., Johnson, J. E., Mcmahon, A. P., & Takada, S. (1997) Wnt signaling required for expansion of neural crest and CNS progenitors. *Nature*: 389(6654), 966-970.

Florez, J. C., Jablonski, K. A., Bayley, N., Pollin, T. I., de Bakker, P. I., Shuldiner, A. R., Knowler, W. C., Nathan, D. M. & Altshuler, D. (2006) TCF7L2 polymorphisms and progression to diabetes in the Diabetes Prevention Program. *The New England Journal of Medicine*: 355(3), 241-250.

Galli, L. M., Barnes, T. L., Secrest, S. S., Kadowaki, T. & Burrus, L. W. (2007) Porcupine-mediated lipid-modification regulates the activity and distribution of Wnt proteins in the chick neural tube. *Development (Cambridge, England)*: 134(18), 3339-3348.

Gama, A., Paredes, J., Gärtner, F., Alves, A. & Schmitt, F. (2008) Expression of E-cadherin, P-cadherin and β-catenin in canine malignant mammary tumours in relation to clinicopathological parameters, proliferation and survival. *The Veterinary Journal*: 177(1), 45-53.

Gillick, A., & Spiegle, M. (1987) Dacarbazine treatment of malignant melanoma in a dog. *Canadian Veterinary Journal*: 28, 204.

Gong, Y., Slee, R. B., Fukai, N., Rawadi, G., Roman-Roman, S., Reginato, A. M., Wang, H., Cundy, T., Glorieux, F. H., Lev, D., Zacharin, M., Oexle, K., Marcelino, J., Suwairi, W., Heeger, S., Sabatakos, G., Apte, S., Adkins, W. N., Allgrove, J., Arslan-Kirchner, M., Batch, J. A., Beighton, P., Black, G. C., Boles, R. G., Boon, L. M., Borrone, C., Brunner, H. G., Carle, G. F., Dallapiccola, B., De Paepe, A., Floege, B., Halfhide, M. L., Hall, B., Hennekam, R. C., Hirose, T., Jans, A., Jűppner, H., Kim, C. A., Keppler-Noreuil, K., Kohlschuetter, A., LaCombe, D., Lambert, M., Lemyre, E., Letteboer, T., Peltonen, L., Ramesar, R. S., Romanengo, M., Somer, H., Steichen-Gersdorf, E., Steinmann, B., Sullivan, B., Superti-Furga, A., Swoboda, W., van den Boogaard, M. J., van Hul, W., Vikkula, M., Votruba, M., Zabel, B., Garcia, T., Baron, R., Olsen, B. R. & Warman, M. L. (2001) LDL receptor-related protein 5 (LRP5) affects bone accrual and eye development. *Cell*: 107(4), 513-523.

Gross, T. L., Ihrke, P. J., Walder, E. J. & Affolter, V. K. (2005) In Skin diseases of the dog and cat: clinical and histopathologic diagnosis, 2nd ed. Blackwell publishing: Oxford 813-836.

Haass, N. K., Smalley, K. S. M., Li, L. & Herlyn, M. (2005) Adhesion, migration and communication in melanocytes and melanoma. *Pigment Cell Research*: 18(3), 150-159.

Hamderson, B. R. & Fagotto, F. (2002) The ins and outs of APC and beta-catenin nuclear transport. *EMBO reports*: 3(9), 834-839.

Han, J. I., Kim, D. Y. & Na, K. J. (2009) Increased expression of MET and RON receptor tyrosine kinases in canine cutaneous melanotic tumor. *Journal of Veterinary Clinics*: 26(5), 429-432.

Han, J. I., Kim, D. Y. & Na, K. J. (2010) Dysregulation of the Wnt/β-catenin signaling pathway in canine cutaneous melanotic tumor. *Veterinary Pathology*: 47(2), 285-291.

Hausmann, G., Banziger, C. & Basler, K. (2007) Helping Wingless take flight: how WNT proteins are secreted. *Nature reviews*: 8(4), 331-336.

He, X., Semenov, M., Tamai, K. & Zeng, X. (2004) LDL receptor-related proteins 5 and 6 in Wnt/beta-catenin signaling: arrows point the way. *Development (Cambridge, England)*: 131(8), 1663-1677.

Hovanes, K., Li, T. W., Munguia, J. E., Truong, T., Milovanovic, T., Lawrence Marsh, J., Holcombe, R. F. & Waterman, M. L. (2001) Beta-catenin-sensitive isoforms of lymphoid enhancer factor-1 are selectively expressed in colon cancer. *Nature Genetics*: 28(1), 53-57.

Hsieh, J. C., Lee, L., Zhang, L., Wefer, S. & Brown, K. (2003) Mesd encodes an LRP5/6 chaperone essential for specification of mouse embryonic polarity. *Cell*: 112(3), 355-367.

Huang, H. & He, X. (2008) Wnt/beta-catenin signaling: new (and old) players and new insights. *Current opinion in cell biology*: 20(2), 119-125.

Jho, E. H., Zhang, T., Domon, C., Joo, C. K., Freund, J. N. & Costantini, F. (2002) Wnt/beta-catenin/Tcf signaling induces the transcription of Axin2, a negative regulator of the signaling pathway. *Molecular and Cellular Biology*: 22(4), 1172-1183.

Kimelman, D. & Xu, W. (2006) beta-catenin destruction complex: insights and questions from a structural perspective. *Oncogene*: 25(57), 7482-7491.

Kinzler, K. W., Nilbert, N. C., Vogelstein, B., Bryan, T. M., Levy, D. B., Smith, K. J., Preisinger, A. C., Hamilton, S. R., Hedge, P., Markhan, A., Carlson, M., Joslyn, G., Groden, J., White, R., Miki, Y., Miyoshi, Y., Nishisho, I. & Nakamura, Y. (1991) Identification of a gene located at chromosome 5q21 that is mutated in colorectal cancers. *Science*: 251(4999), 1366-1370.

Koenig, A., Bianco, S. R., Fosmire, S., Wojcieszyn, J., and Modiano, J. F. (2002) Expression and significance of p53, Rb, p21/waf-1, p16/ink4a, and PTEN tumor suppressors in canine melanoma. *Veterinary Pathology*: 39(4), 458-472.

Komekado, H., Yamamoto, H., Chiba, T. & Kikuchi, A. (2007) Glycosylation and palmitoylation of Wnt-3a are coupled to produce an active form of Wnt-3a. *Genes to Cells*: 12(4), 521-534.

Korinek, V., Barker, N., Morin, P. J., van Wichen, D., de Weger, R., Kinzler, K. W., Vogelstein, B. & Clevers, H. Constitutive transcriptional activation by a beta-catenin-Tcf complex in APC -/- colon carcinoma. *Science*: 275(5307), 1784-1787.

Lammi, L., Arte, S., Somer, M., Jarvinen, H., Lahermo, P., Thesleff, I., Pirinen, S. & Nieminen, P. (2004) Mutations in AXIN2 cause familial tooth agenesis and predispose to colorectal cancer. *American Journal of Human Genetics*: 74(5), 1043–1050.

Larue, L. & Beermann, F. (2007) Cutaneous melanoma in genetically modified animals. *Pigment Cell Research*: 20(6), 485-497.

Larue, L., and Delmas, V. (2006) The WNT/β-catenin pathway in melanoma. *Frontiers in Biosciences*: 11, 733-742.

Lee, E., Salic, A., Kruger, R., Heinrich, R. & Kirschner, M. W. (2003) The roles of APC and Axin derived from experimental and theoretical analysis of the Wnt pathway. *PLoS Biology*: 1(1), E10.

Little, R. D., Carulli, J. P., Del Mastro, R. G., Dupuis, J., Osborne, M., Folz, C., Manning, S. P., Swain, P. M., Zhao, S. C., Eustace, B., Lappe, M. M., Spitzer, L., Zweier, S., Braunschweiger, K., Benchekroun, Y., Hu, X., Adair, R., Chee, L., FitzGerald, M. G., Tulig, C., Caruso, A., Tzellas, N., Bawa, A., Franklin, B., McGuire, S., Nogues, X., Gong, G., Allen, K. M., Anisowicz, A., Morales, A. J., Lomedico, P. T., Recker, S. M., Van Eerdewegh, P., Recker, R. R. & Johnson, M. L. (2002) A mutation in the LDL-receptor-related protein 5 gene results in the autosomal dominant high-bone-mass trait. *American Journal of Human Genetics*: 70(1), 11-19.

Liu, W., Dong, X., Mai, M., Seelan, R. S., Taniguchi, K., Krishnadath, K. K., Halling, K. C., Cunningham, J. M., Boardman, L. A., Qian, C., Christensen, E., Schmidt, S. S., Roche, P. C., Smith, D. I. & Thibodeau, S. N. (2000) Mutations in AXIN2 cause colorectal cancer with defective mismatch repair by activating beta-catenin/TCF signaling. *Nature Genetics*: 26(2), 146-147.

Logan, C. Y. & Nusse, R. (2004) The Wnt signaling pathway in development and disease. *Annual Review of Cell and Developmental Biology*: 20, 781-810.

Longstreet, J. (1988) Cutaneous malignant melanoma and ultraviolet radiation: a review. *Cancer Metastasis Reviews*: 7(4), 321-333.

Luo, W., Peterson, A., Garcia, B. A., Coombs, G., Kofahl, B., Heinrich, R., Shabanowitz, J., Hunt, D. F., Yost, H. J. & Virshup, D. M. (2007) Protein phosphatase 1 regulates assembly and function of the beta-catenin degradation complex. *The EMBO Journal*: 26(6), 1511-1521.

MacDonald, B. T., Yokota, C., Tamai, K., Zeng, X. & He, X. (2008) Wnt signal amplification via activity, cooperativity, and regulation of multiple intracellular PPPSP motifs in the Wnt co-receptor LRP6. *The Journal of Biological Chemistry*: 283(23), 16115-16123.

Mani, A., Radhakrishnan, J., Wang, H., Mani, A., Mani, M. A., Nelson-Williams, C., Carew, K. S., Mane, S., Najmabadi, H., Wu, D. & Lifton, R. P. (2007) LRP6 mutation in a family with early coronary disease and metabolic risk factors. *Science*: 315(5816), 1278-1282.

Mayr, B., Schaffner, G., and Reifinger, M. (2003) N-ras mutations in canine malignant melanomas. *Veterinary Journal*: 165(2), 169-171.

Meier, F., Nesbit, M. & Hsu, M. (2000) Human melanoma progression in skin reconstructs. Biological significance of bFGF. *The American Journal of Pathology*: 156(1), 193-200.

Moore, A. S. (1993) Recent advances in chemotherapy for nonlymphoid malignant neoplasms. *Compendium on Continuing Education for the Practicing Veterinarian*: 15, 1039-1050.

Muller, H., Samanta, R. & Wieschaus, E. (1999) Wingless signaling in the *Drosophila* embryo: zygotic reguirements and the role of the frizzled genes. *Development*: 126(3), 577-86.

Nelson, W. J. & Nusse, R. (2004) Convergence of Wnt, β-catenin, and cadherin pathways. *Science*: 303(5663), 1483-7.

Niemann, S., Zhao, C., Pascu, F., Stahl, U., Aulepp, U., Niswander, L., Weber, J. L. & Muller, U. (2004) Homozygous WNT3 mutation causes tetra-amelia in a large consanguineous family. *American Journal of Human Genetics*: 74(3), 558-563.

Nishisho, I., Nakamura, Y., Miyoshi, Y., Miki, Y., Ando, H., Horii, A., Koyama, K., Utsunomiya, J., Baba, S. & Hedge, P. (1991) Mutations of chromosome 5q21 genes in FAP and colorectal cancer patients. *Science*: 253(5020), 665-669.

Oates, N. A., van Vliet, J., Duffy, D. L., Kroes, H. Y., Martin, N. G., Boomsma, D. I., Campbell, M., Coulthard, M. G., Whitelaw, E. &Chong, S. Increased DNA methylation at the AXIN1 gene in a monozygotic twin from a pair discordant for a caudal duplication anomaly. *American Journal of Human Genetics*: 79(1), 155-162.

Ogilvie, G. K., Obradovich, J. E., Elmslie, R. E. (1991) Efficacy of mitoxantrone against various neoplasms in dogs. *Journal of the American Veterinary Medical Association*: 198(9), 1618-1621.

Omholt, K., Platz, A., Ringborg, U., Hansson, J. (2001) Cytoplasmic and nuclear accumulation of β-catenin is rarely caused by ctnnb1 exon 3 mutations in cutaneous malignant melanoma. *International Journal of Cancer*: 92(6), 839-842.

Rassnick, K. M., Ruslander, D. M., Cotter, S. M. (2001) Use of carboplatin for treatment of dogs with malignant melanoma: 27 cases (1989-2000). *Journal of the American Veterinary Medical Association*: 218(9), 1444-1448.

Rawlings, N. G., Simko, E., and Bebchuk, T. (2003) Localization of integrin αvβ3 and vascular endothelial growth factor receptor-2 (KDR/Flk-1) in cutaneous and oral melanomas of dog. *Histology and Histopathology*: 18(3), 819-826.

Roose, J., Huls, G., van Beest, M., Moerer, P., van der Horn, K., Goldschmeding, R., Loqtenberg, T. & Clevers, H. (1999) Synergy between tumor suppressor APC and the beta-catenin-Tcf4 target Tcf1. *Science*: 285(5435), 1923-1926.

Rothwell, T. L. W., Howlett, C. R., Middleton, D. J., Griffiths, D. A., and Duff, B. C. (1987) Skin neoplasms of dogs in Sydney. *Australian Veterinary Journal*: 64(6), 161-164.

Sanders, D. S. A., Blessing, K., Hassan, G. A. R., Bruton, R., Marsden, J. R. & Jankowski, J. (1999) Alterations in cadherin and catenin expression during the biological progression of melanocytic tumours. *Molecular Pathology*: 52(3), 151-157.

Sato, A., Kojima, T., Ui-Tei, K., Miyata, Y. & Saigo, K. (1999) Dfrizzled-3, a new *Drosophila* Wnt receptor, acting as an attenuator of Wingless signaling in wingless hypomorphic mutants. *Development*: 126(20), 4421-4430.

Satoh, S., Daigo, Y., Furukawa, Y., Kato, T., Miwa, N., Nishiwaki, T., Kawasoe, T., Ishiguro, H., Fujita, M., Tokino, T., Sasaki, Y., Imaoka, S., Murata, M., Shimano, T., Yamaoka, Y. & Nakamura, Y. (2000) AXIN1 mutations in hepatocellular carcinomas, and growth suppression in cancer cells by virus-mediated transfer of AXIN1. *Nature Genetics*: 24(3), 245-250.

Shin, I. M. & Herlyn, M. (1993) Role of growth factors and their receptors in the development and progression of melanoma. *The Journal of Investigative Dermatology*: 100(2 Suppl), 196S-203S.

Smith, S. H., Goldschmidt, M. H. & McManus, P. M. (2002) A comparative review of melanocytic neoplasm. *Veterinary Pathology*: 39(6), 651-678.

Spiegelman, V. S., Slaga, T. J., Pagano, M., Minamoto, T., Ronai, Z. & Fuchs, S. Y. (2000) Wnt/beta-catenin signaling induces the expression and activity of betaTrCP ubiquitin ligase receptor. *Molecular Cell*: 5(5), 877-882.

Stadeli, R., Hoffmans, R. & Basler, K. (2006) Transcription under the control of nuclear Arm/beta-catenin. *Current Biology*: 16(10), R378-385.

Su, Y., Fu, C., Ishikawa, S., Stella, A., Kojima, M., Shitoh, K., Schreiber, E. M., Day, B. W. & Lie, B. (2008) APC is essential for targeting phosphorylated-catenin to the SCF (beta-TrCP) ubiquitin ligase. *Molecular Cell*: 32(5), 652-661.

Sun, T. Q., Lu, B., Feng, J. J., Reinhard, C., Jan T. N., Fantl, W. J. & Williams, L. T. (2001) PAR-1 is a Dishevelled-associated kinase and a positive regulator of Wnt signaling. *Nature Cell Biology*: 3(7), 628-636.

Takacs, C. M., Baird, J. R., Hughes, E. G., Kent, S. S., Henchabane, H., Paik, R. & Ahmed, Y. (2008) Dual positive and negative regulation of wingless signaling by adenomatous polyposis coli. *Science*: 319(5861), 333-336.

Takada, R., Satomi, Y., Kurata, T., Ueno, N., Norioka, S., Kondoh, H., Takao, T. & Takada, S. (2006) Monounsaturated fatty acid modification of Wnt protein: its role in Wnt secretion. *Developmental Cell*: 11(6), 791-801.

Tamai, K., Zeng, X., Liu, C., Zhang, X., Harada, Y., Chang, Z. & He, X. (2004) A mechanism for Wnt coreceptor activation. *Molecular Cell*: 13(1), 149-156.

Tang, A., Eller, M. S., Hara, M., Yaar, M., Hirohashi, S., & Gilchrest, B. A. (1994) E-cadherin is the major mediator of human melanocyte adhesion to keratinocytes in vitro. *Journal of Cell Science*: 107(Pt 4), 983-992.

Thamm, D. H., Huelsmeyer, M. K., Mitzey, A. M., Qurollo, B., Rose, B. J. & Kurzman, I. D. (2010) RT-PCR-based tyrosine kinase display profiling of canine melanoma: IGF-1 receptor as a potential therapeutic target. *Melanoma Research*: 20(1), 35-42.

Toomes, C., Bottomley, H. M., Jackson, R. M., Towns, K. V., Scott, S., Mackey, D. A., Craig, J. E., Jiang, L., Yang, Z., Trembath, R., Woodruff, G., Gregory-Evans, C. Y., Gregory-Evans, K., Parker, M. J., Black, G. C., Downey, L. M., Zhang, K. & Inglehearn, C. F. (2004) Mutations in LRP5 or FZD4 underlie the common familial exudative vitreoretinopathy locus on chromosome 11q. *American Journal of Human Genetics*: 74(4), 721-730.

Umbhauer, M., Djiane, A., Goisset, C., Penzo-Mendez, A., Riou, J. F., Boucaut, J. C. & Shi, D. L. (2000) The C-terminal cytoplasmic Lys-Thr-X-X-X-Trp motif in frizzled receptors mediates Wnt/beta catenin signaling. *EMBO Journal*: 19(18), 4944-4954.

Vail, D. M. & MacEwen, E. G. (2000) Spontaneously occurring tumors of companion animals as models for human cancer. *Cancer Investigation*: 18(8), 781-792.

von Euler, H., Sadeghi, A., Carlsson, B., Rivera, P., Loskog, A., Segall, T., Korsgren, O. & Tötterman, T. H. (2008) Efficient adenovector CD40 ligand immunotherapy of canine malignant melanoma. *Journal of Immunotherapy*: 31(4), 377-384.

Wehrli, M., Dougan, S. T., Caldwell, K., O'Keefe, L., Schwartz, S., Vaizel-Ohayon, D., Schejter, E., Tomlinson, A. & DiNardo, S. (2000) arrow encodes an LDL-receptor-related protein essential for Wingless signaling. *Nature*: 407(6803), 527-530.

Willert, J., Epping, M., Pollack, J., Brown, P. & Nusse, R. (2002) A transcriptional response to Wnt protein in human embryonic carcinoma cells. *BMC Developmental Biology*: 2, 8.

Willert, K., Brown, J. D., Danenberg, E., Duncan, A. W., Weissman, I. L., Reya, T., Yates, J. R. 3rd. & Nusse, R. (2003) Wnt proteins are lipid-modified and can act as stem cell growth factors. *Nature*: 423(6938), 448-452.

Woodhead, A. D., Setlow, R. B. & Tanaka, M. (1999) Environmental factors in nonmelanoma and melanoma skin cancer. *Journal of Epidemiology*: 9(6 Suppl), S102-S114.

Woods, C. G., Stricker, S., Seemann, P., Stern, R., Cox, J., Sherridan, E., Roberts, E., Springell, K., Scott, S., Karbani, G., Sharif, S. M., Toomes, C., Bond, J., Kumar, D., Al-Gazali, L. & Mundlos, S. (2006) Mutations in WNT7A cause a range of limb malformations, including Fuhrmann syndrome and Al-Awadi/Raas-Rothschild/Schinzel phocomelia syndrome. *American Journal of Human Genetics*: 79(2), 402-408.

Xing, Y., Clements, W. K., Kimelman, D. & Xu, W. (2003) Crystal structure of a beta-catenin/axin complex suggests a mechanism for the beta-catenin destruction complex. *Genes & development*: 17(22), 2753-2764.

Xu, Q., Wang, Y., Dabdoub, A., Smallwood, P. M., Williams, J., Woods, C., Kelly, M. W., Jiang, L., Tasman, W., Zhang, K. & Nathans, J. (2004) Vascular development in the retina and inner ear: control by Norrin and Frizzled-4, a high-affinity ligand-receptor pair. *Cell*: 116(6), 883-895.

Yanagawa, S., van Leeuwen, F., Wodarz, A., Klingensmith, J. & Nusse, R. (1995) The disheveled protein is modified by wingless signaling in *Drosophila*. *Genes & Development*: 9(9), 1087-1097.

Zeng, X., Huang, H., Tamai, K., Zhang, X., Harada, Y., Yokota, C., Almeida, K., Wang, J., Doble, B., Woodgett, J., Wynshaw-Boris, A., Hsieh, J. C. & He, X. (2008) Initiation of Wnt signaling: control of Wnt coreceptor Lrp6 phosphorylation/activation via frizzled, disheveled and axin functions. *Development (Cambridge, England)*: 135(2), 873-877.

Zeng, X., Tamai, K., Doble, B., Li, S., Huang, H., Habas, R., Okamura, H., Woodgett, J. & He, X. (2005) A dual-kinase mechanism for Wnt co-receptor phosphorylation and activation. *Nature*: 438(7069), 873-877.

Zhai, L., Chaturvedi, D. & Cumberledge, S. (2004) Drosophila Wnt-1 undergoes a hydrophobic modification and is targeted to lipid rafts; a process that requires Porcupine. *The Journal of Biological Chemistry*: 279(32), 33220-33227.

4

Improving Diagnosis by Using Computerized Citometry

Valcinir Bedin
UNICAMP-FTESM-BWS-Pele Saudável
Brazil

1. Introduction

Melanoma is the most aggressive skin neoplasm [1] affecting not only adults but also children and adolescents [2]. Traditional methods of study have been applied to achieve the best diagnosis in order to recommend the best treatment [3]. The aim of this chapter is to contribute with new technologies to improve this diagnosis.

Cutaneous melanoma arises from the transformation of epidermal melanocytes, whose main function is the production of melanin, the pigment that gives skin photoprotection [4,5]. The epidermal melanocytes also act as sensory and regulatory cells through induction of neuroendocrine and immunomodulatory, thereby maintaining skin homeostasis [6]. The human melanocytes, in adulthood, are normally quiescent and mitotic activity may present with mild action of specific external stimuli such as ultraviolet radiation and wound healing [5,6]. This proliferative activity specifically requires delicate control of the cell cycle and changes in their regulatory signals can result in uncontrolled cell division and may represent the beginning of the process of malignant transformation [5]. The process of malignant transformation of melanocytes is likely multifactorial and results from complex interactions between genetic, constitutional and environmental [7] ,

Cutaneous melanoma is a cancer that allows the study of cellular events relevant to malignant transformation, because its natural history shows progressive stages of tumor aggressiveness, according to their ability to infiltrate the dermis [7,8,9,10, 11.12]. This feature of the tumor based on the fact that the transition from radial growth pattern for the vertical growth pattern with infiltration of the dermis is a major milestone in several biological properties of the tumor, including its ability to metastasize [11].

As in most human malignancies, the development of melanoma results from disruption of the integrity of the genome of melanocytes, which induces sustained instability, caused by chromosomal abnormalities, which will determine the characteristics of these neoplastic cells [7,8,11]. The genesis of the genome involves dynamic changes produced by mutations that determine gain of function of oncogenes or loss of function of tumor suppressor genes [13]. This process occurs in stages, determining the progressive transformation of normal cells into neoplastic cells [13].]

For the purposes of prognosis, one of the most modern assessment takes into account the concept of "micro-stage." The four major types of melanoma are lentigo malignant melanoma, acral lentiginous melanoma, superficial spreading melanoma and nodular melanoma [5].

The lentigo maligna melanoma has irregular margins and usually occurs on sun-exposed areas in older patients. The acral lentiginous occurs on the hands and feet and often shows massive invasion occurs when the vertical growth phase. The most common among Caucasians is the surface of melanoma, which affects the trunk and extremities. These lesions have varied colors. Nodular melanoma is highly pigmented and grows rapidly to make the micro staging of melanoma is important in determining the level of invasion Clark or Breslow thickness measurement (top of the granular layer of the epidermis to the deepest extent of tumor) . The association between clinical-pathological correlation and microscopic measurements are useful in assessing prognosis [1.14].

It is essential to obtain a biopsy in order to have a histopathologic diagnosis of pigmented skin lesion. The excision biopsy is the procedure of choice in the removal of a lesion with suspected melanoma. The sentinel lymph node biopsy is an innovation that has helped the prognosis [15].

Over 95% of melanomas involving the skin belong to one of four major types, but there is a small but important group of cutaneous melanomas can be classified as unusual variants. Many of these variants have distinct histopathological features: they include desmoplastic melanoma, neurotropic melanoma, pedunculated melanoma, metastatic melanoma, amelanotic melanoma, melanoma that arises on a benign nevus, melanoma regressive ("invisible") and melanoma cells in a balloon. Other lesions may simulate melanoma histopathologically. Some techniques for histopathology, and immuno histochemistry with markings for S-100 protein, vimentin, keratin, and HMB-45, can help distinguish these lesions from true melanoma [1].

Therefore, through the last two decades, many other morphological and biological factors are still being investigated, as some morphometric characteristics, number of nucleolar organizer regions [16, 17], expression of p53 protein, indicative of the rate of apoptosis, [18] as expression of bcl-2 protein, [19] expression of adhesion molecules [20] and markers of cell proliferation [21]. However, the computerized morphometric analysis has been little studied and our evaluation o is that the morphometric assessment may contribute greatly to our knowledge of these tumors and their degree of aggressiveness.

Some techniques of histopathology, as the expression of PCNA, p53, Bax and Bcl-X, have been used to differentiate malignancies [22]. Immunohistochemistry staining with markings for S-100 protein, vimentin, keratin, and HMB-45, can help distinguish benign lesions from true melanoma .

Other prognostic markers, however, which are not yet used in daily practice, might add important information and thus improve prognosis, treatment, and survival. Therefore a search for new prognostic factors is desirable. For this purpose, traditional or new immunohistochemical markers, gene expression arrays, comparative genomic hybridization and mutational profiling have been applied [22-31]. Most of these techniques are sophisticated and expensive, requiring specially equipped laboratories with a trained staff, Detailed morphological analysis of the nuclei in histological or cytological preparations can give important information on cell physiology and, furthermore, can be of considerable great diagnostic and prognostic importance [32-42].

Physiologic or pathologic changes of the cell accompany changes of the chromatin arrangement. In particular, neoplastic growth induces important modifications, not only of the DNA, but also of the composition and distribution of the histone and non-histone nuclear proteins, thus provoking alterations of the distribution of heterochromatin in the nucleus. Nuclear texture features have been studied as prognostic markers in neoplasias .

The resources available in commercial softwares are usually restricted to basic morphometric parameters such as diameter, area and perimeter, which cannot adequately measure texture features of nuclei.
The most common way to process the images has the principle to work with them directly, as we do, that is, concentrating the work on the intensity and distribution of gray levels at each point of the figure. These methods are referred to as spatial methods. Thus, the information can be removed, such as distance between two points, areas, angles, [43] count of elements such as cells, nuclei, mitosis, and others. The image analysis by the computer can predict survival in patients with malignancy with a high degree of accuracy and with less subjectivity than visual examination [44]. However, no quantitative pathology must be understood as a synonym for self diagnosis or that the responsibility of the pathologist should be taken on computer applications. For over 30 years, several experimental systems were developed for the prescreening of cytological preparations, including the use of techniques of image processing [45]. Despite the large number of algorithms, yet none of the systems resulted in clinically acceptable commercial product. Images of stained cells are heterogeneous and complex, and can be difficult to classify them due to the large number of cellular aggregates and overlays. The automatic processing of images and quantification of morphological characteristics of cells have a double benefit. First, the process can allow automated screening and second, to take the diagnostic criteria more objective and reproducible. [46]. The parameters of image analysis can be used with the advantage of stimulating small changes in the cellular substance that are not obvious to the human eye, or are invisible or are difficult to include a qualifying description [47]. There are structures seen in optical and electron microscopy that could not be readily classified by using simple parameters such as length, area and circumference, especially if their general appearance can be described by textural characteristics.
More recently studies have been made that combined computer technology and histology. A few of these works can be listed. The use of automated microscopy epiluminescente [48] and the use of multiple cytometric markers such as DNA microdensitometry, cariometry, AgNOR and MIB1-Ki67 [49] for evaluation of malignancy in pigmented lesions. Tissue count analysis of histological sections of melanoma associated with the size of the mask [50], evaluation of components of skin biopsy using the CART (classification and regression trees) [51] and association of clinic and anatomy of melanocytic skin cancer by analyzing image dermoscopy [52]. Mijovic Z, Mihailovic D, 2002, [53] used discriminant analysis of variables kariometric to distinguish between malignant melanocytic skin lesions and benign lesions. The fractal dimension of clones of K1735 melanoma in mice was studied by Aham et al [54].
Some studies have been made in distinguishing benign pigmented lesions from melanoma. Oka et al in 2004 [55] presented a study showing dermoscopic parameters for the differentiation of melanoma with Clark's nevus, using linear discriminant analysis. Rubegni et al in 2001 [56] differentiating pigmented Spitz nevus and melanoma by digital dermoscopy and discriminant analysis. An automated method for the mmunohistochemical quantification and fractal analysis was presented i by Gerges et al in 2004 [57]. The vascularization and the fractal dimension of the dermoepidermal interface in guttate and plaque psoriasis was studied by Uhoda et al [58] in 2005. Cytomorphometric parameters and the metastatic potential of uveal and cutaneous melanoma, compared with prognostic factors, was developed by Pereira FB et al in 2001 [59]. The resources available in commercial software (eg, KS-300) are restricted to basic morphometric parameters such as

diameter, area, perimeter [60], which in itself helps to objectify, but can not "measure" sets more morphological complexes, for example, the texture of nuclei.
Whereas a digital one core is composed of pixels with gray levels forming a pattern, texture nuclear depends on the spatial relationship of each pixel with neighboring pixels in the nucleus. Thus the texture measures can be studied as statistical properties of an image.

2. Texture and biological function

The texture is a characteristic that describes the generic appearance of part of an image and appearance is often expressed as soft, sandy, regular, coarse, granular, etc. [35]. The texture of the image "equivalent" to histological or cytological tissue is closely related to physiological and pathophysiological disorder of the body, which is the basis of microscopic analysis. The chromatin texture of nuclei is related to epigenetic changes, such as methylation or histone modification, remodeling profoundly nuclear architecture characteristic of each type of tissue. Physiological or pathological changes can still influence this process, explaining the wide variety of chromatin structure [61, 62, 63, 64].
Therefore, the study of nuclear texture has become increasingly important for histopathology and cytopathology. Deshabhoina et al in 2003 [45] published a study which used the texture image to separate melanoma and seborrheic keratosis. Another study focused on the detection of pigment network and applying dermoscopic images using texture analysis [66]. The size, shape and texture of the nuclei are of fundamental importance in cytological evaluation of malignancy [67, 68].
Traditionally, analysis of histological and cytological textures are made by the opinion of "expert" [69, 70, 71, 72] specialist trained in microscopic analysis [73, 74, 75, 76, 77, 78, 79, 80]. This type of evaluation, however, contains a strong subjective component, which explains the considerable degree of disagreement among experts in all fields of histopathology and cytopathology [81, 82, 83, 84, 85, 86, 87]. Christropher & Hotz 2004 [88] show that subjectivity in their study. This explains the attempts to "objectify" the diagnostic process, using mathematical tools applied in the analysis of microscopic images [89].
Pilot studies demonstrated the utility of such techniques for objective differentiation of cells in various malignancies [90, 91, 92]
Texture descriptors have shown great utility in nuclear medicine [.93, 94, 95] Image analysis
To face this problem new parameters have been established, such as entropy, symmetry parameters (contour and surface) and the application of graph theory [96] A stylish alternative to texture is that which examines the composition of the image as sums of sines and cosines. One of the first such attempts was the use of Fourier transform. In 1808, Joseph Fourier proposed to the Paris Academy of Sciences of the whole curve could be irregular as a sum of periodic functions. Already in 1809, Gauss, studying the properties of this transformation has created an algorithm able to calculate it accurately and with greater performance at a time when there was not even calculators. This algorithm was used on one computer for the first time only by Cooley in 1969 in a program written in Fortran. Thus, spectral analysis has become practical using the fast Fourier transform (FFT).
The Fourier transforms have been used in various fields such as crystallography and communication theory, conducting, respectively, three-dimensional analysis and data compression. More recently, Fourier transforms were used for the identification and classification of paintings based on the observation that particular characteristics of a painting can be more easily removed if the two-dimensional spectrum is examined, rather than the original painting.

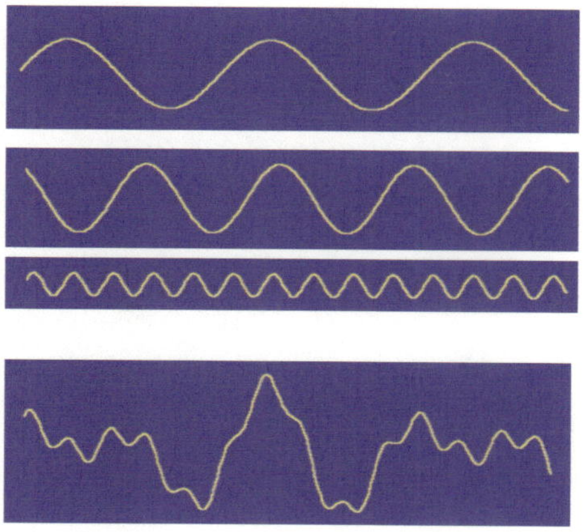

Fig. 1. Fast Fourier Transform.

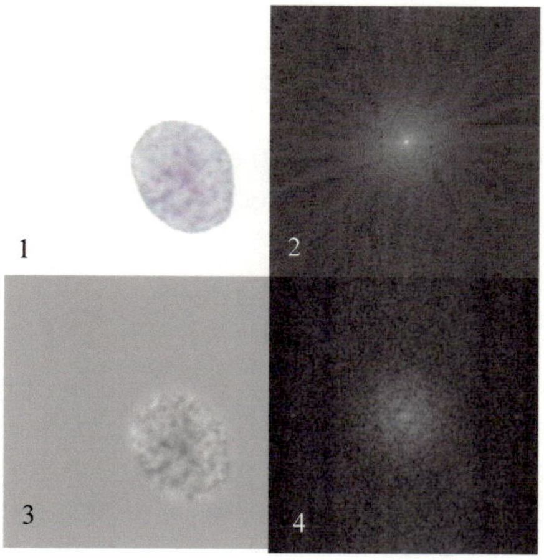

Fig. 2. Fast Fourier Transform.

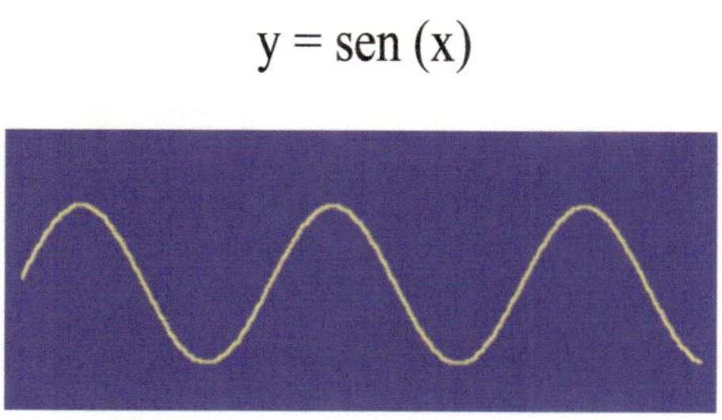

Fig. 3. Taking the square wave from sine.

Fast Fourier Transform

$$F(u,v) = \frac{1}{N}\sum_{x=0}^{M-1}\sum_{y=0}^{N-1} f(x,y)e^{-i2\pi\left(\frac{ux+vy}{N}\right)}$$

Fig. 4. Sum of sines.

The analysis of Fourier transform images of the space domain to the frequency, generally assumed that the frequency is a measure of periodic repetition of some event. In image processing, the spatial frequency is a measure that expresses the rate of change of brightness (gray levels, usually between 0 and 255) occurring in a sequence of points. High spatial frequencies correspond to the details of that brightness varies rapidly [97]. Low spatial frequencies represent slow changes of brightness. The frequency distribution of the image represents the frequency and directional interference. The Fourier texture features can be calculated from the distribution of frequencies in different regions of the transformed space.

3. Core subjected to Fourier transform

Computer analysis of images is a breakthrough in the study of pathology since, through this method, we have more precision in diagnoses that are made today and we can proceed in diagnoses not previously possible. Another advantage of the method is that it is able to reduce the influence of subjectivism in the diagnosis, reducing potential human error.
The barrier to the spread of this method is its high cost, either in the acquisition of proper equipment and in the design and development of computer programs .There is also the cost of implementation of the procedure.
Few studies were found in the literature that used the Fourier transform for histological and all could be improved. Banda-Ganboa in 1993 [98] studied cervical cells using this instrument. As he had not enough technology to eliminate the effects of the troubled border he could not study the chromatin but only the nuclear contour. Smith in 1999 [99] successfully demonstrated that the Fourier transform can sort the histological architecture of prostate tumors in 97.2% accuracy on Gleason grading in the histological images and 88.6% in the drawings made by hand. He used the method of similarity between the images processed and employed no pre-processing technique. De Vries [100] in 2000 studied the organization in cases of dermal eclerodermia. Clark in 2001 [101] explained the transparency of the cornea demonstrating ultrastructural differences between the connective tissue of the cornea and sclera through the Fourier transform of images from electron microscopy. In 2002 a study showed the importance of the Shannon entropy [102] in image analysis. Still another study this year showed the characteristics between the elastotic tissue from patients

with different skin types [103]. Another study showed the difference between keloids and hypertrophic scars [104] utilizing texture analysis and, with more resources, the authors improve their work [105]. The relationship between the texture of chromatin and phenotype in acute leukemia were studied with image analysis in 2005 [106]. In 2007 the method was used in a study showing no difference between aggressive and non-aggressive subtypes of basal cell carcinoma [107]. In 2008, Adam et al [108] improved on his previous work showing that the pre-processing of images improves the texture analysis of nuclear chromatin based on Fourier transform. This year the same group published another study showing that dichotomization of continuous data may be a bug in studies of prognostic factors.

4. Fractal dimension

For centuries, the objects and concepts of philosophy and Euclidean geometry were considered as those that best describe the world in which we live. The discovery of non-Euclidean geometries introduced new objects that represent certain phenomena of the universe, as happened with fractals. Thus, it is now known that these objects depict forms and phenomena of nature. The idea of fractals has its origins in the work of some scientists between 1857 and 1913. This work has made known some objects, cataloged as "demons" that was supposed to have no scientific value. In 1872, Karl Weierstrass found an example of a function with the property to be continuous throughout its domain, but nowhere differentiable. The graph of this function is presently called fractal. In 1904, Helge von Koch, not satisfied with the very abstract and analytical definition of Weierstrass, gave a more geometric definition of a similar function, now known as Koch snowflake (or Koch snowflake), which is the result of endless additions triangles to the perimeter of an initial triangle. Each time new triangles are added, the perimeter grows, and inevitably approaches infinity. Thus, the fractal covers a finite area within an infinite perimeter.

There were also many other works related to these figures, but that science could only be developed fully from the 60s of the twentieth century, with the aid of the emerging computer technology. One of the pioneers to use this technique was Benoit Mandelbrot, a French mathematician born in Poland, who discovered fractal geometry in the 70s of the twentieth century, and so named from the Latin adjective fractus, frangere the verb, which means breaking .

Fractal geometry is the branch of mathematics that studies the properties and behavior of fractals. It describes many situations that can not be explained easily by classical geometry, and were in science, technology and computer generated art. The conceptual roots of fractals dating from attempts to measure the size of objects for which traditional definitions based on Euclidean geometry fail [109].

A fractal (formerly known as monster curve) is a geometric object that can be divided into parts, each of which resembles the original object. It is said that fractals have infinite detail, are generally self-similar and independent of scale. In many cases a fractal can be generated by a repeating pattern, typically a recurring process or interactive.

In order to introduce the idea that size is not necessarily entirely, Mandelbrot used the following example:

What is the size of a ball of string? Mandelbrot replied that this depends on the point of view. Seen from a great distance, the ball is no more than a point with zero size. Viewed more closely, the ball seems to occupy a peripheral space, thus taking three dimensions.

Seen more closely, the thread becomes visible, and the object it is in fact one-dimensional, though that size is only clew around itself so that it occupies a three-dimensional space. The notion of how many numbers are needed to specify a point continues to be useful. From far away, there is no need - the point is the only thing that exists. Closer, it takes three. Closer still, one is enough - any particular position along the wire is single, much as the cord is coiled up. Computers, with their power of calculation and graphical representations that can run, are responsible for bringing back these "monsters" to life, generating almost instantly on the monitor and fractals with their bizarre shapes, their artistic designs or detailed landscapes and scenery.

Most of the objects of study in pathology have a complex structural characteristic and the complexity of their structures, for example, the irregularity of the margins of a tumor, remains at a constant level, despite a large range of magnifications. These structures also have patterns that repeat themselves in different increases, a property called the scale of self similarity. This has important implications for measurements of parameters such as length or area, since, in this case, the Euclidean measures can be invalidated. The fractal geometry system overcomes the limitations of Euclidean geometry for these objects and measurement of fractal dimension gives an index of their spatial properties. The fractal dimension (FD) can be measured using image analysis systems, splitters, and methods of dilation of the pixel. Some uses include fractal analysis of DNA coding and spatial extent of the property of tumors, vessels and neurons. Fractal concepts have also been incorporated into models of biological processes, including epithelial cell growth, vascular growth, periodontal diseases and viral infections.

An important aspect of texture analysis is the determination of fractality, since this feature characterizes the complexity of a structure not revealed by classical morphometry based on Euclidean geometry. Recent studies have shown the fractal nature of nuclear chromatin and of the surrounding nucleoplasmic space [110-112]. Fractals are self-similar structures, i.e. they exhibit similar features at different magnifications, in a scale-invariant manner. Previous studies have shown that fractal characteristics of nuclear chromatin are of prognostic importance in neoplasias [113-116]. Therefore our group prove that the fractal dimension of nuclear chromatin measured in routinely stained histological preparations of melanomas can be of prognostic survival value.

There are studies showing the application of FD of nuclear chromatin as a prognostic factor in lymphoblastic leukemia [117], to measure irregularities of the nuclei and glandular margins in order to distinguish benign from malignant lesions [118], to measure margins infiltrated by malignant tumors [119] to access tumor angiogenesis [93] and for measuring the distribution of collagen tissue. Fractal geometry was also applied to access the irregular distribution of chromatin in malignant cells [120]. In the future the fractal geometry can help in diagnosis, in understanding the pathogenesis and its management of injuries. It may also provide new perspectives on disease processes.

In a study carried by our group [109], a method for measuring the surface roughness was used in which a video image of the surface area is formed and divided into a group of regions covering the entire video image. Each region had the same size. A fractal dimension value is calculated for each region. The values of fractal dimensions of the regions are subjected to an average fractal dimension associated with a size of a particular region. The steps of partition, and average calculation is repeated for each region added, and each had a unique and equal size. When all the average values of fractal dimension were placed as a function of a regional size is set straight. The combination of the descending line and the

point where this straight line intercepts the y-axis indicates the surface roughness of that area.
Sakar et al [121] in 1992, described that,in order to determine the fractal dimension (FD), one should have a value of x and y coordinates correspond to the dimensions of an image type MxM, where we have 2 M pixels. The coordinate z denotes the gray level of pixels. Thus, the pair x, y indicate the position and height of the image area in the gray level.

5. Image acquisition

Image acquisition may be performed with a digital camera with high resolution (12 megapixels) and an oil immersion objective (x100). The images must be saved in uncompressed bitmap format 24-bit color. At least 150 nuclei from each tumor, chosen at random, must be acquired in each case, by the same operator, at best focus, ie, the focus on the sharp contours are presented in most of the perimeter of the nuclear membrane.

a. Only cores must be acquired with characteristics of melanoma cells, ignoring any other cells of the field.
b. Core with no creases, folds and crevices.
c. Nuclei with no overlap of any structure, for example, bubbles, precipitation of dye or other nuclei.

The nuclei must be then converted to a gray scale, 8 bit, by calculating the luminance. Finally calculate the following parameters for each core :

- Core Area
- Greater rope
- Mean transverse diameter
- Form factor
- Fractal dimension of chromatin

After normalization of the histogram of gray value (Albrechtsen) for each core a pseudo three-dimensional image is created with the z axis defined by the gray level of each pixel, thereby transforming the texture of chromatin stained with hematoxylin-eosin in a rough surface (Fig. 9). The fractal dimension (FD) of the surface of the pseudo 3-D images is calculated using a special software.
According to Sarkar et al, one must fill the space with cubes and count the number of intersections with irregular surface. This procedure is repeated with smaller or larger cubes. In a log-log diagram type for each of these procedures the number of intersections is placed against the size of the cubes. The fractal dimension can thus be obtained by the slope of the linear regression line.

6. Parameters extracted

To prepare the image to be transformed to calculate the fractal dimension tit is converted to gray scale by calculating the luminance and the white background is replaced by the average luminance of the nucleus. The following is accomplished the removal of sharp discontinuities of the edges of the core, using the technique of softening [80].

7. Greater rope

The relevance of tumor thickness, Clark's level and the mitotic rate are well known prognostic factors in the literature [23,24].

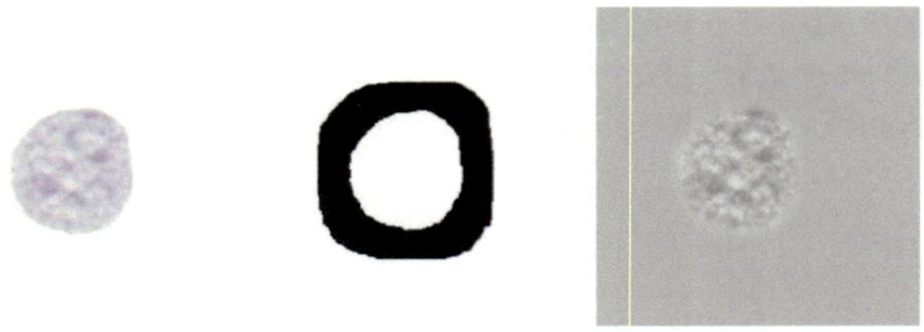

Fig. 5. Softening of core borders.

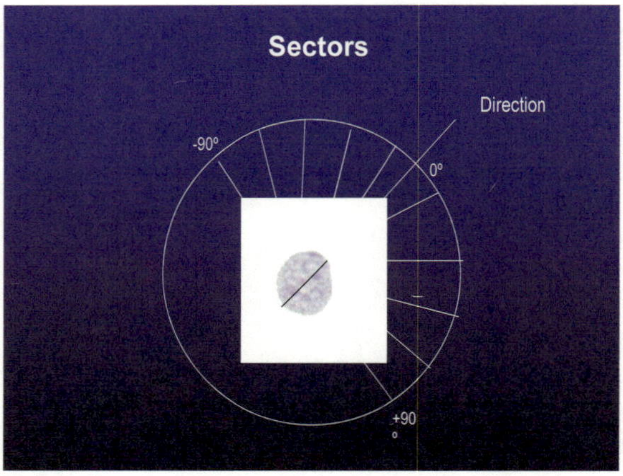

Fig. 6. Direction of the biggest rope.

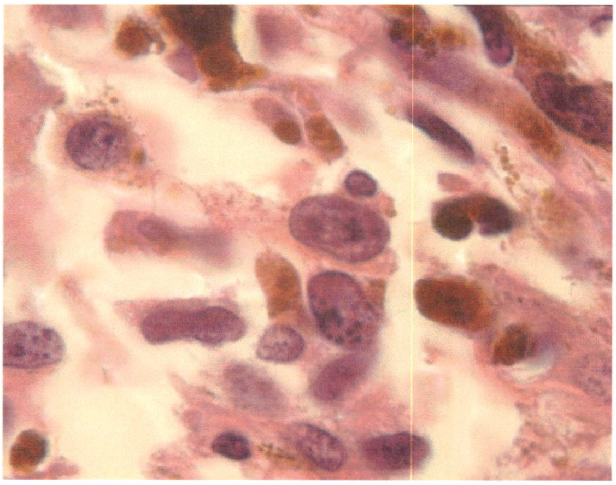

Fig. 7. Melanoma - HE.

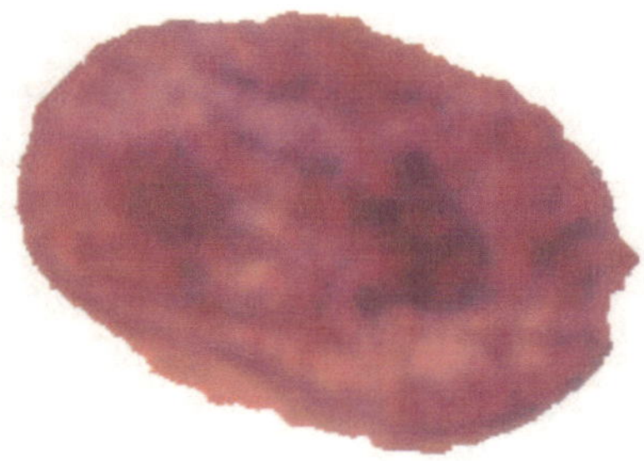

Fig. 8. Segmented core.

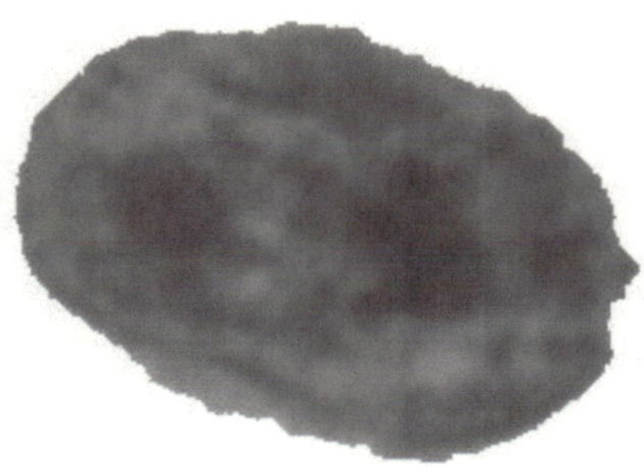

Fig. 9. Core grayscale.

Fig. 10. Pseudo 3D image.

The main emphasis of our investigation has been to test karyometic variables being as prognostic factors.

The use of computerized image analysis has contributed to an objective description of melanoma cells and decreased substantially inter-observer variation. Objective measurement of nucleolar organizer regions (AgNORs), proliferating cell nuclear antigen (PCNA) and Ki-67, nuclear DNA content or karyometric variables such as chromatin compactness, and nuclear size and shape, have been used for differential diagnosis between melanomas and several forms of melanocytic nevi [122-125].

Karyometric differences between benign and malignant melanocytic lesions reflect alterations at the genetic and epigenetic level during the progression from common melanocytic nevi to dysplastic nevi to melanoma. This process involves dynamic changes in the genome produced by mutations through gain of oncogene function or loss of action of tumor suppressor genes. But many additional alterations of gene expression can be found during tumor progression, passing from the radial to the vertical growth phase and finally to the metastatic phenotype [23]. Abnormalities in mitotic regulators such as RASSF1A and Aurora kinases promote chromosomal instability on melanoma cells [126]. Comparative genomic hybridization revealed a higher number of genetic alterations in primary melanomas which developed metastases within one year after surgery compared to tumors that did not metastasize [127]. Thus the aggressive behavior of melanoma seems to be associated with an accumulation of multiple genetic alterations.

The nucleus is organized at three hierarchical levels: the organization of nuclear processes, the higher-order organization of the chromatin fiber, and the spatial arrangement of genomes within the nuclear space. Structure and function interact mutually in a dynamic way. There is increasing evidence for self-organization of nuclear architecture and function at all levels of organization leading to a high degree of structural complexity in the mammalian cell nucleus [128]. Chromatin is separated into two distinct conformations: euchromatin, which is uncondensed and the much denser heterochromatin, which is considered to be transcriptionally less active. Recent investigations are challenging this concept, demonstrating that chromatin structure is correlated with gene density, rather than activity. According to them, decondensed chromatin is representing gene-rich and condensed chromatin gene-poor regions [128]. Mascolo et al [129] demonstrated that overexperession of the chromatin assembly factor-1 which promotes histone incorporation into chromatin, was associatied with a higher risk to develop metastases. Based on these studies we may hypothesize that the chromatin organization of aggressive melanomas with an increased number of genetic and epigenetic alterations should be different from those with a more benign clinical course. The characteristics of the nuclear architecture, as seen by the pathologist in routine sections, reflect genomic and non-genomic changes in both the structure of DNA and chromatin[130]. Taking together all these studies, we may expect that changes of nuclear shape, size and chromatin texture would accompany tumor progression and the transformation to a more aggressive phenotype.

Our karyometric measurements corroborate this hypothesis. With increasing tumor thickness, i.e. vertical growth, the nuclear area enlarged and the form factor decreased, i.e. the nuclei tended to lose their roundedness. In the univariate Cox regression, nuclear area was also a significantly negative prognostic factor, i.e., the ability to metastasize was higher in melanomas with larger nuclei. This result confirms a previous study, which showed that the mean nuclear volume of primary melanomas with subsequent metastatic course was larger than tumors that did not metastatize [131]. Talve et al [132] observed in aneuploid melanomas a correlation of tumor thickness with nuclear size and increased genetic instability. The nuclear size is also positively correlated with the fractal dimension of the chromatin architecture of the nuclei.

The fractal concept of self-similar structures was introduced by Mandelbrot [133]. Paumgartner et al. [134] applied it to microscopic images in biology and medicine. Grosberg et al [135] postulated that folded polymers should be fractals. During condensation, a polymer is repeatedly subjected to the self-similar process of crumpling, and this applies also to chromatin. Thus, the condensed polymer becomes finally a fractal. In that way a long polymer can be packed in a small volume without entanglements, which facilitates unravelling when necessary and is therefore an advantage for cell physiology [136]. Recent experimental studies showed indirect evidence for the fractal nature of DNA, nuclear chromatin and the surrounding nucleoplasmic space [110-112]. Our results gave evidence for the fractal nature of nuclear chromatin stained by haematoxylin in paraffin sections of melanoma cells.

The question whether a given structure should be considered as fractal, is linked not only to its scaling characteristics, which follow power laws. The goodness-of fit of the linear regression in the log-log plot is essential. The observed values should lie as close as possible on the straight regression line, where the slope gives an estimate of the fractal dimension..

We are measuring the fractal dimension of a rough and irregular surface, The dimension of a plane surface is 2 and that of a cube is 3. In an intuitive way one can interpret the fractal dimension of a rough, "landscape-like" surface as being in between the dimensions of a plane and of the cube, therefore $2 < FD < 3$. The fractal dimension is equivalent to the slope of the regression line which depends on the number of intercepts of the surface with the boxes. A "smoother" surface has less intercepts and therefore a lower FD than a "rougher" surface. The fractal dimension was an independent adverse prognostic factor for survival in malignant melanomas. In other words, melanomas with a "rougher" surface had a bad prognosis. A more aggressive behavior is usually found in genetically unstable neoplasias with a higher number of genetic or epigenetic changes, which provoke a more complex chromatin rearrangement, revealing an increased number of darker and lighter areas.

Previous studies demonstrated an association between higher FD values of the nucleus and worse prognosis in multiple myelomas [116], squamous cell carcinomas of the oral cavity [113] and in squamous cell carcinomas of the larynx [114]

Tumor thickness, nuclear size, mitotic index and fractal dimension have all been positively correlated with each other . Nevertheless, the stepwise procedure in the multivariate Cox regression selected the fractal dimension and the Clark level as independent variables that built up the best proportional hazard model explaining patients' survival. This implies that the complexity of chromatin distribution contains relevant prognostic information which is independent of the Clark level. Since this investigation was based on a relatively small number of patients, it should be followed by confirmatory studies.[109]

The chromatin texture of hematoxylin-eosin stained nuclei in paraffin sections of melanoma cells can be described as a fractal. The increased nuclear fractal dimension found in the more aggressive melanomas is the mathematical equivalent of a greater complexity of their chromatin architecture. We conclude that there is strong evidence that the fractal dimension of the nuclear chromatin texture is a new and promising variable in prognostic models of malignant melanomas [109].

8. References

[1] Creagan ET. Malignant Melanoma: an emerging and preventable medical catastrophe. *Mayo Clin Proc*, 72: 570-574, 1997

[2] de Sa BC, Rezze GG, Scramin AP, Landaman G, Neves RI. Cutaneous melanoma in childhood and adolescence: retrospective study of 32 patients. *Melanoma Res*.2004 Dec; 14 (6):487-92.

[3] Czarnecki D, Staples M, Mar A, et al. Recurrent melanoma skin cancer in southern . *Australia. Int J Dermatol* 1996;35:410-412.

[4] Green CL, Khavari PA. Targets for molecular therapy of skin cancer. *Semin Cancer Biol* 2004; 14:63-9.

[5] Rizos H, Becker TM, Holland EA. Cell cycle regulation in the melanocyte. In: Thompson JF, Morton DL, Kroon BBR, editors. *Textbook of melanoma*. London: Martin Dinitz; 2004. p.13-24

[6] Slominski A, Wortsman J, Nickoloff B, McClatchey K, Mihm MC, Ross JS. Molecular pathology of malignant melanoma. *Am J Clin Pathol* 1998; 110:788-94.

[7] Albino AP, Reed JA, McNutt NS. Molecular biology of cutaneous malignant melanoma. In: De Vita VT Jr, Hellman S, Rosenberg SA, editors. *Cancer: principles and practice of oncology*. 5th ed. Philadelphia: Lippincott Raven; 1997. p.1935-46.

[8] Parmiter RH, Nowell PC. Cytogenetics if nekabicttuc tynirs. *J Invest Dermatol* 1993; 100:2545-85.

[9] Parmiter RH, Nowell PC. Cytogenetics if nekabicttuc tynirs. *J Invest Dermatol* 1993; 100:2545-85.

[10] Su YA, Trent JM. Genetics of cutaneous malignant melanoma. *Cancer Control* 1995; 2:392-7.

[11] Robertson G, Coleman A, Lugo TG. A malignant melanoma tumor suprressor on human chromosome 11. *Cancer Res* 1996; 56:4487-92.

[12] Kim CJ, Reintgen DS, Yeatman TJ. The promise of microarray technology in melanoma care. *Cancer Control* 2002; 9:49-53

[13] Hanahan D, Weinberg RA. The hallmarks of cancer. *Cell* 2000; 100:57-70.

[14] Perdinaro C. Dermatopathologic variants of malignant melanoma. *Mayo Clin Proc*, 72: 273-279, 1997.

[15] Duprat JP, Silva DC, Coimbra FJ, Lima IA, Lima EN, Almeida OM, Brechtbuhl ER, Landman G, Scramin AP, Neves RI. Sentinel lymph node in cutaneous melanoma: analysis of 240 consecutive cases. *Plasti reconstr surg*. 2005 Jun; 115(7) 1944-51.

[16] Lorand-Metze I, Meira DG, Lima CSP, Vassallo J, Metze K. The differential diagnosis between aplastic anemia and hypocellular myelodysplasia in patients with pancytopenia. *Journal of Hematology:* 84:562-563 (1999).

[17] Metze K, Lobo AN, Lorand-Metze I. Nucleolus organizer regions (agnors) and total tumor mass are independent prognostic parameters for treatment-free period in chronic lymphocytic leukemia. *Int. J. Cancer Pred Oncol:* 89, 4410-443 (2000).

[18] Jahoda CAB, Reynolds AJ, Chaponnier C, Forester JC, Gabbiani G. Smooth muscle alpha-actin is a marker for hair follicle dermis in vivo and in vitro. J *Cell Sci* 1991;99:627-36.

[19] Hall PA, Levison DA. Assessment of cell proliferation in histological material (Review). *J Clin Pathol* 1990; 43:184-92

[20] Weinstein GD, Frost P. Cell proliferation in human basal cell carcinoma. *Cancer Res* 1970;30:727-8.

[21] Grimwood RE, Ferris CF, Mercill DB, Huff JC. Proliferating cells of human basal cell carcinoma are located on the periphery of tumor nodules. *J Invest Dermatol* 1986;86:191-4

[22] Sampaio-Goes FC, Oliveira DT, Dorta RG, Nonogaki S, Landman G, Nishimoto IN, Kowalski LP. Espression of PCNA, p53, Bax, and Bcl-X in oral poorly differentiated and basaloid squamous cell carcinoma: Relationship with prognosis. *Head Neck,* 2005.Aug 31

[23] Carlson JA, Ross JS, Slominski AJ: New techniques in dermatopathology that help to diagnose and prognosticate melanoma. *Clinics in Dermatology* 2009, 27:75-102.

[24] Gimotty PA, Botbyl J, Soong SJ, Guerry D: A population-based validation of the American Joint Committee on Cancer melanoma staging system. *J Clin Oncol* 2005, 23:8065-75.

[25] de Sá BC, Fugimori ML, Ribeiro Kde C, Duprat Neto JP, Neves RI, Landman G: Proteins involved in pRb and p53 pathways are differentially expressed in thin and thick superficial spreading melanomas. *Melanoma Res* 2009, *19*(3):135-41.

[26] Neto DS, Pantaleão L, de Sá BC, Landman G: Alpha-v-beta3 integrin expression in melanocytic nevi and cutaneous melanoma. *J Cutan Pathol* 2007, *34*(11):851-6.

[27] Bachmann IM, Ladstein RG, Straume O, Naumov GN, Akslen LA: Tumor Necrosis is associated with increased alphavbeta3 integrin expression and poor prognosis in nodular cutaneous melanomas. *BMC Cancer* 2008, *8:*362

[28] Winklmeier A, Poser I, Hoek KS, Bosserhoff AK: Loss of full length CtBP1 expression enhances the invasive potential of human melanoma. *BMC Cancer* 2009, *9:*52

[29] Sousa JF, Esperafico EM: Suppression subtractive hybridization profiles of radial growth phase and metastatic melanoma cell lines reveal novel potential targets. *BMC Cancer* 2008, *8:*19.

[30] Kaufmann S, Kuphal S, Schubert T, Bosserhoff AK: Functional implication of Netrin expression in malignant melanoma. *Cell Oncol* 2009, *31*(6):415-22.

[31] Metze K, Ferreira RC, Adam RL, Leite NJ, Ward LS, de Matos PS: Chromatin texture is size dependent in follicular adenomas but not in hyperplastic nodules of the thyroid. *World J Surg* 2008, *32*(12):2744-6.

[32] Ferreira RC, de Matos PS, Adam RL, Leite NJ, Metze K: Application of the Minkowski fractal dimension for the differential diagnosis in thyroid Follicular neoplasias. *Cellular Oncology* 2006, *28:*5-6.

[33] Mello MRB, Metze K, Adam RA, Pereira FG, Magalhães MG, Machado Lorand-Metze I: Phenotypic subtypes of acute lymphoblastic leukemia associated with different nuclear chromatin texture. *Analytical and Quantitative Cytology and Histology* 2008, *30:*175-184.

[34] Moro-Rodríguez E, Figols J, Alvira M, Uranga-Ocio JA, García-Poblete E: 13 GFAP and alpha1a-AR staining and nuclear morphometry of oligodendrogliomas by confocal microscopy and image analysis: useful parameters for predicting survival in oligodendrogliomas. *Diagn Pathol* 2008, *15*(3 Suppl 1):S26.

[35] Adam RL, Leite NJ, Metze K: Image preprocessing improves Fourier-based texture analysis of nuclear chromatin. *Anal Quant Cytol Histol* 2008, *30*(3):175-84.

[36] Metze K, Lorand-Metze IG: Interpretation of the AgNOR pattern in hematologic cytology. *Acta Haematol* 1993, *89*(2):110-2.

[37] Li LX, Crotty KA, Palmer AA, Kril JJ, Stankovic R, Scolyer RA, McCarthy SW: Differentiating benign nevi from malignant melanoma using DNA microdensitometry and karyometry and maturation: a zonal comparison, correlation and multivariate analysis. *Anal Quant Cytol Histol* 2002, *24*:234-43.

[38] Li LX, Crotty KA, Palmer AA, Kril JJ, Scolyer RA, Thompson JF, McCarthy SW: Argyrophilic staining of nucleolar organizer region count and morphometry in benign and malignant melanocytic lesions.*Am J Dermatopathol* 2003, *25*(3):190-7.

[39] Cia EMM, Trevisan M, Metze K: Argyrophilic nucleolar organizer region (AgNOR) technique: a helpful tool for differential diagnosis in urinary cytology.

[40] Lorand-Metze I, Carvalho MA, Metze K: Relationship between morphometric analysis of nucleolar organizer regions and cell proliferation in acute leukemias.*Cytometry* 1998, *32*:51-56.

[41] Jondet M, Agoli-Agbo R, Dehennin L: Automatic measurement of epithelium differentiation and classification of cervical intraneoplasia by computerized image analysis. *Diagn Pathol* 2010, *5*:7.

[42] Adam RL, Silva RC, Pereira FG, Leite NJ, Lorand-Metze I, Metze K: The fractal dimension of nuclear chromatin as a prognostic factor in acute precursor B lymphoblastic leukemia. *Cell Oncol* 2006, *28*(1-2):55-9.

[43] Montironi R, Scarpelli M, Lopez-Beltran A, Mazzucchelli R, Alberts D, Ranger-Moore J, Bartels HG, Hamilton PW, Einspahr J, Bartels PH: Chromatin phenotype karyometry can predict recurrence in papillary urothelial neoplasms of low malignant potential. *Cell Oncol* 2007, *29*(1):47-58

[44] CanzonierI V, Monfardini S, Carbone A. Defining prognostic factors in malignancies through image analysis. *American Journal of Clinical Pathology*. 1995. 103: 195-8.

[45] Haralick RM, Shanmugan K, Dinstein I. Texture features for image classification. *IEEE Transactions on Systems, Man and Cybernetics* 3: 610-21, 1973.

[46] Morris JA. Information and observer disagreement in histopathology. *Histopathology*. 1994. 25:123-8.

[47] Stephenson TJ. Image analysis. *Journal of Pathology*. 1992. 166(1) 83-7.

[48] Gerger A, Pompl R, Smolle J. Automated epiluminescence microscopy - tissue counter analysis using CART and 1-NN in the diagnosis of melanoma .*Skin research and technology* 9 (2): 105-110 May 2003.

[49] Li LXL, Crotty KA, Scolyer RA, Thompson JF, Kril JJ, Palmer AA, McCarthy SW. Use of multiple cytometric markers improves discrimination between benign and malignant melanocytic lesions: a study of DNA microdensitometry, karyometry, argyrophilic staining of nucleolar organizer regions and MIB1-Ki67 immunoreactivity *Melanoma research* 13 (6): 581-586 Dec 2003 .

[50] Smolle J, Gerger A, Weger W, Kutzner H, Tronnier M .Tissue counter analysis of histologic sections of melanoma: Influence of mask size and shape, feature selection, statistical methods and tissue preparation .*Analytical cellular pathology* 24 (2-3): 59-67 2002

[51] Kahofer P, Hofmann-Wellenhof R, Smolle J, Gerger A .Tissue counter analysis of tissue components in skin biopsies - Evaluation using CART (Classification and regression trees).*American journal of dermatopathology* 25 (3): 215-222 JUN 2003.

[52] Kahofer P, Hofmann-Wellenhof R, Smolle J. Tissue counter analysis of dermatoscopic images of melanocytic skin tumours: preliminary findings. . *Melanoma research* 12 (1): 71-75 Feb 2002

[53] Mijovic Z, Mihailovic D. Discriminant analysis of image karyometric variables in benign and malignant melanocytic skin lesion .*Analytical and quantitative cytology and histology* 24 (6): 314-316 Dec 2002

[54] Ahammer H, Devaney TTJ, Tritthart HA .Fractal dimension of K1735 mouse melanoma clones and spheroid invasion in vitro.*European Biophysics Journal with Biophysics Letters* 30 (7): 494-499 DEC 2001.

[55] Oka H, Tanaka M, Kobayashi S, Argenziano G, Soyer HP, Nishikawa T. Linear discriminant analysis of dermoscopic parameters for the differentiation of early melanomas from Clark naevi .*Melanoma research* 14 (2): 131-134 Apr 2004

[56] Rubegni P, Ferrari A, Cevenini G, Piccolo D, Burroni M, Perotti R, Peris K, Taddeucci P, Biagioli M, Dell'Eva G, Chimenti S, Andreassi L. Differentiation between pigmented Spitz naevus and melanoma by digital dermoscopy and stepwise logistic discriminant analysis . *Melanoma research* 11 (1): 37-44 Feb 2001.

[57] Gerger A, Bergthaler P, Smolle J .An automated method for the quantification and fractal analysis of immunostaining. *Cellular oncology* 26 (3): 125-134 2004.

[58] Uhoda I, Pierard GE, Pierard- Franchimont C, Arrese JE, Goffin V, Nikkels A, Paquet P, Quatresooz P. Vascularity and fractal dimension of the dermo-epidermal interface in guttate and plaque-type psoriasis. *Dermatology* 210 (3): 189-193 2005

[59] Pereira FB, Burnier MN, Shibata H, Wang B, Carey C...Cytomorphometric parameters and the metastatic potential of cutaneous and uveal melanoma - A comparison with prognostic factors. *American journal of dermatopathology* 23 (4): 304-307 Aug 2001

[60] True LD. Morphometric applications in anatomic pathology. *Human Pathology*. 1996. 27 (5)450-67.

[61] Cremer T, Albiez H, Bolzer A, Kohler D, Kupper K, Stefan M et al. From chromosome territories to a functional nuclear architecture. *Cellular Oncology* 27: 105–6, 2005.

[62] Gilbert N. Chromatin architecture of the human genome. *Cellular Oncology* 27: 106–7, 2005.

[63] Misteli T. Fundamental principles of nuclear architecture in cancer. *Cellular Oncology* 27: 107, 2005.

[64] Orr JA, Maxwell P, Diamond J, Hamilton P. W. Histone acetylation induces chromatin reorganization and altered gene expression in prostate neoplasia. *Cellular Oncology* 27: 107–8, 2005.

[65] Deshabhoina SV, Umbaugh SE, Stoecker WV, Moss RH, Srinivasan SK .Melanoma and seborrheic keratosis differentiation using texture features.*Skin Research and Technology*. 9 (4): 348-356 NOV 2003

[66] Anantha M, Moss RH, Stoecker WV. Detection of pigment network in dermatoscopy images using texture analysis .*Computerized medical imaging and graphics* 28 (5): 225-234 jul 2004

[67] Bedin V. Parâmetros de textura de cromatina como fator prognóstico em carcinoma basocelular. Campinas, 2004. *Dissertação – Mestrado* – Universidade Estadual de Campinas.

[68] Adam RL. Análise espectral usando a Transformada de Fourier Discreta para o estudo de núcleos celulares: Elaboração de Programa e aplicação no desenvolvimento do coração. *Dissertação – Mestrado* - Universidade Estadual de Campinas, 2002.
[69] Auada MP, Adam RL, Leite NJ, Puzzi MB, Cintra ML, Rizzo WB, Metze K. Texture analysis of the epidermis based on fast Fourier transformation in Sjögren-Larsson syndrome.*Anal Quant Cytol Histol.* 2006 Aug;28(4):219-27
[70] Chapman JA, Miller NA, Lickley HL, Qian J, Christens-Barry WA, Fu Y, Yuan Y, Axelrod DE. Ductal carcinoma in situ of the breast (DCIS) with heterogeneity of nuclear grade: prognostic effects of quantitative nuclear assessment. *BMC Cancer.* 2007 Sep 10;7:174
[71] de Troya-Martín M, Blázquez-Sánchez N, Fernández-Canedo I, Frieyro-Elicegui M, Fúnez-Liébana R, Rivas-Ruiz F. Dermoscopic study of cutaneous malignant melanoma: descriptive analysis of 45 cases; *Actas Dermosifiliogr.* 2008 Jan-Feb;99(1):44-53.
[72] Diaz G, Zucca A, Setzu MD, Cappai C. Chromatin pattern by variogram analysis. *Microsc Res Tech.* 1997 Nov 1;39(3):305-11
[73] Doudkine A, Macaulay C, Poulin N, Palcic B. Nuclear texture measurements in image cytometry. *Pathologica* 87: 286-99, 1995.
[74] Guillaud M, Adler-Storthz K, Malpica A, Staerkel G, Matisic J, Van Niekirk D, Cox D, Poulin N, Follen M, Macaulay C. Subvisual chromatin changes in cervical epithelium measured by texture image analysis and correlated with HPV. *Gynecol Oncol.* 2005 Dec;99(3 Suppl 1):S16-23. Epub 2005 Sep
[75] Huisman A, Ploeger LS, Dullens HF, Poulin N, Grizzle WE, Van Diest PJ. Development of 3D chromatin texture analysis using confocal laser scanning microscopy. *Cell Oncol.* 2005;27(5-6):335-45.
[76] Huisman A, Ploeger LS, Dullens HF, Jonges TN, Belien JA, Meijer GA, Poulin N, Grizzle WE, Van Diest PJ. Prostate tissue using chromatin texture analysis in 3-D by confocal laser scanning microscopy. *Prostate.* 2007 Feb 15;67(3):248-54.
[77] Isitor GN, Thorne R. Comparison between nuclear chromatin patterns of digitalized images of cells of the mammalian testicular and renal tissues: an imaging segmentation study. *Comput Med Imaging Graph.* 2007 Mar;31(2):63-70. Epub 2006 Dec 1
[78] Karaçali B, Tözeren A. Automated detection of regions of interest for tissue microarray experiments: an image texture analysis. *BMC Med Imaging.* 2007 Mar 9;7:2
[79] Makarov DV, Marlow C, Epstein JI, Miller MC, Landis P, Partin AW, Carter HB, Veltri RW. Using nuclear morphometry to predict the need for treatment among men with low grade, low Using nuclear morphometry to predict the need for treatment among men with low grade, low stage prostate cancer enrolled in a program of expectant management with curative intent. *Prostate.* 2008 Feb 1;68(2):183-9.
[80] Mello MR, Metze K, Adam RL, Pereira FG, Magalhães MG, Machado CG, Lorand-Metze I. Phenotypic subtypes of acute lymphoblastic leukemia associated with different nuclear chromatin texture. *Anal Quant Cytol Histol.* 2008 Apr;30(2):92-8
[81] Rode M, Flezar MS, Kogoj-Rode M, Krasovec M. Image cytometric evaluation of nuclear texture features and DNA content of the reticular form of oral lichen planus. *Anal Quant Cytol Histol.* 2006 Oct;28(5):262-8.

[82] Sabo E, Beck AH, Montgomery EA, Bhattacharya B, Meitner P, Wang JY, Resnick MB. Computerized morphometry as an aid in determining the grade of dysplasia and progression to adenocarcinoma in Barrett's esophagus. *Lab Invest.* 2006 Dec;86(12):1261-71.

[83] Scarpelli M, Montironi R, Tarquini LM, Hamilton PW, López Beltran A, Ranger-Moore J, Bartels PH. Karyometry detects subvisual differences in chromatin organisation state between non-recurrent and recurrent papillary urothelial neoplasms of low malignant potential. *J Clin Pathol.* 2004 Nov;57(11):1201-7

[84] Scheurer ME, Guillaud M, Tortolero-Luna G, Mcaulay C, Follen M, Adler-Storthz K. Human papillomavirus-related cellular changes measured by cytometric analysis of DNA ploidy and chromatin texture. *Cytometry B Clin Cytom.* 2007 Sep;72(5):324-31

[85] Schmid K, Angerstein N, Geleff S, Gschwendtner A. Quantitative nuclear texture features analysis confirms WHO classification 2004 for lung carcinomas. *Mod Pathol.* 2006 Mar;19(3):453-9

[86] Veltri RW, Miller MC, Isharwal S, Marlow C, Makarov DV, Partin AW. Prediction of prostate-specific antigen recurrence in men with long-term follow-up postprostatectomy using quantitative nuclear morphometry. *Cancer Epidemiol Biomarkers Prev.* 2008 Jan;17(1):102-10.

[87] Wiltgen M, Gerger A, Wagner C, Bergthaler P, Smolle J. Evaluation of texture features in spatial and frequency domain for automatic discrimination of histologic tissue. *Anal Quant Cytol Histol*; 29(4): 251-63, 2007 Aug.

[88] Christopher MM, Hotz CS Cytologic diagnosis: expression of probability by pathologists. .*Vet Clin Pathol.* 2004;33(2):84-95

[89] Metze K, Adam RL. Quantification in histopathology - some pitfalls. *Brazilian Journal of Medical and Biological Research* 38: 141-3, 2005.

[90] Adam RL, Ribeiro E, Metze K, Leite NJ, Lorand-Metze I. Morfometric and granulometric features of erytroblasts as a diagnostic tool of hematologic diseases. *Cytometry* 59 (1): 46, 2004.

[91] Adam RL, Leite NJ, Carvalho RB, Silva PV, Metze K. Granulometric Residues as a diagnostic tool in cytology. *Cytometry* 59 (1): 63, 2004

[92] Metze K, Adam RL, Silva PV, Carvalho RB, Leite NJ. Analysis of chromatin texture by pinkus' approximate entropy. *Cytometry* 59(1): 63, 2004.

[93] Metze K, Bedin V, Adam RL, Cintra ML, Souza EM, Leite NJ. Parameters derived from the Fast Fourier Transform are predicitve for the recurrence of basal cell carcinoma. *Cellular Oncology* 27: 137, 2005.

[94] Metze K.; Piaza AC, Iaza AA, Adam RL, Leite NJ. Texture analysis of AgNOR stained nuclei in lung cancer. *Cellular Oncology* 27: 137-8, 2005b.

[95] Metze K, Ferreira RC, Adam RL, Leite NJ, Ward LS, De Matos PS. Chromatin Texture is Size Dependent in Follicular Adenomas But Not in Hyperplastic Nodules of the Thyroid. *World J Surg.* 2008 Sep 12

[96] Wanderley de Souza Filho , tese de mestrado UNICAMP 1999

[97] Adam RL, Leite NJ, Metze K. Spectral analysis using discrete Fourier Transformation for the study of nuclei: software design and application on cardiomyocytes during physiological development. *Analytical Cellular Pathology* 22: 64 – 5, 2001.

[98] Banda-Ganboa H. et al. Spectral Analysis of Cervical Cells using the discrete Fourier Transform. Anal *Cell Pathol* 5 (1993) 85-102.

[99] Smith et al. Similarity measurement method for the classification of architecturally different images.,*Comp Biomed Res* 32 (1999) 1-12.

[100] Vries HJCD, Enomoto DHN, Mrle JV, Zuijlen PPMV, Mekkes JR, Bos JD. Dermal organization in scleroderma. The FFT antd the kaser scatter method objectify fibrosis in nonlesional as well as lesional skin. *Laboratory Investigation*.80:1281-9 2000.

[101] Clark JI. Fourier and Power law analysis of structural complexity in cornea and lens. *Micron* 32(3) 239-249 2001

[102] Metze K, Adam RL, Leite NJ. Are higher order estimates of Shannon´s entropy important for image analysis? *Analytical Cellular Pathology* 24: 194, 2002

[103] Metze K, Gomes Neto A, Adam RL, Gomes AA, Leite NJ, Souza EM, Cintra ML. Texture of dermal elastotic tissue in patients with different phototypes. *Analytical Cellular Pathology* 24: 196, 2002.

[104] Metze K, Silva PVVT, Adam RL, Cintra ML, Leite NJ. Differentiation of keloid and hypertrophic scar by texture analysis. *Analytical Cellular Pathology* 24: 196-7, 2002.

[105] Adam RL, Corsini TCG, Silva PV, Cintra ML, Leite NJ, Metze K. Fractal dimensions applied to thick contour detection and residues - comparison of keloids and hypertrophic scars. *Cytometry* 59 (1): 63-4 2004

[106] Metze K, Silva RC., Adam RL, Leite NJ, Pereira FG, Lorand-Metze I. Relation between chromatin texture and phenotype in acute leukemias. *Cellular Oncology* 27: 112-3, 2005

[107] Metze K, Bedin V, Adam RL, Macedo De Souza E, Cintra ML. 'Recurrent' basal cell carcinomas may represent new primary neoplasias: differences between aggressive and nonaggressive histologic subtypes. *J Plast Reconstr Aesthet Surg*. 2007; 60(4):451-3

[108] Adam RL, Leite NJ, Metze K. Image preprocessing improves Fourier-based texture analysis of nuclear chromatin. *Anal Quant Cytol Histol*. 2008 Jun;30(3):175-84.

[109] Bedin V, Adam RL, de Sá BCS, Landman G, Metze K.. Fractal dimension of chromatin is an independent prognostic factor for survival in melanoma. *BMC Cancer* 2010, 10:260 (5 June 2010)

[110] Lebedev DV, Filatov MV, Kuklin AI, Islamov AKh, Kentzinger E, Pantina R, Toperverg BP, Isaev-Ivanov VV: Fractal nature of chromatin organization in interphase chicken erythrocyte nuclei: DNA structure exhibits biphasic fractal properties. *FEBS Lett* 2005, 579(6):1465-8.

[111] Lieberman-Aiden E, van Berkum NL, Williams L, Imakaev M, Ragoczy T, Telling A, Amit I, Lajoie BR, Sabo PJ, Dorschner MO, Sandstrom R, Bernstein B, Bender MA, Groudine M, Gnirke A, Stamatoyannopoulos J, Mirny LA, Lander ES, Dekker J: Comprehensive mapping of long-range interactions reveals folding principles of the human genome. *Science* 2009, 326:289-293.

[112] Bancaud A, Huet S, Daigle N, Mozziconacci J, Beaudouin J, Ellenberg J: Molecular crowding affects diffusion and binding of nuclear proteins in heterochromatin and reveals the fractal organization of chromatin. *EMBO J* 2009, 28:3785-3798.

[113] Goutzanis L, Papadogeorgakis N, Pavlopoulos PM, Katti K, Petsinis V, Plochoras I, Pantelidaki C, Kavantzas N, Patsouris E, Alexandridis C: Nuclear fractal dimension

as a prognostic factor in oral squamous cell carcinoma. *Oral Oncology*. 2008, 44(4):345-353.

[114] Mashiah A, Wolach O, Sandbank J: Lymphoma and leukemia cells possess fractal dimensions that correlate with their biological features. *Acta Haematologica* 2008, (119):142-150.

[115] Delides A, Panayiotides I, Alegakis A, Kyroudi A, Banis C, Pavlaki A, Helidonis E, Kittas C: Fractal dimension as a prognostic factor for laryngeal carcinoma. *Anticancer Res* 2005, 25(3B):2141-4.

[116] Metze K, Ferro DP, Falconi MA, Adam RL, Ortega M, Lima CP, De Souza AC, Lorand-Metze I: Fractal characteristics of nuclear chromatin in routinely stained cytology are independent prognostic factors in patients with multiple myeloma. *Virchows Archiv* 2009, 455(S1):7-11.

[117] Adam RL, Silva RC, Pereira FG, Leite NJ, Lorand-Metze I, Metze K. The fractal dimension of nuclear chromatin as a prognostic factor in acute precursor lymphoblastic leukemia. *Cell Oncol*. 2006;28(1-2):55-9.

[118] Dev P. Basic principles and applications of fractal geometry in pathology: a review. *Anal Quant Cytol Histol*. 2005 Oct;27(5):284-90

[119] Lee TK, McLean DI, Atkins MS. Irregularity index: a new border irregularity measure for cutaneous melanocytic lesions. *Med Image Anal*;7(1):47-64, 2003

[120] Ferreira RC, De Matos PS, Adam RL, Leite NJ, Metze K. Application of the Minkowski-Bouligand fractal dimension for the differential diagnosis of thyroid follicular neoplasias.*Cell Oncol*. 2006;28(5-6):331-3.

[121] Sakar et al. An Efficient Approach to Estimate Fractal Dimension of Textural Images.*Pattern Recognition*, Vol. 25, No. 9, pp. 1035-1041, 1992

[122] Li LXL, Crotty KA, Scolyer RA, Thompson JF, Kril JJ, Palmer AA, McCarthy SW: Use of multiple cytometric markers improves discrimination between benign and malignant melanocytic lesions: a study of DNA microdensitometry, karyometry, argyrophilic staining of nucleolar organizer regions and MIB1- Ki67 immunoreactivity. *Melanoma Research* 2003, 13:581-586.

[123] Kossard S, WilkinsoN B: Nucleolar organizer regions and image-analysis nuclear morphometry of small-cell (nevoid) melanoma. *Journal of Cutaneous Pathology* 22(2):132-136.

[124] Rieger E, Hofmann-Wellenhof R, Soyer HP, Kofler R, Cerroni L, Smolle J, Kerl H: Comparison of proliferative activity as assessed by proliferating cell nuclear antigen (PCNA) and Ki-67 monoclonal antibodies in melanocytic skin lesions. A quantitative immunohistochemical study. *J Cutan Pathol* 1993, 20:229-36.

[125] Rother J, Jones D: Molecular markers of tumor progression in melanoma. *Curr Genomics* 2009, 10(4):231-9

[126] Balázs M, Adám Z, Treszl A, Bégány A, Hunyadi J, Adány R: Chromosomal imbalances in primary and metastatic melanomas revealed by comparative genomic hybridization. *Cytometry* 2001, 46(4):222-32.

[127] Misteli T: Beyond the Sequence: Cellular Organization of Genome Function. *Cell* 2007, 128(4):787-800. PubMed Abstract

[128] Ilbert N, Boyle S, Fiegler H, Woodfine K, Carter NP, Bickmore WA: Chromatin architecture of the human genome: gene-rich domains are enriched in open chromatin fibers. *Cell* 2004, 118:555-566.

[129] Mascolo M, Vecchione ML, Ilardi G, Scalvenzi M, Molea G, Di Benedetto M, Nugnes L, Siano M, De Rosa G, Staibano S: Overexpression of Chromatin Assembly Factor-1/p60 helps to predict the prognosis of melanoma patients. *BMC Cancer* 2010, 10(1):63.

[130] Rothhammer T, Bosserhoff AK: Epigenetic events in malignant melanoma. *Pigment Cell Res* 20:92-111.

[131] Mossbacher U, Knollmayer S, Binder M, Steiner A, Wolff K, Pehamberger H: Increased nuclear volume in metastasizing "thick" melanomas. *J Invest Dermatol* 1996, 106(3):437-40.

[132] Talve LA, Collan YU, Ekfors TO: Primary malignant melanoma of the skin. Relationships of nuclear DNA content, nuclear morphometric variables, Clark level and tumor thickness. *Anal Quant Cytol Histol* 1997, 19(1):62-74

[133] Mandelbrot BB: Stochastic models for the Earth's relief, the shape and the fractal dimension of the coastlines, and the number-area rule for islands. *Proc Natl Acad Sci USA* 1975, 72(10):3825-3828.

[134] Paumgartner D, Losa G, Weibel ER: Resolution effect on the stereological estimation of surface and volume and its interpretation in terms of fractal dimensions. *J Microsc* 1981, 21(Pt 1):51-63.

[135] Grosberg AY, Nechaev S, Shakhnovich E: The role of topological constraints in the kinetics of collapse of macromolecules. *J Phys France* 49:2095-2100.

[136] McNally JG, Mazza D: Fractal geometry in the nucleus. *EMBO Journal* 2010, 29(1):2-3

5

Modern Techniques for Computer-Aided Melanoma Diagnosis

Maciej Ogorzałek, Leszek Nowak, Grzegorz Surówka and Ana Alekseenko
Jagiellonian University Faculty of Physics, Astronomy and Applied Computer Science
Jagiellonian University Dermatology Clinic, Collegium Medicum
Poland

1. Introduction

During the last two decades we have observed an amazing development of imaging techniques targeted for bio-medical applications. New technologies, devices and equipment combined with sophisticated analysis, visualization and storage algorithms as well as programs designed for acquisition of data, signal processing, database building or data manipulation are now available commercially.

Tremendous advances were also observed in the domain of dermatology. Two types of specialized equipment have been developed for this purpose, namely the dermatoscope and the SIAscope. The dermatoscope or epiluminescence microscope has become a standard tool (Argenziano *et al.* 1998). Connected with a digital camera and lighting equipment providing light with specific wavelengths, it becomes a powerful diagnostic device. The SIAscope can be used to acquire images under different lighting conditions while the standard dermatoscope takes the images under single light wave-length.

Images acquired using dermatoscopes can be stored and analyzed further by digital computers. Some of such applications for clinical use are based on personal computers or laptop platforms (Burroni *et al.* 2004,). Newer versions can be connected even to an iPhone or hand-held device such as a palmtop computer. Several companies produce hardware solutions for dermatologic diagnosis - one of such popular solutions is proposed by DermLite.

In both techniques the digital image serves as a basis for medical analysis and diagnosis of lesions under consideration. As there is a general lack of precision in human interpretation of image content, advanced computerized techniques can assist doctors in the diagnostic process (European Consensus 2009). Several companies offer complex software solutions - let us mention here only a few, such as: Mole Expert, MoleMAX, and DDAX3 (see the websites listed under Dermatoscopic systems in the list of references).

Analysis these solutions, targeted as an aid for the practicing medical doctor, reveals they all contain data storage and manipulation software (multi-media database). Some provide also some basic tools for skin lesion images analysis. Great success in application of the dermoscopic equipment and software could be noted in Australia - one of the courtiers with highest incidence of malignant melanoma registered in the last few years. The Solarscan system has been in use in almost all dermatology clinics across Australia (compare Talbot and Bischof, Menzies *et al.* 2005).

In this chapter we review some of the now standard methods of image processing for melanoma diagnosis and also introduce new identification methods based on color decompositions used in video and TV image processing as well as new spatial and frequency information found in the skin texture. These new methods assume that some neighborhood properties of pixels in dermatoscopic images can be a sensitive probe of different pigmented skin atypia and the melanoma progression. The most promising methods are those decomposing different frequency scales of the texture. Such multi-resolution analysis is well suited to determine distinctive signals characterizing the class of the image. We present also classification analysis of the pigmented skin lesion images taken in white light based on the inductive learning methods proposed by Michalski (AQ). These methods are developed for a computer system supporting the decision making process for early diagnosis of melanoma. Symbolic (machine) learning methods used in our study are tested on two types of features extracted from pigmented lesion images: color/geometric features, and wavelet-based features. Classification performance with the wavelet features, although achieved with simple rules, is very high. Symbolic learning applied to our skin lesion data outperforms other classical machine learning methods.

2. Clinical diagnostic approaches for diagnosis of melanoma

Analyzing the medical literature and textbooks one can find out that there are several standard approaches for analysis and diagnosis of cutaneous lesions (Johr 2002, European Consensus 2009). Let us shortly describe the characteristic features used in each method for classification of lesions.

2.1 Menzies scale

This scale is used to differentiate melanoma lesion from a non-melanoma one. Lack of negative features and the presence of at least one positive attribute suggest that the lesion should be diagnosed as melanoma. The features used for differentiation are presented in table 1.

Negative features	Positive features
• lesion axial symmetry • lesion color symmetry • the presence of one color	blue-white veil numerous brown dots pseudopodia radial streaks discoloration of a scar black dots-globules at the periphery many colors (5 or 6) numerous blue / gray dots extended network

Table 1. Menzies scale feature table.

2.2 Seven-point scale

This scale uses major and minor criteria to grade lesions in scale from 1 to 7. The presence of any major criteria adds two points, one point is for minor criteria. To diagnose a melanoma using this scale the lesion must score at least 3 points. Table 2 contains the scoring criteria.

Criteria	Points
Major	
• atypical net pigmentation	2
• atypical vascular pattern	2
• blue-white veil	2
Minor	
• Irregular streaks(radial streaks)	1
• Irregular pigmentation	1
• irregular spots / globules	1
• areas of regression	1
Score	**< 3** = non melanoma **≥ 3** = suspected melanoma

Table 2. The 7-point scale criteria and scoring table.

2.3 TDS score based on ABCD rule

TDS (**T**otal **D**ermoscopy **S**core) – is a uniform system used for dermatoscopy assessment. Using a linear equation the ABCD rule (Nachbar *et al.* 1994) introduced the option to grade skin lesion depending on the degree of their malignancy. This degree is determined by the TDS value calculated from the following equation:

$$TDS = A * 1{,}3 + B * 0{,}1 + C * 0{,}5 + D * 0{,}5 \quad (1)$$

The ABCD (Asymmetry, Border, Color, Dermoscopic structures) rule is used for diagnosis of skin changes of melanocytic origin. It is used to assess lesion and brings an answer to the question whether it is a mild change, suspicious or malicious. The variables for the equation (1) are determined by visual assessment of: A - lesion shape asymmetry and color asymmetry, B – border shape and sharpness, C – presence of various colors (red, blue-gray, brown, black, white), D – presence of dermoscopic structures such as pigmentation net, regression regions, dots, globules and so on.

2.4 ABCDE rule

The ABCDE (Asymmetry, Border, Color, Diameter, Evolution) (Thomas *et al.* 1998) (Rigel *et al.* 2005) is a rule that evolved on ABCD scale used to calculate TDS value. According to this rule, the lesion is suspicious if visual assessment of the lesion is positive on any of the following features: A - lesion shape asymmetry and color asymmetry, B – border shape and sharpness, C – presence of various colors (red, blue-gray, brown, black, white), D – diameter of the lesion is greater than 6mm, E – elevation of lesion has grown over short period of time, or lesion has evolved rapidly.

3. Definitions and discussion of measures of performance in the diagnosis process

Skin cancer is a fast developing disease of modern society, reaching 20% increase of diagnosed cases every year. In Central Europe the incidence rate is 10-14 per 100,000 population and in Southern Europe the incidence is 6-10 per 100,000; in the USA 10-25 per 100,000; and in Australia, where the highest incidence is observed, 50-60 per 100,000.

Dermatoscopy is primary and commonly used method of diagnostics for nearly thirty years. This method is non-invasive and requires great deal of experience to make correct diagnosis. As described in (Menzies *et al.* 2005) only experts have 90% sensitivity and 59% specificity in skin lesion diagnosis, as shown in table 3. The result of strict compliance with the instructions should be similar to this document. Specificity and sensitivity are indexes calculated from the following equations:

$$Sensitivity = \frac{TruePositive}{TruePositive + FalseNegative} \tag{2}$$

$$Specificity = \frac{TrueNegative}{TrueNegative + FalsePositive} \tag{3}$$

	Sensitivity	Specificity
Experts	90%	59%
Dermatologists	81%	60%
Trainees	85%	36%
General practitioners	62%	63%

Table 3. Sensitivity and specificity.

Variables like TP, TF, FN and FP are described in table 4. That is why computer aided diagnostic gains more popularity every year and more complex algorithms are being developed. Some of this algorithms use: colorimetric and geometric analysis, statistical differentiation based on knowledge databases of diagnosed cases (supplied with most video and photo dermatoscopes).

	Actually Abnormal	Actually Normal
Diagnosed as Abnormal	True Positive (TP)	False Positive (FP)
Diagnosed as Normal	False Negative (FN)	True Negative (TN)

Table 4. Diagnosing possibilities.

The diagnostician has to perform difficult classification task and take the decision of telling the patient that he is in good health or not, basing on available information obtained in the process of clinical examination.

It is possible to apply computerized image processing, feature extraction and classification methods to improve diagnosis process and assist the physician in making the decision.

4. Construction of image classifiers

In process of images classification a number of classification methods (Chan *et al.* 1999) can be used. For the dermoscopic image differentiation, classification algorithms such as Artificial Neural Networks (Park *et al.* 2004) and Support Vector Machines (Wu *et al.* 2008) are used. Support Vector Machines (in short: SVM) are commonly used with four types of kernels: linear, polynomial, radial and sigmoid (Chang *et al.* 1998), each for different classification effectiveness. As for classification using Artificial Neural Networks (in short NN), the radial basis function is preferred. NN are composed of simple elements (neurons)

that are inspired by biological nervous systems. These neurons are working in parallel creating a network that is trained to perform connections between elements. Before NN can be used for classification, the network need to be trained, so that when it is given certain input it will respond with desired output.
Radial basis function, known also as Gaussian function is used often due to its strong classification power. RBF consists of two layers as shown in figure 1. First layer is a hidden radial basis layer of S1 neurons.

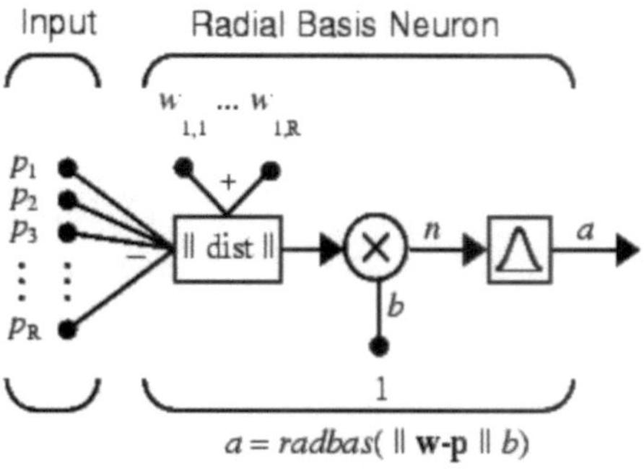

Fig. 1. Radial Basis Function Neural Network.

The second layer is a linear basis layer of S2 neurons. In figure 1 presents a NN working with Radial Basis Functions.
Conventional neural networks are performing empirical risk minimization where network weights are determined by minimizing the error between actual and desired outputs. SVM are based on the structural risk minimization where the parameters are optimized by minimizing classification error (see http://www.kernel-machines.org/).

5. Image acquisition process and image pre-processing

While working with digital images of any kind, the image acquisition is always the first step of image analysis process. Image acquisition is a stage, at which images are collected in order to create certain data set, which is later analyzed to see if any of the gathered images share similar features or contain any of the predefined features, or meet previously defined assumption.

5.1 Image acquisition

Dermoscopic images are basically digital photographs/images of magnified skin lesion, taken with conventional camera equipped with special lens extension. The lens attached to the dermatoscope acts like a microscope magnifier with its own light source that illuminates the skin surface evenly. There are various types of dermoscopy equipment, but all of them use the same principle and allow registering skin images with x10 magnification and above. Due to light source integrated into dermatoscope lens, there happens to be problem with skin reflections. To counteract this problem, a liquid is used as a medium layer between the lens and the skin. In modern dermatoscope the liquid is not necessary, because of the polarized light source that removes the reflection problem.
Digital images acquired using photo dermatoscope are sufficiently high resolution to allow for precise analysis in terms of differential structures appearance. Dermatologist can create

accurate documentation of gathered images, opening a path for computer analysis, where images are processed in order to extract information that can later be used to classify those images.

5.2 Image preprocessing

Before analysis of any image set can take place, pre-processing should be performed on all the images. This process is applied in order to make sure that all the images are consistent in desired characteristic. When working with dermatoscopic images, pre-processing can cover number of features like: image illumination equalization, color range normalization, image scale fitting, or image resolution normalization. This can be dependent on defined prerequisites and methods applied in post processing.

An example of elementary operation such as image normalization is the resolution matching. Assuming that the image size in pixels is given, and all images are in the same proportion (e.g. aspect ratio of 4:3), it is easy to find the images of smallest resolution and then scale the larger images to match the size of the smallest one. This operation allows calculating the features like lesion dimensions, lesion border length and lesions area coverage. It is possible to normalize the other parameters like color palette normalization, color saturation normalization, normalization of color components, and so on. Very common operation in preprocessing is color components normalization, known as the histogram equalization.

Image histogram is the distribution of colors values in between extreme colors used in the palette. Assuming the situation where the brightest points of the grayscale image are not white and the darkest points are not black, performing histogram equalization will redistribute all the colors of the image in a way that brightest spot of the processed image will be color and the darkest regions of the image will become black. Figure 2 illustrates the results of histogram equalization performed on a dermoscopic image.

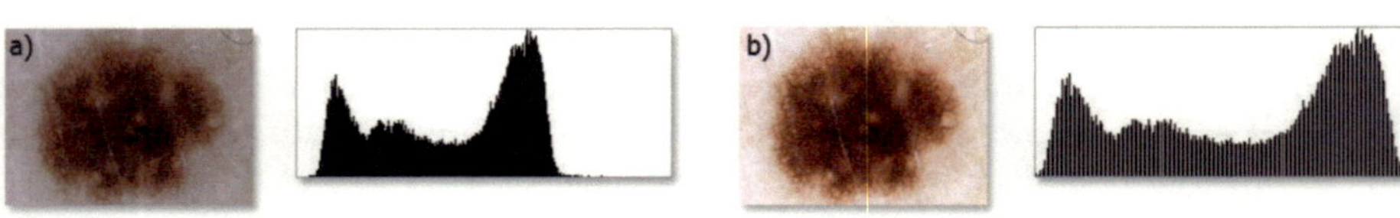

Fig. 2. a) original image and its corresponding histogram, b) image after histogram equalization and its corresponding histogram.

Normalized image is characterized by better brightness, sharpness and color depth, thereby allowing easier separation the lesion area from the background (skin color). Applying histogram equalization operation allows for better differentiation of image detail, and thus improves the efficiency of features extraction. Histogram equalization can be performed for each of the color components separately, or on all of the components at once.

5.3 Filters

Filtering an image consists of application of a certain transformation or an algorithm to image data in order to modify certain part of it. The most common task of a filter is to separate redundant information from the relevant data. By using simple filters it is possible to sharpen image, blur image, change color, etc. Applying more complex filters is possible to

enhance more important sections of the image. An example for this can be strengthening particles or detection edges.
In image processing one certain transformation is most notable, namely the binarization. It is a point transformation that is one of the basic operations used when processing any image. This operation based on gray-scale image and given threshold value will outputs a binary image, which uses only two colors (black and white) to represent data. To achieve the binary image a threshold needs to be defined. This threshold is used to determine which points of the original image will be converted to black and which to white. The binarization process is illustrated by figure 3. Having a binary image allows performing various operations like measuring the length, performing segmentation, determining the number of elements, etc. Binary image is easy to work with, as most operations are fast to perform and do not require long computing time. It is quite easy to analyze the shape of objects, calculate symmetry, or find the center of weight of an object.

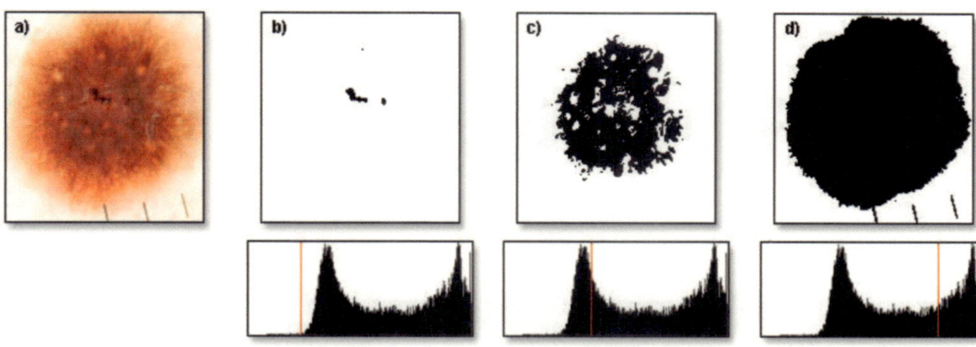

Fig. 3. a) original image, b) binarized image using threshold value of 60, c) binarized image using threshold value of 100, d) binarized image using threshold value of 200.

A simple example illustrating the idea of using filters in dermoscopic images can be the removal of artifacts such as hair (figure 4). To do this, a maximum filter can be applied on a binary image. Maximum filter process each point of an image and calculate its surrounding (neighborhood) in determined distance, then the maximum value is entered in the output image. As a result, the small details of the image are removed depending on the neighborhood size. The use of this filter on the single object will reduce it in size.

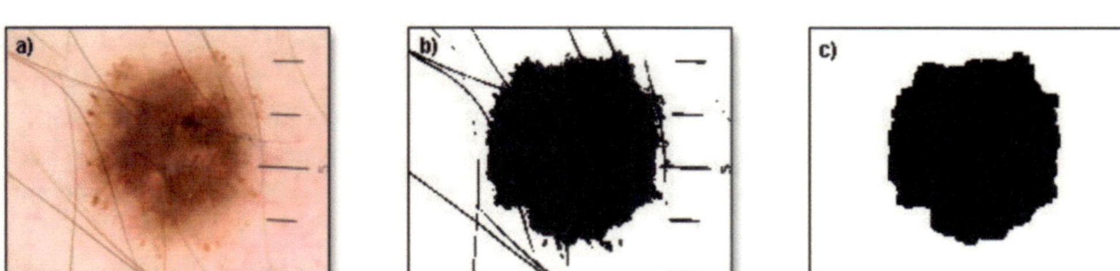

Fig. 4. Hair removal. a) original image, b) binarized image, c) image with removed artifacts.

Performing binarization on dermoscopic image can sometimes create errors in output, may it be due to poor illumination of the corners, or hairs on the image. Dealing with unevenly illuminated image is another practical example of filtering unwanted data from dermoscopic image. For this purpose a specific algorithm is used and results of its application can be viewed in figure 5. This algorithm's task is to check whether there is an object in the middle of the image, and then whether each of the corners of the image contains different object in contact with the edges of the image. If it happens that all image corners contain objects then they are removed. Condition for the proper removal of redundant objects is that on the image, there must be at least two different objects, and each of the points in the corners must be a part of one of the objects. If all conditions are met, the filter removes all points belonging to object in contact with the corners of the image. This filter can only work with images that cover entire lesion. If image contains only a fragment of the lesion, this filter will not modify the input image.

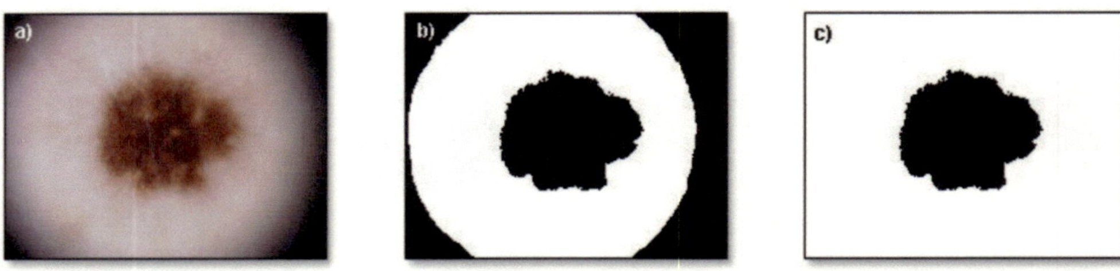

Fig. 5. Filtering of vigneting artefacts. a) original image, b) binarized image, c) image with filtered corners.

6. Numerical methods for image analysis

Several types of image analysis can be done in an automatic way. Specifically geometric features and color features/decompositions can be easily performed and are found in many commercial image analysis and dermoscope accompanying programs.

6.1 Geometric features

Many attempts have been made to automate the process of dermoscopic image feature extraction, and a number of algorithms have been developed to do this. Most common geometric features that are calculated are lesion dimensions, borders shape, lesion symmetry and color symmetry lesion area. More complex problem like various differential structures recognition still exist and is a subject of current image processing research.

Calculation the dimensions of lesion on the dermoscopic image is an easy task. The easiest way to determine the surface size is to count all points that are marked as the lesion on the binary image achieved in process of binarization. The sum of these points and its percentage cover of an image lesion image can be used as variables in classification process. These two factors can be used to calculate other factors like various color coverage of the lesion.

Border length of the lesion is another feature that is easily calculated from a binary mask of the dermoscopic lesion image. Border length can be calculates simply by counting all boundary points on binary lesion mask. It is possible to estimate how irregular the border is by comparing it to the lesion size, e.g. circular lesion would have shorter border length comparing to irregular lesion of the same size.

The symmetry of the lesion is an important factor in diagnostic process. Calculating symmetry value as a geometrical feature requires more complex operations, as it is necessary to estimate proper axis of symmetry. This task can proved to be complicated, even with the manual axis alignment. The examples images for determining the symmetry axis are illustrated in figure 6.

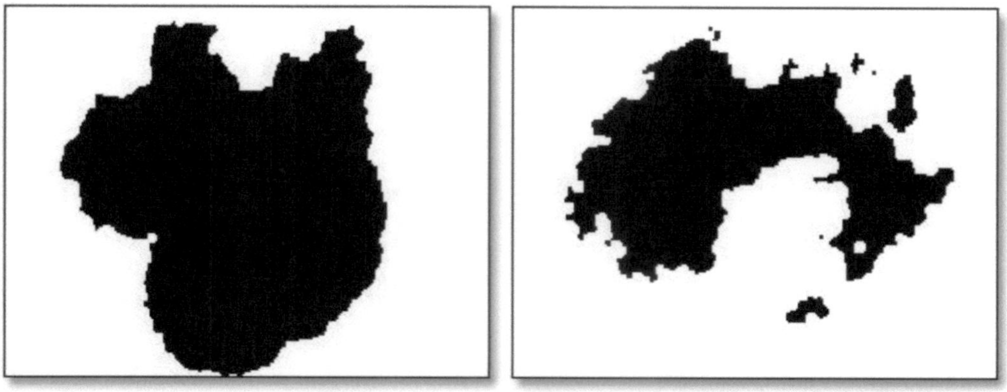

Fig. 6. Examples of lesion shapes.

Using the algorithm of smallest bounding box estimation prove to be effective way to determine the symmetry axis for various lesion shapes. Symmetry axis for calculated bounding rectangle is used as the symmetry axis for the lesion. As shown on the figure 7.

Calculating the value of the symmetry is very simple and is done by checking if every point of the lesion on one side of the symmetry axis has its corresponding point on the other side of this axis. Symmetry is calculated separately for vertical and horizontal axis, and then the average value is subtracted from the lesion size value. The percentage of asymmetry can be calculated from this data and later used in the classification process.

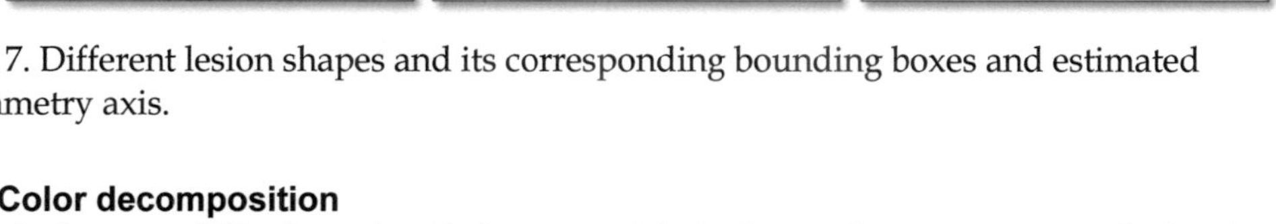

Fig. 7. Different lesion shapes and its corresponding bounding boxes and estimated symmetry axis.

6.2 Color decomposition

Skin lesions are difficult to classify because of their short color ranges, instead of real-world images (Deng et al., 2001). Malignant melanoma is a kind of skin cancer that has some characteristic color groups like: black, blue-grey, red, light brown, dark brown and skin color. These colors appear on images and can depend on cancer progress stage, lesion depth and blood vessels. These colors are also used in melanoma diagnosis scales like ABCD.

Typically in digital images we use RGB (additive) or CMYK (subtractive) color representations.

There exists however several other decompositions used in video or TV coding. These color decompositions have not been used so far for melanoma diagnosis - they were first proposed as useful features in our works (Ogorzałek *et al.* 2009, 2010). Typical melanoma image color decompositions are shown in two color spaces in figure 8. It can be easily seen that in the second picture the points representing colors are grouped in two areas and thus could be distinguished/classified very easily.

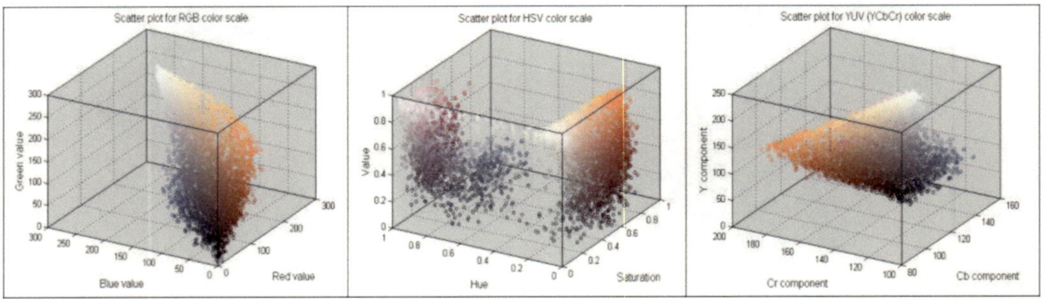

Fig. 8. Three different color decompositions of dermoscopic image. Every point corresponds to a region of the images. HSV decomposition (middle picture) gives the best classification possibilities.

6.3 Image segmentation

Image segmentation is performed in two steps: color quantization and spatial segmentation. In the first step image is quantized to several region classes. Quantization is done in color space only. After that a class-map is created by their belonging to the corresponding color class. Second step is spatial segmentation is performed on created class-map. Color similarity is in second step not taken into consideration. The next step is objects extraction (Liu *et al.* 2005). Described method extracts borders from a segmented image. By using these borders objects in the image can be extracted. Object extraction is done by a region growing algorithm. This is the most time consuming part of presented method. The result of the segmentation process is illustrated in figure 9.

Each object is represented in four color spaces: RGB, HSV, NTSC and YCbCr. Every color space is represented by few variables like: red, green and blue in RGB. There are 12 color spaces features.

7. Analysis of images based on Wavelet transformations

Our database of dermoscopic images (2272x1704, 24bit) collected with Minolta Dimage Z5 camera with epiluminescence lens consisted of 78 cases of melanoma and 80 cases of dysplastic nevi (taken at the same conditions). The selection to the categories: melanoma (label=1) and dysplastic nevus (label=0) was done on the grounds of biopsy and histopathologic examination (Żabińska-Płazak *et al.* 2005).

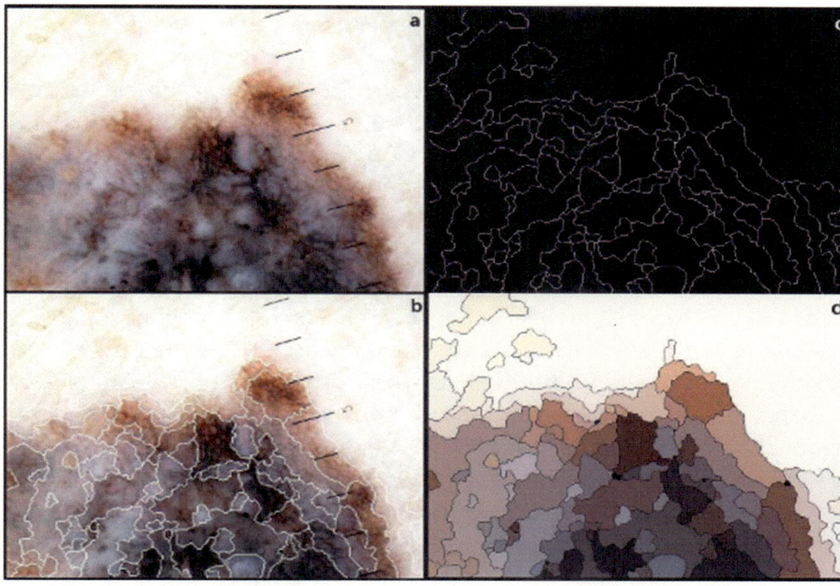

Fig. 9. a) original image, b) initial segmentation of the image, c) binary segmentation mask, d) final image segmentation.

The preparation stage for geometric/coloristic feature set (Fikrle *et al.* 2006) (Ogorzałek *et al.* 2009) was done in the following way:

All the images were scaled to 800x600 pixels, normalized in the quantization depth by a histogram correction, and removed the background (in dermoscopic images 'background' means skin of normal complexion). Identification of the mole spot was done by color indexing i.e. reduction of the quantization depth. Then artifacts like obscuration of the image corners or a pitch on the lesion were extracted. In the end with opening/closing operations (and binarization when required) we got an output form of the lesion image.

The preparation stage for the wavelet-based features (Patwardhan *et al.* 2003, 2005) (Surówka *et al.* 2006) was done in the following way:

Since the wavelet decomposition downscales the input image by a factor of 2 in rows or columns every iteration, the width and length had to be powers of 2, so the source images were filled with black pixels in due number of rows and columns. In order to apply any transform on the picture, the compressed image (JPG) must be changed into a 2D matrix of numbers. The usual way of extracting the numerical values of pixels consists in changing the RGB representation into a one-dimension color index.

7.1 Wavelet-based features

Skin texture analysis based on the multiresolution wavelet-based decomposition of the dermoscopic images is a new method to obtain valuable features for melanoma and dysplastic nevus classification. Wavelet transforms have been widely studied as tools for a multi-scale pattern recognition analysis. Wavelets are functions well localized both in space and frequency. The wavelet theory is closely related to the theory of digital filtering (Kadiyala *et al.* 1999, Mallat 1989) so the properties of the decomposition filters (the choice of the basis, degree of regularity, and the sub-bands of interest) play an important role in texture characterization.

Performance of the wavelet analysis of images depends on various factors:

- For feature extraction it is important to choose between recursive decomposition of the low-frequency branch (Mallat 1989) (the pyramidal algorithm) and, on the other hand, a more selective tree-structured analysis where the further decomposition is applied to the output of any channel (Patwardhan *et al.* 2003, Chang *et al.* 1993). The latter is advocated by observations that the significant sub-bands of the pigmented skin texture are those in the middle frequency range (Patwardhan *et al.* 2003, 2005).
- The decomposition should be performed over an optimal finite range of resolutions (Chang *et al.* 1993, Mallat 1989). This issue addresses the problem of the wavelet order.
- Different wavelet bases have diverse impact on the texture classification (Kadiyala *et al.* 1999). They have certain constraints and should, in principle, be orthonormal (energy preserving, non-redundant). Biorthogonal (near orthogonal) bases can produce, on the other hand, more compact and symmetric wavelets and the requirement for orthogonality is not superior (Mallat 1989).
- Images are two-dimensional signals so separable or non-separable sampling is possible. In the former case a one-dimensional decomposition algorithm is applied to the rows and to the columns of the image. The resulting signal is a tensor product of the separate 1D filter. The non-separable case, on the contrary, is based on lattice sampling. Both representations have advantages and disadvantages.

Unfortunately, up to now only a limited number of the aforementioned possibilities have been tested on skin dermoscopic textures (Patwardhan *et al.* 2005, Patwardhan *et al.* 2003, Surówka *et al.* 2006). Since skin textures are signals consisting mainly of middle frequency bands it has been shown that the most adequate approach to the wavelet-based multiresolution analysis is the concept of wavelet packets (Chang *et al.* 1993). In this approach an image is decomposed along dominant frequency channels forming a parent-child structure of a tree. A certain path of the tree is chosen according to the average energy content of the channel referenced to the highest energy of a channel on the same decomposition level. The determined subbands form a feature set for classification. Such an approach is shown in (Chang *et al.* 1993). The main bias of the method in (Chang *et al.* 1993) is the threshold value of the channel energy that triggers subsequent decompositions. Since features used for selection of melanoma and dysplastic lesions are clustered into rough sets, the structure of the tree may be affected by an arbitrary choice of the threshold. In the adaptive wavelet-based tree structure analysis (ADWAT) (Patwardhan *et al.* 2003, 2005) decision about the further decomposition of the channel is taken by statistical analysis of average energy, maximum energy ratio and fractional energy ratio among all the features at each level of decomposition. The resulting tree structured models of melanoma and dysplastic nevus are patterns for semantic comparison with unknown skin lesion images. The sensitivity and specificity of this method is further improved by introducing Gaussian and Bell shaped fuzzy clustering of the features (Patwardhan *et al.* 2005). Work (Surówka *et al.* 2006) is based on the idea presented in (Patwardhan *et al.* 2003) to perform a tree-like selective wavelet analysis of the skin lesion images. Unlike in (Patwardhan *et al.* 2003) the feature set is built from all of the analyzed channels and the decision to include a given branch of the tree does not come from ADWAT. Instead, all the wavelet based features are input to the Ridge classification model (Merkwirth), which determines a minimum-bias optimal vector of features. Those selected features can be used in various machine-learning methods.

After the preparation stage described earlier, the 2D=1Dx1D wavelet transform was applied to the values of pixels extracted from the discussed dermatoscopic images. The class of the filter was Daubechies 3 (Daubechies 1992) and its efficient algorithm was taken from (Numerical Recipes in C 1999). The choice for the filter was made concerning simplicity, performance and possible comparisons with (Patwardhan *et al.* 2003).
One iteration of the wavelet algorithm produces 4 subimages which can be considered as LL, LH, HL and HH filters, where L and H denote the respective low-pass and high-pass filters. One subimage is a product of the wavelet transform acting on each raw and then on each column of the parent image. Each iteration reduces half of the rows and half of the columns from the parent image. The algorithm presented in (Numerical Recipes in C 1999) is a pyramidal one i.e. it decomposes the image along the LL band in each iteration. An example of the decomposition process with 3 iterations is shown in figure 10. Here the smooth and the detail part resulting from any iteration can be easily recognized.

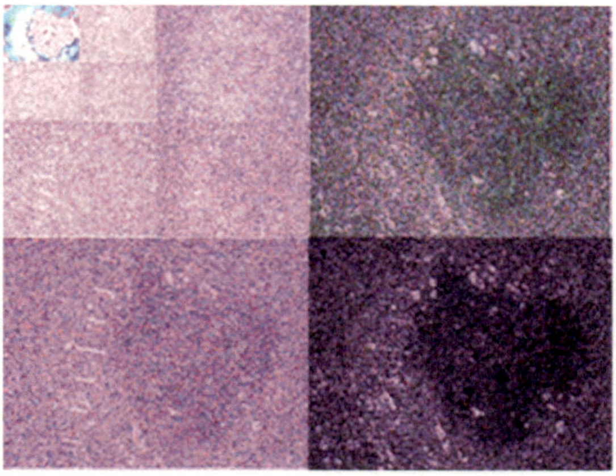

Fig. 10. Multi-band images i.e. a set of images of the same mole from its different frequency segments. Here recursive decomposition of the low-pass band takes place. For the sequence of the pyramid see next figure. Note that the luminosity of this summary image is offset otherwise it would be too dark for a presentation

According to the idea of the wavelet analysis, we adapted the pyramidal algorithm to a selective analysis of any sub-band of the parent image. Altogether 3 iterations were calculated. The proper sequence of filters in that decomposition is shown below. Every iteration has the same arrangement of filters with (sub) labels denoting 1=low-low, 2=low-high, 3=high-low and 4=high-high sub-band.

1	2
3	4

1.1	1.2	2.1	2.2
1.3	1.4	2.3	2.4
3.1	3.2	4.1	4.2
3.3	3.4	4.3	4.4

1.1.1	1.1.2	1.2.1	1.2.2	2.1.1	2.1.2	2.2.1	2.2.2
1.1.3	1.1.3	1.2.3	1.2.4	2.1.3	2.1.4	2.2.3	2.2.4
1.3.1	1.3.2	1.4.1	1.4.2	2.3.1	2.3.2	2.4.1	2.4.2
1.3.3	1.3.4	1.4.3	1.4.4	2.3.3	2.3.4	2.4.3	2.4.4
3.1.1	3.1.2	3.3.1	3.3.2	4.1.1	4.1.2	4.2.1	4.2.2
3.1.3	3.1.4	3.3.3	3.3.4	4.1.3	4.1.4	4.2.3	4.2.4
3.2.1	3.2.2	3.4.1	3.4.2	4.3.1	4.3.2	4.4.1	4.4.2
3.2.3	3.2.4	3.4.3	3.4.4	4.3.3	4.3.4	4.4.3	4.4.4

Fig. 11. Sequence of the pyramid construction.

Following the original idea (Chang *et al.* 1993) and its extended applications (Patwardhan *et al.* 2003, 2005) a feature set at a given level of decomposition was built. One iteration (resulting in 4 subimages) produced 11 coefficients calculated from the energy of the pixels (e_1, e_2, e_3, e_4), the maximum energy ratio (e_i/e_{max}, i=any three out of four except the subimage with the maximum energy) and the fractional energy ratio ($e_1/(e_2+e_3+e_4)$ + its two permutations). Term 'energy' means here the sum of the absolute values of the pixels, where M and N denote the actual dimensions of the sub-image.
Energy is calculated according to the following equation:

$$e = \frac{1}{MN}\sum_{m=1}^{M}\sum_{n=1}^{N}|f(m,n)| \qquad (4)$$

Since the algorithm is applied to the image recursively, the number of coefficients amounts to (1+4+16)x11=231. Numbers 1, 4 and 16 in this calculation mean here the number of sub-images to filter in each iteration.
In the approaches presented in (Patwardhan *et al.* 2003, 2005) the calculated features were discriminated according to their distributions within a particular channel. Only features that generated bimodal distributions separating melanoma and dysplastic images were kept in the feature set. All other were rejected. In (Surówka *et al.* 2006) the features were not used to control the development of the tree structure signatures. Instead, all 231 coefficients were accepted as potentially significant discriminating signals.
Since the number of dermatoscopy images taken to the analysis was limited and the 231 coefficients affect the classification in a different way, one can additionally pre-select the coefficients by their importance. The criterion was to maximize the classification performance of 20 and then10 most significant features. In (Surówka *et al.* 2006) the selection was twofold and was done in a Matlab toolbox ENTOOL (Merkwirth). First one Ridge regression model with 40 penalty vectors was used to determine an optimal representation of the images in a numeric form. Ridge regression constructs a linear model $\hat{y} = X\beta + \beta_0$ (X-data matrix, y-vector of categories), but instead of minimizing the sum of squared residuals $(y - X\beta + \beta_0)^T (y - X\beta + \beta_0)$, it minimizes the regularized loss function (Tikhonov regularization): $RSS_{pen.} = (y - X\beta + \beta_0)^T (y - X\beta + \beta_0) + \lambda\beta^T\beta$
The additional penalty $\lambda\beta^T\beta$ shrinks the regression coefficients $\hat{\beta}$ towards zero, thereby moderately increasing bias while considerably decreasing variance of the constructed models. The penalty parameter $\lambda \geq 0$ controls the amount of shrinkage and can be used to fine tune the bias-variance tradeoff. For this study, the optimal ridge penalty λ is automatically determined by Leave-One-Out Cross Validation on each training fold individually. To apply ridge regression to a binary classification problem, training outputs were coded as $y = 1$ (melanoma), $y = 0$ (dysplastic) and a threshold of 0.5 was applied to discriminate between both classes when doing predictions. Prior to the model construction, input variables were normalized by removing the mean and dividing by the standard deviation for each variable separately. Ten most significant features are presented below. They were obtained from a statistical analysis in ENTOOL (see Merkwirth). Indices denote the subchannels of the three different decomposition levels.
The ROC curve below presents the classification performance of 10 most significant features derived with help of 100 Ridge regression models. AUC is 95%.

average energy	$e_{4.1.2}, e_{2.1.1}, e_{3.3.2}, e_{3.3.1}$
maximum energy ratio	$e_{1.2.2} / e_{1.2.1}, e_{4.2} / e_{4.1}, e_{4.3} / e_{4.1}$
fractional energy ratio	$e_{1.2.2} / (e_{2.3.1} + e_{2.3.2} + e_{2.3.4}), e_{3.1.1} / (e_{3.1.2} + e_{3.1.3} + e_{3.1.4})$

Table 5. coefficients calculated from the energy (the sum of the absolute values of the pixels): e_1, e_2, e_3, e_4, the maximum energy ratios: (e_i/e_{max}, i=any three out of four except the subimage with the maximum energy), and the fractional energy ratios ($e_1/(e_2+e_3+e_4)$ + its two permutations).

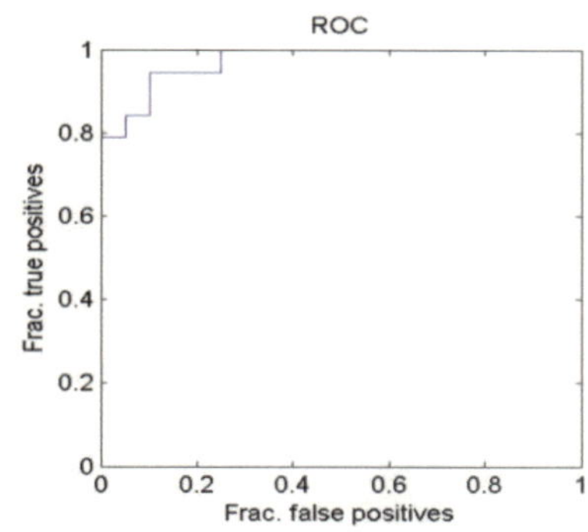

Fig. 12. ROC curve presenting the classification performance of 10 most significant features derived with help of 100 Ridge regression models. AUC is 95%.

Following are the sets of images no which the system was tested:

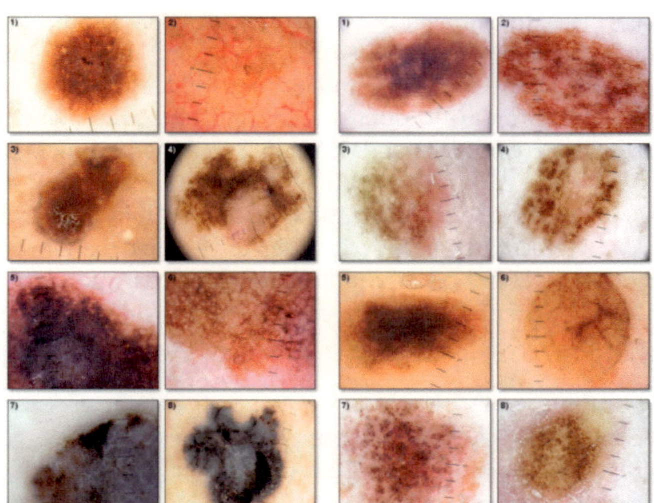

Fig. 13. Selected images from two data sets used for testing. On the left melanoma images on the right dysplasty images.

7.2 Discussion

Classification models constructed using wavelet-based tree structure decomposition of the dermoscopy images are reported in the literature (Chang *et al.* 1993), (Patwardhan *et al.* 2003,

2005). In (Chang *et al.* 1993) channel decomposition is determined based on the ratio of the average energy of that channel to the highest average energy of a channel at the same level of decomposition. The decomposition is performed if this ratio is above a predefined threshold value. In the learning phase tree-like topologies of both classes are produced. In the testing phase unknown images are decomposed with the thresholds set in the learning phase to build tree structures that are classified due to the Mahanalobis distance from the known patterns. The maximum performance obtained is TPF=70% and FPF=20% for the learning phase of 15M+15D and the testing phase 10M+15D (M=melanoma, D=dysplastic nevus). Arbitrary selection of the maximum energy thresholds is the main drawback of this method.

In the ADWAT method (Patwardhan *et al.* 2003), like in this work, different combinations of channel energy ratios over a given decomposition level are used as additional features and a statistical analysis of the feature data (not solely the maximum energy) is used to find the threshold values. Based on histograms of the features only linearly separable and bimodally distributed features between image classes are further decomposed. The thresholds are selected to optimally partition the two image classes. In the testing phase unknown skin lesion images are semantically compared with the tree structure of the melanoma and the dysplastic nevus class.

Results from (Patwardhan *et al.* 2005) for the ADWAT method read: TPF=86.66%, FPF=11.11%, and the method itself is more robust than (Chang *et al.* 1993). Such results are cited for 15M+15D in the learning phase and 15M+45D in the testing phase.

In (Patwardhan *et al.* 2005) an extended ADWAT method is reported. In this approach three classes are defined: melanoma, dysplastic nevus and suspicion lesion. Unknown images are classified as melanoma only if the tree structure completely matches the pattern assigned to the melanoma image class. Incomplete tree structures are assigned to the suspicious lesion class and their trans-illumination images are analyzed in the second step. The trans-illumination images are taken in 580nm and 680nm light by the Nevoscope tool in an illumination mode that provides lesion depth and structural information. For the learning/testing scheme of 15M+15D and 15M+45D this method yields TPF=93.33% and FPF=8.88%.

When additionally fuzzy membership partitions of the melanoma and dysplastic lesion images by the Bell or Gaussian membership function are applied, better results are obtained: TPF=100% and FPF=4.44% (FPF=17.77%) for the Gauss (Bell) partition functions.

8. Machine learning of wavelet-based features of melanoma

We experimentally apply to the dermoscopic images the main global machine learning methods, namely neural networks, and support vector machines. They serve as a generalization engine in the classification task.

The selected machine learning methods were tested over the same set of samples (78 cases of melanoma + 80 cases of dysplastic nevus). Due to small statistics of individuals, for each classifier we applied the n-fold cross validation test to gain a reasonable estimation of its accuracy. The n-fold cross validation method randomly divides the set of all available patterns into n subsets. N different models are then trained using data from n−1 sets and validated using the remaining one (the holdout fold). The procedure is repeated for each of the n folds. Accuracy of both classifiers was measured by means of the Receiver Operating Characteristics (ROC) (Receiver operating characteristic (ROC) analysis 1998). The ROC curve shows the sensitivity, i.e. ratio of correctly identified melanoma lesions, in relation to the specificity, i.e. ratio of correctly identified dysplastic nevi. For the aforementioned methods we cite the area under the ROC curve (AUC) as the key indicator of the performance.

8.1 Neural network binary classifier

The MLP neural network classifier is easy in implementation and provides stable solutions. The topology of the network was subject to tests to determine an optimal configuration for maximizing its performance (both quality of the classifier and minimal training time).

The examined three-layer feed-forward back-propagated neural network had the following architecture. The input layer was composed of ten linear-output neurons with constant unity weights. The hidden layer made of ten neurons and an output layer formed by one neuron had logistic-like activation functions. In one training cycle some 150 000 iterations were performed until the network could classify the input with a defined precision.

To evaluate features according to their rank, which was crucial in effective teaching of the neural network, prior to the training of the neural network, the number of features was reduced by the Ridge model to twenty and ten (out of 231) most discriminating ones, to avoid the network overtraining effect.

The classifier was trained on the ten selected features. Ten most significant features selected with help of the Ridge linear model yielded sensitivity (TPF) of 89.2% and specificity (1-FPF) of 90% (Surówka *et al.* 2006). The cross validation set was shifted between the training runs. Bimodal distribution of the MLP-classified lesions is displayed in figure 14. As we can see, correctly identified lesions are those distributed around 1 on the ordinate and around 0 for the other ones. On average the classification performance yields sensitivity (true positive fraction) of 89.2% and specificity (1-false positive fraction) of 90%.

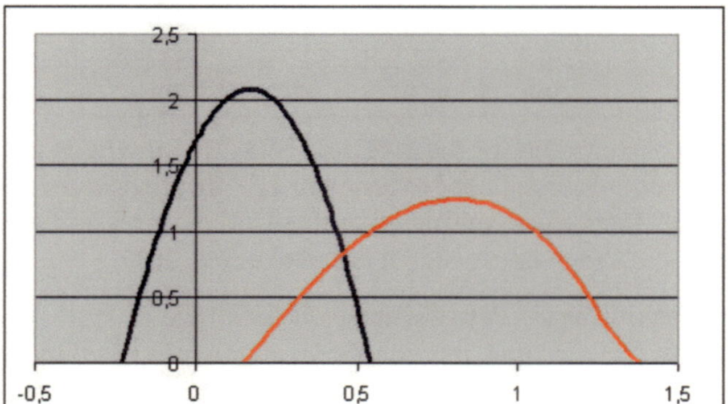

Fig. 14. Distribution of the recognized image classes. Input tags on the abscissa are: 1=melanoma, 0=dysplastic.

Lack of full separability of the two categories exhibits, as the major factor, the generalization error. Yet the inherent fuzzy nature of both feature sets also plays a role. The magnitude of both effects can be estimated by comparing appropriate performance factors above.

Due to statistics of our database we decided to perform experimentation with the oversampling technique. The image data were limited to the pigmented spot of the mole (background-free) and divided into 64x64 blocks of pixels. Each block was decomposed with the Daubechies-3 wavelets for all possible subbands of frequency (3 iterations). When the blocks were treated as individual images the accuracy of the feature set was estimated by AUC=87.8%. Segments grouped to their parent images yielded AUC=91.4%. This method appeared not to significantly improve the accuracy of the MLP-classifier and was a burden for our computational resources.

8.2 Support Vector Machine - C-SVM algorithm

The Support Vector Machine (SVM) technique (Vapnik *et al.* 1997, 1998) is well suited to search for an optimal binary classifier. In the Support Vector Machine approach input vectors are mapped into higher dimensional space to identify a hyperplane that best separates the positive and negative samples i.e. maximizes the margin between two classes. This principle is more intuitive than the MLP 'black box' approach. Since we cannot expect perfect separation of melanoma and dysplastic lesion images, the C-SVM algorithm was employed with the RBF kernel implemented in the osu-svm-3.0 toolbox for Matlab (Chang). The input data set was processed by scaling the values of each feature to [−1, 1]. The C-SVM approach with the radial base kernel (RBF) appeared to yield very good performance. Taking into consideration the whole feature set (231) the result for the scaled data was TPF=94.7% and (1-FPF)=95%. The most efficient discrimination between class melanoma and dysplastic nevus was found for the parameters C = 512 and = 0.000244, which were fixed by a grid search over the full parameter space. The feature set limited by the same Ridge model (Surówka *et al.* 2006) to the 10 most discriminating features yields a TPF=84.2% and (1-FPF)=85%, which is a very good result taking into account the reduction in the feature space. Tests with the polynomial kernel were not stable and yielded worse results.
In table 6 we show results of the above mentioned methods tested on the same data set.

	MLP	SVM RBS	
#attributes	10	231	10
TPF	89.2%	94.7%	84.2%
1-FPF	90%	95%	85%

Table 6. Classification performance of the MLP and SVM RBS methods tested on our data set. The quality of the methods is quoted in terms of TPF (true positive fraction) and FPF (false positive fraction). Tests were conducted with all 231 features and with 10 most important selected by the Ridge linear model (Surówka *et al.* 2006).

It must be stressed that unlike in (Patwardhan *et al.* 2005) we do not take advantage of any specialized instruments (Nevoscope) and our lesion images are taken in white light only.

9. Comparison of standard methods and feature sets with the new proposed approaches

Classification of the pigmented skin lesion images can vary from linear models through MLP, SVM, k-NN, to ensembles of models. Applicability of symbolic methods of classification to the problem of early detection of melanoma has not been thoroughly tested yet. However, one can show that inductive classification based on symbolic rules and knowledge inference (Meyrowitz *et al.* 1993) can be both simple and comprehensive for human understanding, and yield high classification performance to compare with 'black box' machine learning methods.

Symbolic methods of classification generate symbolic/declarative information about the classes. It is done usually by classification rules or sets/chains of notions/ideas inferred from the learning cases. On the contrary, classical numeric approaches as neural networks, fuzzy sets or genetic algorithms produce complex, less comprehensive (interpretable) knowledge (Michalski *et al.* 2006).

In this approach we study the classification methods developed by Michalski and applied in his software tool AQ21 (Michalski *et al.* 2006, Wojtusiak 2005). The learning phase of this classification i.e. construction of descriptions of the classes is the most important for the knowledge induction (Michalski 2004). In this step all positive and no negative examples form a description of a class (in the simplest way as an alternative of positive values and negation of counter-examples). Then such a definition is subject to maximally specific generalization to be able to classify new unknown examples (by elimination/addition of selectors, value range extension, value range closure, resolution, or negation extension). In the theory of Michalski class definitions should obey two conditions: completeness (each member of the class should comply with the class description), and consistency (if an object fulfills its class description, it cannot belong to other classes). Assigning an object to its proper class according to the generated rules can be represented in the form $D :\gg Y$ (*D*-description of class *Y*), where the description is a disjunction (an alternative) of the complexes: $D = C_1 \vee C_2 \vee \ldots C_n$. Such a form eliminates inseparable or incomplete descriptions by precedence of the class whose object membership probability is the biggest.

Reduction of the description, which is the goal of this calculus, leads to the maximum detailed set of complexes (called a star). To focus on the most promising candidate descriptions a heuristic LEF function (Lexicographic Evaluation Functional) is used.

Out of the lesion images the following features were extracted (altogether 45 features):

Set A: Geometry: area, perimeter, roundness, aspect ratio, fullness ratio, symmetry, border length, bounding rectangle.

Colors: average values and standard deviations, min, max for components {R,G,B}, {H,S,V}, {Y,Cr,Cb}, weighted color transforms, gray-blue, white, black, number of colors, area percentage.

Distributions: distance of the centre of gravity of a color component from the lesion centre of gravity and the bounding rectangle centre of gravity, zone: whitish, reddish, light-brown, dark-brown.

Set B: For wavelet features the (1D)x(1D) Daubechies wavelet packets (Mojsilovic *et al.* 2000) were applied sto the indexed images. An efficient pyramidal algorithm (Mallat 1989) (Chang *et al.* 1989) was adapted into a tree structure multi-level filter. In each iteration of the wavelet algorithm four subimages were produced: LL (upper left), LH (upper right), HL (lower left) and HH (lower right), where L and H denote the respective low- and high-pass filters (Porter *et al.* 1996). One iteration produced 11 coefficients calculated from energies of the four subimages (e1, e2, e3, e4), the maximum energy ratio (ei/emax, i=any three out of four except the subimage with the maximum energy) and the fractional energy ratio (e1/(e2+e3+e4) + its three permutations), where the term energy means the sum of the absolute values of the pixels normalized by the total number of pixels in the (sub)image (Patwardhan et al. 2003, 2005). Altogether 3 iterations were done yielding (1+4+16)*11=231 features. Both feature sets have been used separately.

AQ21 implements methods of the Attributional Calculus (Michalski 2004), so prior to the learning stage all continuous domains of the features have to be digitized by invoking the built-in ChiMerge algorithm (ChiMerge 5) (Kerber 1992). Since we had 231 features in the wavelet domain we decided to pre-select the most relevant ones. For feature selection we used the simplified 'Promise' method (Baim 1982) available in AQ21.

Pseudo-code of the simplified Promise algorithm looks as follows:

```
P = 0
For each value of the attribute v_i
    S = {examples : e = v_i}
    Find class C that has the largest number of examples in S
    P = P+ #C ∩ S /#S
Return P
```

The 'Attribute_selection_threshold' parameter defining the minimum attribute discriminatory power was experimentally set to 0.9. This value limited our feature set B to less than 10 attributes out of 231.

The AQ21 program was run in two different learning modes: Theory Formation (TF) and Approximate Theory Formation (ATF) (Wojtusiak 2005). In the TF mode, learned rules are complete and consistent, whereas the ATF consists of rules optimized according to the *Q* measure that reads: $Q(R,w) = compl(R)^{w} \bullet cons(R)^{(l-w)}$, where the optimization parameter w may cause a loss of completeness (compl) and/or consistency (*cons*) but may increase the predictive power of the learned rule (*R*).

Due to limited statistics of individuals (78+80) the classification accuracy was tested by the n-fold cross validation: (testing(1M+1D)/learning(the rest of M and D).

A summary of other AQ21 settings used in our experiments are presented below.

Learning phase:

Consequent=[class=],*
MaxRule=1,
Cross_validation=80.

Testing:

Method=atest,
Threshold=0.5,
Eval_of_conjunction=min, Eval_of_disjunction=max,
Eval_of_selector=strict.

Overall results obtained for feature set A and B are shown in table 7. In case of multiple instances due to cross validation we quote below the average predictive accuracy as 1- (#errors+#no_class + #both_classes) /(#iterations).

	TF	ATF
Feature set A	88%	93%
Feature set B	94%	100%

Table 7. Results of the AQ21 classification in feature set A and B

From table 6 we can see the quality of both feature sets. Our working hypothesis was that the geometric/colorimetric features, as more prone to local distortions/artifacts and also more sensitive to the segmentation process (Ogorzałek *et al.* 2009), should yield worse results than the wavelet-based signals which reproduce frequency modes of the skin lesion of melanoma and dysplastic-like origin. On this stage of work we cannot answer the question if the wavelet features carry better signals of melanoma than other direct measures, or they are just less biased by the image analysis process. However in view of the fact, that early stages of melanoma do not reveal apparent structures of malignancy it seems, that wavelet bases may probe those inherent signals.

Another conclusion is that methodology of Approximate Theory Formation (ATF) seems to fit the best to the inherent fuzzy nature of benign and malignant skin lesion images.
However comparison of the feature sets was not the primary goal of our study. Output generated from the tests includes learned rules consisting of selectors with a feature name, relation and the value/range. This is the full knowledge we can get from the symbolic classification methodology. We can observe the learned rules, and see the meaning and precedence of features (Meyrowitz *et al.* 1993). For instance from the feature set B we get an example rule:

[class=1]

 # Rule 1

<-- *[co188_M=0.421220..0.446530,0.520865..0.525190,0.596670..0.640195,0.642360..0.793450 : 78,0,100%,78,0,100%]*

This rule gives a range of values where the selector "col88" (which corresponds to a fractional energy ratio $e_{2,3,4}/(e_{2,3,1}+e_{2,3,2},+e_{2,3,3})$ has the total predictive power for the class "melanoma". Of course this feature can be interpreted not only in terms of energy, but also structural interpretation may be deduced. The same analysis for the feature set A gives less predictive (94%) and more complex rules with some primary features like: "average level of red" and „symmetry" (Ogorzałek *et al.* 2009).
Comparisons with other machine learning methods tested on the same data set and analysis of the published results show that performance of the presented approach may be better than other learning methods and is promising in view of further research with better statistics of the melanoma data (Sboner *et al.* 2003)(Burroni 2004)(Surówka *et al.* 2007).

10. Performance analysis

78 (80) dermoscopy images of the melanoma (dysplastic) lesions, all confirmed by histological examinations, have been classified using a wavelet-based set of features. Discriminant power of those features has been determined by either Ridge regression models, or the 'promise' algorithm, and generalized in a three-layer back-propagated neural network/support vector machine, and by the Attributional Calculus.
Our results, presented in table 6 and table 7, confirm that neighborhood properties of pixels in dermoscopy images record the melanoma progression and together with the selected machine learning methods may be important diagnostic aids. Especially the inductive learning approach (AQ21, table 7) shows great classification potential.
The present accuracy of the classifiers is a promising factor for the further research in the field, especially considering the fact that all dermoscopy images were taken in white light without any specialized instruments. The constructed model of features for melanoma and dysplastic lesions can evolve, after some fine-tuning and improvements, to a computer-aided diagnostic system.
In future work, the most important factor is increase in statistics of the dermoscopic images. This is the most critical factor due to low rate (1-2%) of melanoma patients in the population (~1500) examined for the sake of this study.
Diversity of images should also cast a light on the role of image acquisition and quality.
Since the features of melanoma and dysplastic nevus form two joint sets, it would be reasonable to study soft membership functions to categorize the members of classification. Another interesting aspect that has not been investigated is considering the class melanoma as a few subsets of different morphology.
Last but not least, probing different bases of the wavelet decomposition should explain the role of the basis for optimal selection of the feature set.

11. Acknowledgment

This work has been supported by the Polish Ministry of Science and Higher Education research grant N N518 419038 "Application of Computational Intelligence Techniques in Analysis of Images for Computer-Assisted Melanoma Diagnosis".

12. References

Argenziano, G., Fabbrocini, G., Carli, P., DeGiorgi, V., Sammarco, P., Delfino, M. (1998): Epiluminescence *Microscopy for the Diagnosis of Doubtful Melanocytic Skin Lesions.* Arch. Dermatl. 134, 1563–1570

Baim P., (1982), *The PROMISE Method For Selecting Most Relevant Attributes For Inductive Learning Systems,* Reports of the Intelligent Systems Group, ISG 82-1, UIUCDCS-F-82-898, Department of Computer Science, University of Illinois, Urbana, September

Burroni, M., Corona, R., Dell'Eva, G., Sera, F., Bono, R., Puddu, P., Perotti, R., Nobile, F., Andreassi, L., Rubegni, P. (2004): *Melanoma Computer-Aided Diagnosis: Reliability and Feasibility Study.* Clin. Cancer Res. 10, 1881–1886

Carli, P., DeGiorgi, V.,Massi, D., Giannotti, B. (2000): *The Role of Pattern Analysis and the ABCD rule of dermoscopy in the detection of histological atypia in Melanocytic Naevi.* British J. Dematol. 143, 290–297

Chan, H.P., Sahiner, B., Wagner, R.F., Petrick, N. (1999): *Classifier Design for Computer-Aided Diagnosis: Effects of Finite Sample Size and on Mean Performance of Classical and Neural Network Classifiers.* Med. Phys. 26, 2654–2668

Chang C.C., Lin C.J., LIBSVM: a library for support vector machines, Available from: http://www.csie.ntu.edu.tw/cjlin/libsvm

Chang C.C., Lin C.J., (1998), *Training - support vector classifiers: theory and algorithms, Receiver operating characteristic (ROC) analysis* in Basic principles and applications in radiology, European Journal of Radiology vol. 27, 1998, pp. 88-94.

Chang T., Kuo C.C.J., (1993) *Texture Analysis and Classification with Tree-Structured Wavelet Transform,* IEEE Transactions on Image Processing, vol. 2, 429-441.

Daubechies I., (1992), *Ten Lectures on Wavelets,* S.I.A.M., Philadelphia, *Numerical Recipes in C,* The art of scientific computing, PWN 1999, pp. 591 - 606.

Deng Y., Manjunat B.S. (2001). *Unsupervised segmentation of color-texture regions in images and video,* IEEE Transactions on Pattern Analysis and Machine Intelligence

Diepgen, T.L., Eysenbach, G. (1998): *Digital Images in Dermatology and the Dermatology Online Atlas on the World Wide Web.* J. Dermatol. 25(12), 782–787

Dreiseitl, S., Ohno-Machado, L., Kittler, H., Vinterbo, S., Billhards, H., Binder, M.A. (2001): *Comparison of Machine Learning Methods for the Diagnosis of Pigmented Skin Lesions.* J. Biomed. Inform. 34, 28–36

European Consensus-based Interdisciplinary Guideline (2009), Developed by the Guideline Subcommittee of the European Dermatology Forum, Available from: http://www.euroderm.org/download/guideline_on_malignant_melanoma-aktuell-2.pdf

Fikrle T., Pizinger K., (2006) *Digital analysis of dermatoscopical images of 260 melanocytic skin lesions; perimeter/area ratio for the differentiation between malignant melanomas and melanocytic nevi,* Eur. Acad. Derm.Vener., 21.

Grzymala-Busse, P., Grzymala-Busse, J.W., Hippe, Z.S. (2001): *Melanoma prediction using data mining system LERS.* In: Computer Software and Applications Conference, COMPSAC 2001, pp. 615–620

Hall, P.N., Claridge, E., Smith, J.D. (1995): *Computer Screening for Early Detection of Melanoma: Is there a Future?* British J. Dermatol. 132, 325–328

Iyatomi, H., Oka, H., Hasimoto, M., Tanaka, M., Ogawa, K. (2005): *An Internet-based Melanoma Diagnostic System - Toward the Practical Application,* Proceedings CIBCB '05, pp.1-4

Johr, R.H. (2002): *Dermoscopy: Alternative Melanocytic Algorithms - The ABCD Rule of Dermatoscopy, Menzies Scoring Method, and 7-Point Checklist,* Clinics in Dermatology (Elsevier), vol. 20, pp. 240–247

Kadiyala M., DeBrunner V., (1999), *Effect of wavelet bases in texture classification using a tree structured wavelet transform,* 33 Asilomar Conference on Signals, Systems, and Computers, 2: 1292-1296.

Kerber R., (1992) *Chimerge: Discretization for Numeric Attributes",* Proceedings of the Tenth National Conference on Artificial Intelligence , AAAI Press, pp. 123-128.

Liu Y., Zhang D., Lu G., and Ma Y., (2005) *Region-based image retrieval with high-level semantic color names,* IEEE Proceedings of the Multimedia Modeling Conference, pp. 180–187

Mallat S.G., (1989), *A Theory for Multiresolution Signal Decomposition: The Wavelet Representation,* IEEE Transactions on pattern analysis and machine intelligence, vol. 11: 674-693.

Menzies S.W. (1999): Automated Epiluminescence Microscopy: Human vs Machine in the Diagnosis of Melanoma. Arch. Dermatol. 135, 1538–1540

Menzies S.W., Leanne Bischof, Hugues Talbot, *et al.* (2005) *The Performance of SolarScan. An Automated Dermoscopy Image Analysis Instrument for the Diagnosis of Primary Melanome.* Archive of Dermatology, pp. 1388-1396.

Merkwirth Ch., ENTOOL Statistical classification toolbox for MATLAB, Available from: http://zti.if.uj.edu.pl/~merkwirth/entool.htm

Meyrowitz A.L., Chipman S. (ed.), (1993), Fundations of knowledge acquisition, Kluwer Academic Publishers.

Michalski R. S., Kaufman K., Pietrzykowski J., Wojtusiak J., Mitchell S. and Seeman W. D., (2006), *Natural Induction and Conceptual Clustering: A Review of Applications,* Reports of the Machine Learning and Inference Laboratory, MLI 06-3, George Mason University, Fairfax, VA

Michalski R. S., (2004), *Attributional Calculus: A Logic and Representation Language for Natural Induction,* Reports of the Machine Learning and Inference Laboratory, MLI 04-2, George Mason University, Fairfax, VA, 2004.

Mojsilovic A., Popovic M. V., Rackov D. M., (2000), *On the selection of an optimal wavelet basis for texture characterization,* IEEE Transactions on Image Processing, vol. 9, pp. 2043-2050.

Nachbar F., Stolz W., Merkle T., Cognetta A.B., Vogt T., Landthaler M., Bilek P., Braun-Falco O., Plewig G. (1994), *The ABCD rule of dermatoscopy. High prospective value in the diagnosis of doubtful melanocytic skin lesions,* Journal of the American Academy of Dermatology, vol. 30, p. 551-559

Ogorzałek M., Surówka G., L. Nowak, and Merkwirth Ch., (2010) *Computational intelligence and image processing methods for applications in skin cancer diagnosis,* in Biomedical Engineering Systems and Technologies, Communications in Computer and Information Science, vol.52, pp. 3-20.

Ogorzałek M., Surówka G., L. Nowak, and Merkwirth Ch., (2009) *Computational intelligence and image processing methods for applications in skin cancer diagnosis,* Lect. Notes, Comp. Sci.,

Park S. B., Lee J. W. and Kim S. K., (2004), *Content-based image classification using neural network,* pp. 287-300, Pattern Recognition

Patwardhan S. V., Dai S., Dhawan A. P., (2005), *Multi-spectral image analysis and classification of melanoma using fuzzy membership based partitions*, Computerized Medical Imaging and Graphics, vol. 29, 2005, pp. 287-296.

Patwardhan S. V., Dhawan A. P., Relue P. A., (2003), *Classification of melanoma using tree structured wavelet transforms*, Computer Methods and Programs in Biomedicine, vol. 72, 2003, pp. 223-239.

Porter R., Canagarajah N., (1996), *A Robust Automatic Clustering Scheme for Image Segmentation Using Wavelets*, IEEE Transactions on Image Processing, vol 5, pp. 662-665.

Rigel D.S., Friedman R.J., Kopf A.W., Polsky D. (2005), *ABCDE--an evolving concept in the early detection of melanoma*, Archives of Dermatology, vol. 141, no.8, pp. 1032-1034

Sboner A. et al., (2003), *A multiple classifier for early melanoma diagnosis*, Artificial Intelligence in Medicine, vol. 27, pp. 29-44.

Schmid-Saugeon, P., Guillod, J., Thiran, J.-P. (2003), *Towards a Computer-aided diagnosis System for Pigmented Skin Lesions*. Computerized Medical Imaging and Graphics, pp. 65–78

Surówka G., Merkwirth Ch., Żabińska-Płazak E., Graca A., (2006) *Wavelet based classification of skin lesion images*, Bio-Algorithms and Med Systems, vol. 2 no. 4, pp. 43-50.

Surówka G., K. Grzesiak-Kopeć, (2007) *Different Learning Paradigms for the Classification of Melanoid Skin Lesions Using Wavelets*, Proc. of. EMBC07, Lyon

Talbot H. and Bischof L. *An overview of the Polartechnics SolarScan melanoma diagnosis algorithms*, http://itee.uq.edu.au/~aprs/wdic2003/CDROM/33.pdf

Thomas L., Tranchand P., Berard F., Secchi T., Colin C., Moulin G., (1998), *Semiological Value of ABCDE Criteria in the Diagnosis of Cutaneous Pigmented Tumors*, Dermatology vol. 197 p.11-17

Wojtusiak J., (2005) *AQ21 User's Guide*, Reports of the Machine Learning and Inference Laboratory, MLI 04-3, George Mason University, Fairfax, VA

Wu Y. C., Lee S. Y. and Yang C. J. (2008), *Robust and efficient multiclass SVM models for phrase pattern recognition*, Pattern Recognition, pp. 2874–2889

Vapnik V., (1998) *Statistical Learning Theory*, New York, NY: Springer-Verlag

Vapnik V., Golowich S. and Smola A., (1997) *Support vector method for function approximation, regression estimation, and signal processing*, in M. Mozer, M. Jordan and T. Petsche, Advances in Neural Information Processing Systems 9, Cambridge, MA, MIT Press, 1997, pp. 281-287.

Żabińska-Płazak E., Wojas-Pelc A., Dyduch G., (2005), *Videodermatoscopy in the diagnosis of melanocytic skin lesions*, Bio-Algorithms and Med-Systems, vol. 1, , pp. 333-338.

Dermatoscopes descriptions e.g. available from : DermLite
http://www.dermlite.com/cms/en/products/handheld-products.html DermLite connection for iPhone 4 http://www.dermlite.com/cms/

Dermatoscopic system descriptions e.g. available from :
http://moleexpert.com/;
http://www.dermamedicalsystems.com/index.php?menu_id=1;
http://www.fotofinder.de/dermatoskopie.html
http://www.fotofinder.de/dermatoskopie/software.html;
http://www.moleanalyzer.com/;
MoleMAX/PhotoMAX
http://www.dermamedicalsystems.com/derma/MoleMaxII%20engl_.pdf
DBDermo-Mips/DDAX Software http://www.ddax3.com/eng/index.html

6

Investigation of Relations Between Skin Cancer Lesions' Images and Their Reflectance and Fluorescent Spectra

Petya Pavlova[1], Ekaterina Borisova[2], Lachezar Avramov[2],
Elmira Petkova[3] and Petranka Troyanova[3]
[1]*Technical University Sofia, branch of Plovdiv*
[2]*Institute of Electronics, Bulgarian Academy of Sciences, Sofia,*
[3]*University Hospital "Queen Giovanna-ISUL", Sofia,*
Bulgaria

1. Introduction

Biomedical optics is one of the fastest growing areas of research. The non-ionizing nature of light applied for investigation and detection of abnormalities in human tissues make this area very attractive for development of new diagnostic techniques and modalities (Wang, 2007). The optical spectra provide biochemical and morphological information about the tissue under investigation based on its absorption, reflectance, fluorescence and elastic scattering properties (Wang, 2007; Tuchin, 2002). Many techniques based on the recent progress in optics have been developed for biomedical applications. Fluorescence, absorption and diffuse scattering spectroscopy have been widely applied as probes acquiring information about physical, chemical, or physiological processes in the tissues. These methods have been proposed to be used by the medical community in view of extending the capabilities of the standard diagnostic modalities that have already been introduced in the clinical practice, as x-ray, magnetic resonance and ultrasound imaging.

Laser-induced autofluorescence spectroscopy (LIAFS) could be utilized to quantify differences between normal and abnormal tissues *in vivo,* thus providing an appropriate method for detection of pathological lesions in real time. Diffuse reflectance spectroscopy (DRS) also allows distinguishing between pathological areas and normal tissue surroundings. In recent years, there has been growing interest in the combined use of laser-induced autofluorescence and reflectance spectroscopy to differentiate diseased from normal surrounding tissue - mainly for detection and differentiation of cancerous and pre-cancerous changes in human body.

Laser-induced autofluorescence spectroscopy is very promising from a technical point of view due to the easy coupling with optical fibres for delivering the excitation light to every part of the human body without significant losses of light power, as is the case of incoherent light sources, as well as because of the possibility to use information from naturally occurring endogenous fluorophores, without adding external fluorescent markers. LIAFS is also notable among the other non-invasive diagnostic techniques, as it offers real-time detection and differentiation of the lesion investigated with promising precision, selectivity and specificity (Bigio, 1997; Bachmann, 2006). The fluorescent technique is widely applied to cutaneous lesions' investigations, including erythema (Sinichkin, 1998), psoriasis, vitiligo (Borisova, 2000), and skin cancer (Wang, 2006; Troyanova, 2006). This method yields information about the biochemical composition of the tissue under study.

On the other hand, diffuse reflectance spectroscopy is mainly providing morphological information concerning the tissues. The scattering intensity and spectral distribution of the signals detected could give information about the scatterers' size and distribution (cells, nuclei, etc.). Most of the tissue pathologies, including tumours, exhibit significant architecture changes on a cellular and sub-cellular level. The elastic scattering of light penetrating into the tissues depends on this alteration in their architecture, so that the back-scattered signals detected could be used for determining pathological structural changes occurring in the organ under study (Morant, 2003). As the diffuse reflectance signal detected is a superposition of diffuse scattering and absorption from tissues pigments, the resultant spectrum on the tissue surface reveals also information about the main absorbers in the biological tissues, such as haemoglobin and melanin in the skin and its pathologies. To benefit fully from reflectance spectroscopy's advantages, one needs to relate the spectral features with the morphology and biochemical composition of the tissue investigated. (Tuchin, 2002, Borisova, 2006).

Combination of fluorescence and reflectance optical techniques could rapidly improve the sensitivity and specificity of cutaneous tumours' diagnosis (Borisova, 2008). Using imaging analysis techniques in the processing of fluorescence and reflectance spectral data received from cutaneous pathologies could further improve the diagnostic accuracy (Borisova, 2008).

Our work is a stage in the development of methods for skin cancer diagnostics on the basis of optical spectra. The preliminary analysis showed that the spectra of lesions differ from those obtained from normal tissue, with the differences observed depending on the type of pathology. A more "damaged" tissue changes the colouring more intensively. If a lesion' area could be localised correctly, it would provide more precise information about this lesion's structure. In addition, not only does the intensity value of the reflected/emitted light vary from patient to patient, but it also depends on the position of the tested area inside a given lesion. We proposed that the variations in the reflected/emitted value of the light could be caused by two possible reasons:

- different degree of "damaging" – lesion stage of development, and
- different thickness of the suspicious lesion area.

The specific features of the spectra are suitable for the development of a hybrid diagnostic algorithm (including both image and spectra) for detection and discrimination of different type of tissue damaging. We applied this approach to studying skin cancer in an attempt to separate the melanoma from benign and dysplastic melanin-pigmented lesions. The ultimate goal of the investigation is developing a reliable technique for predicting the type and level of skin damaging and the stage of its progress.

2. Basic theory

2.1 Image processing

The aim of image processing is obtaining an image with a value of the lightness of pixels, which depends on the saturation of the damaged tissue. CIE.Lab is a standard for estimating of colours using features of the illuminating light source.

The system presents the colours as relative lightness and chromaticity that consist of two components: a - a red- green axis, and b - a yellow-blue axis. The other parameter -

chroma, is calculated as the distance of the particular chromaticity from the centre of the area (Fig. 1) and corresponds to the visible saturation of the colours.

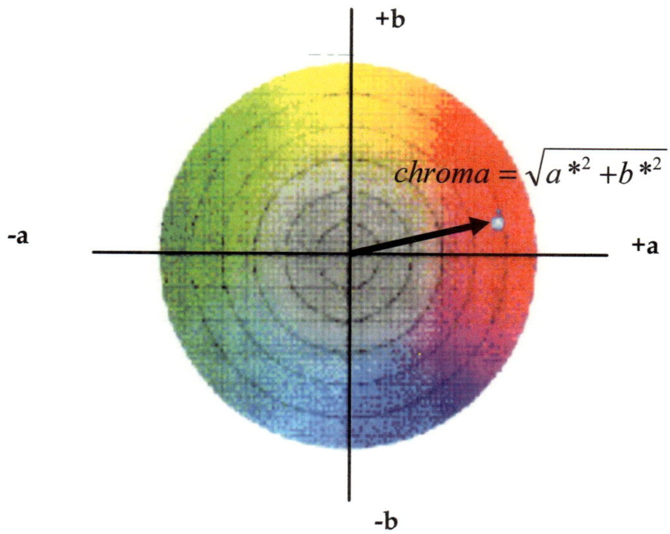

Fig. 1. Chromaticity diagram and chroma distance in the Lab system.

If we use another coloured light to illuminate the object, all the visible colours would change. However, the calculated coordinates (eq. (1)) in the Lab chromaticity area will keep their position, since the colour of the source becomes achromatic.

$$
\begin{aligned}
L &= 116.f(Y / Y_n) - 16 \\
a^* &= 500.[f(X / X_n) - f(Y / Y_n)] \\
b^* &= 200.[f(Y / Y_n) - f(Z / Z_n)]
\end{aligned}
\quad (1)
$$

$$chroma = \sqrt{a^{*2} + b^{*2}}$$

where $f(t) = t^{1/3}$ for $t > 0{,}008856$ and $f(t) = 7{,}787.t + 16 / 116$ otherwise.
Here X_n, Y_n and Z_n are the CIE XYZ three stimulus values of the reference white point.
If we use another colour as a "referent white", all available colours' coordinates would be changed, but the white point again will be at the centre of the chromaticity area with no saturation. Thus, if the healthy skin colour is used as a "referent white" point, all changes of the pigmentation could be described by chroma. Applying this to digital images, the colour of the tissues transforms to grey levels and the areas whose colour differs from the "healthy" one will occur with higher intensity. However, the images consist of pixels whose RGB signals measure relatively and reproduce the colorimetrical features of the objects. Concerning equations (1), a transformation from RGB to XYZ is needed to obtain the Lab parameters and chroma. The relation depends on the chosen area of Locus that needs to be converted and are established for several more frequently used spaces - sRGB, AdobeRGB, ProPhoto etc. given as values of the coefficients c_{ij} in equation (2).

$$\begin{bmatrix} X \\ Y \\ Z \end{bmatrix} = \begin{bmatrix} c_{11} & c_{12} & c_{13} \\ c_{21} & c_{22} & c_{23} \\ c_{31} & c_{32} & c_{33} \end{bmatrix} \cdot \begin{bmatrix} R \\ G \\ B \end{bmatrix} \quad (2)$$

Applying these transformations to images of lesions we achieve a decrease in the saturation of the healthy skin surrounding the damaged one. The sequenced linear contrast stretching of the whole image improves the visibility of the tested area by highlighting the saturated pixels and allowing the lesion localization. The saturation could be imaged by transforming each pixel's chromaticity to a grey level presenting their chroma.

2.2 Spectra processing

The aim of the processing is to highlight the peculiarities of the distribution obtained from suspicious tissues. We used a simple technique developed for the reflected spectra also described in monograph about chromatic monitoring [ed Jones, 2008] that ensures a comparison between the healthy and the tested unhealthy tissues' spectra. We calculated the ratio "healthy skin" to "tested skin" spectrum (Fig. 2)

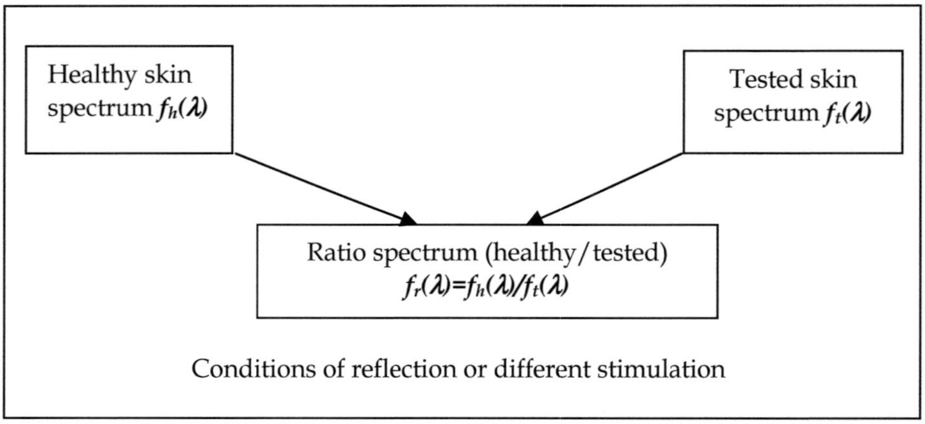

Fig. 2. Scheme of spectra processing.

The result is a new distribution, which is a straight line if the two spectra are proportional to each other, or otherwise may have any other shape. This gives rise to a possibility to overcome the ambiguities resulting from the different patients' states and to extract only the peculiarities common for the disease.

3. Experimental set up

In our investigation we used images and spectra of melanin-pigmented cutaneous benign lesions obtained from 30 patients, dysplastic nevi - obtained from 18 patients, and lesions of malignant melanoma obtained from 27 patients.

The images were obtained from simple photographs taken by a photo camera and processed by a specially prepared computer program that transforms the colour parameters by the sRGB standard. The fluorescent spectra were obtained using three different excitation sources with maxima of the emitted light at 365, 385, and 405 nm, respectively. The emitted fluorescence is registered by a fibre optic micro spectrometer (USB4000, "Ocean Optics,"

Inc., Dunedin, USA). A high-sensitivity linear CCD detected the reflected light dispersed by a grating with 600 lines/mm, with the total spectral resolution of the micro spectrometer being approximately 2 nm. The same device was used for registering the reflectance spectra. All spectra were limited into the range of visible light between 420 and 780 nm. The intensity and shape of the curve of reflected/emitted spectra in different conditions could be estimated in the cases of different patients and different points of obtaining the spectra inside of the lesion.

The results were analysed based on two criteria:

- Significant signal level dependence on the reflection and excitation light wavelength,
- Coincidence of the shape of the spectra ratios obtained from different patients and different points of registering depending on the diagnosis.

4. Results and discussion

4.1 Benign nevus

Figure 3 shows the initial image of a benign nevus lesion, the image of healthy tissue used for obtaining the values of $X_nY_nZ_n$ parameters, and the grey "chroma" image after processing. The damaged area is inhomogeneous. The pixels that pertain to it could be extracted by simply setting a threshold to the grayscale. One could expect that spectra registered from the central and the peripheral area of the spot should be similar in shape and level.

Figure 4 shows the reflected and emitted spectra of the central area obtained from three different patients denoted by P1, P2 and P3. The intensity of the reflected light changes from patient to patient, but, as it is seen, the curves have similar shape. In what concerns the intensity of the emitted spectra, a higher level is present in the case of stimulation with the wavelength of 385 nm. Figure 5 shows the reflected and fluorescent spectra of the central and peripheral areas and the spectra of the healthy areas. The comparison of the shapes of these spectra allows us to suggest that only 385 nm is suitable for seeking similarity. Concerning the reflected spectra, the shape of the curves does not depend on the positions. This fact is confirmed by the spectra ratio given in figure 6.

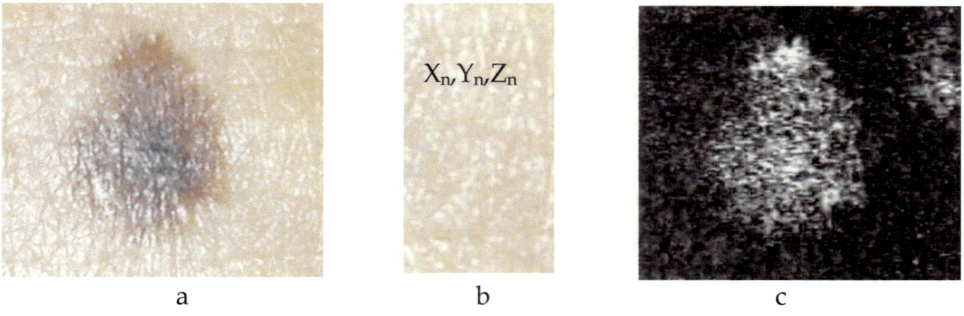

Fig. 3. Benign nevus. Initial image-a, healthy area-b and the "chroma" image after processing- c.

The suggestion that the spectra do not depend on the position inside of the lesion is valid for the intensity in practically all cases of fluorescence; this holds true for the shapes only if stimulation is carried out at 385 nm. Similarity is present in the shapes of the reflected spectra only, but not in their intensity.

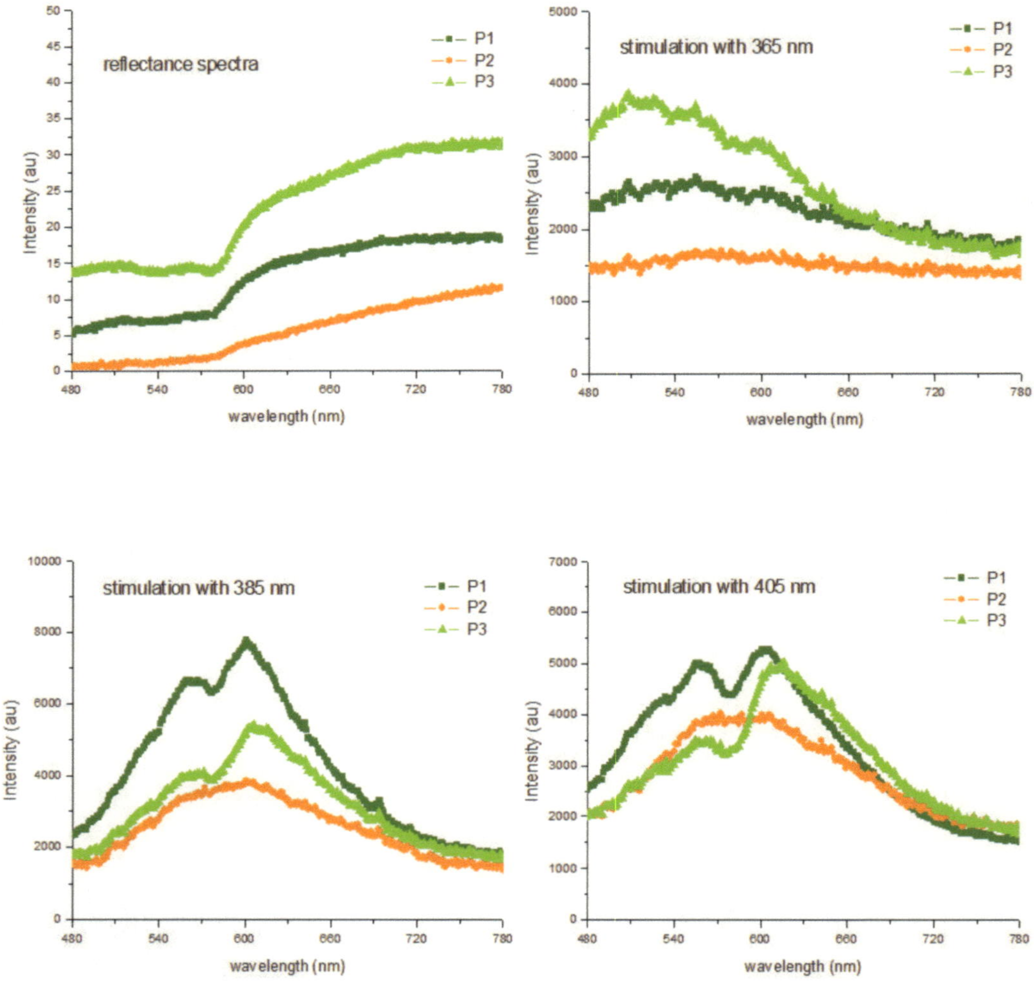

Fig. 4. Reflected and fluorescent spectra of the central area obtained from different patients in dependence on the wavelength of stimulation for benign nevus diagnose

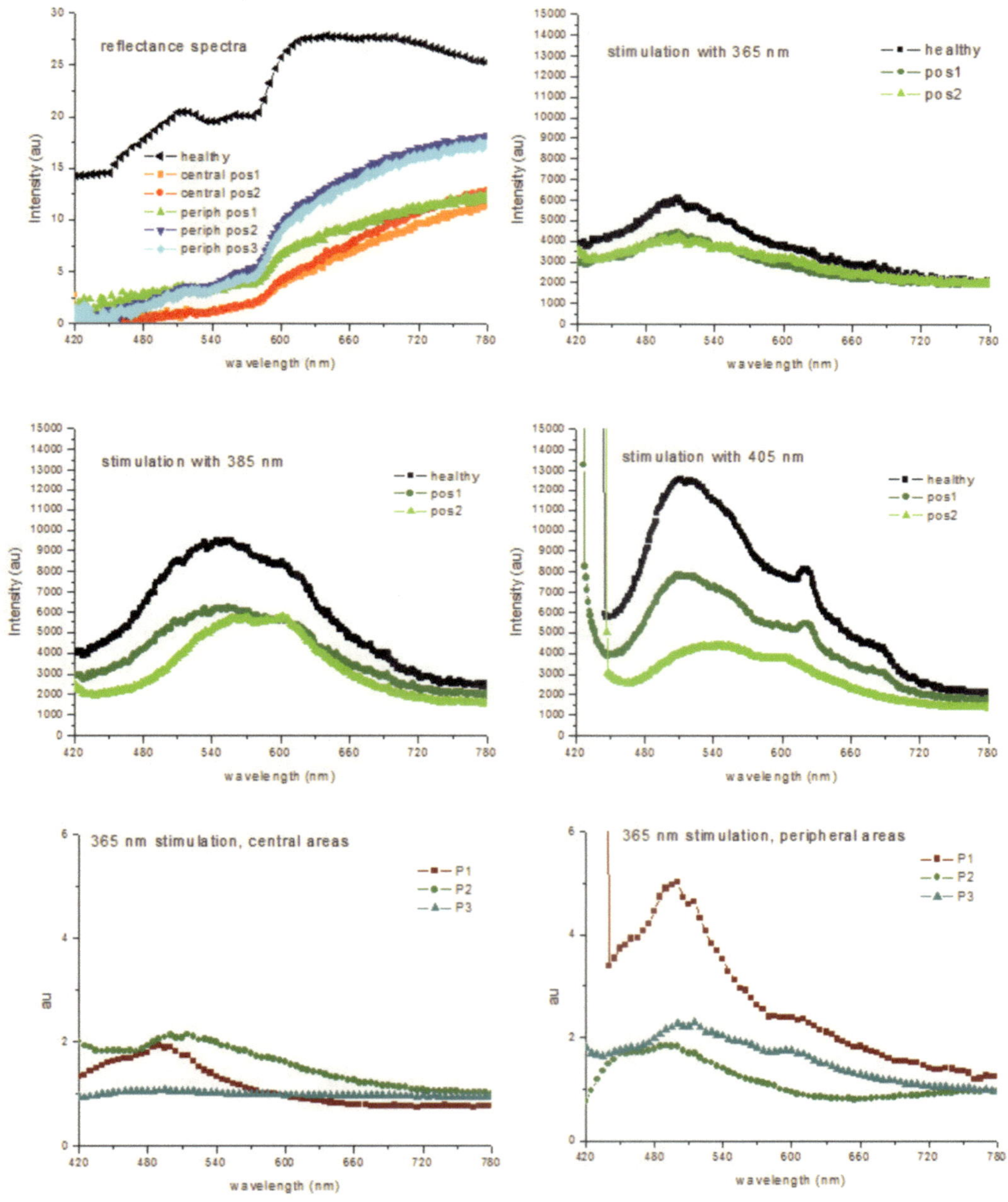

Fig. 5. Reflected and fluorescent spectra of several points in dependence on the wavelength of stimulation for benign nevus diagnose.

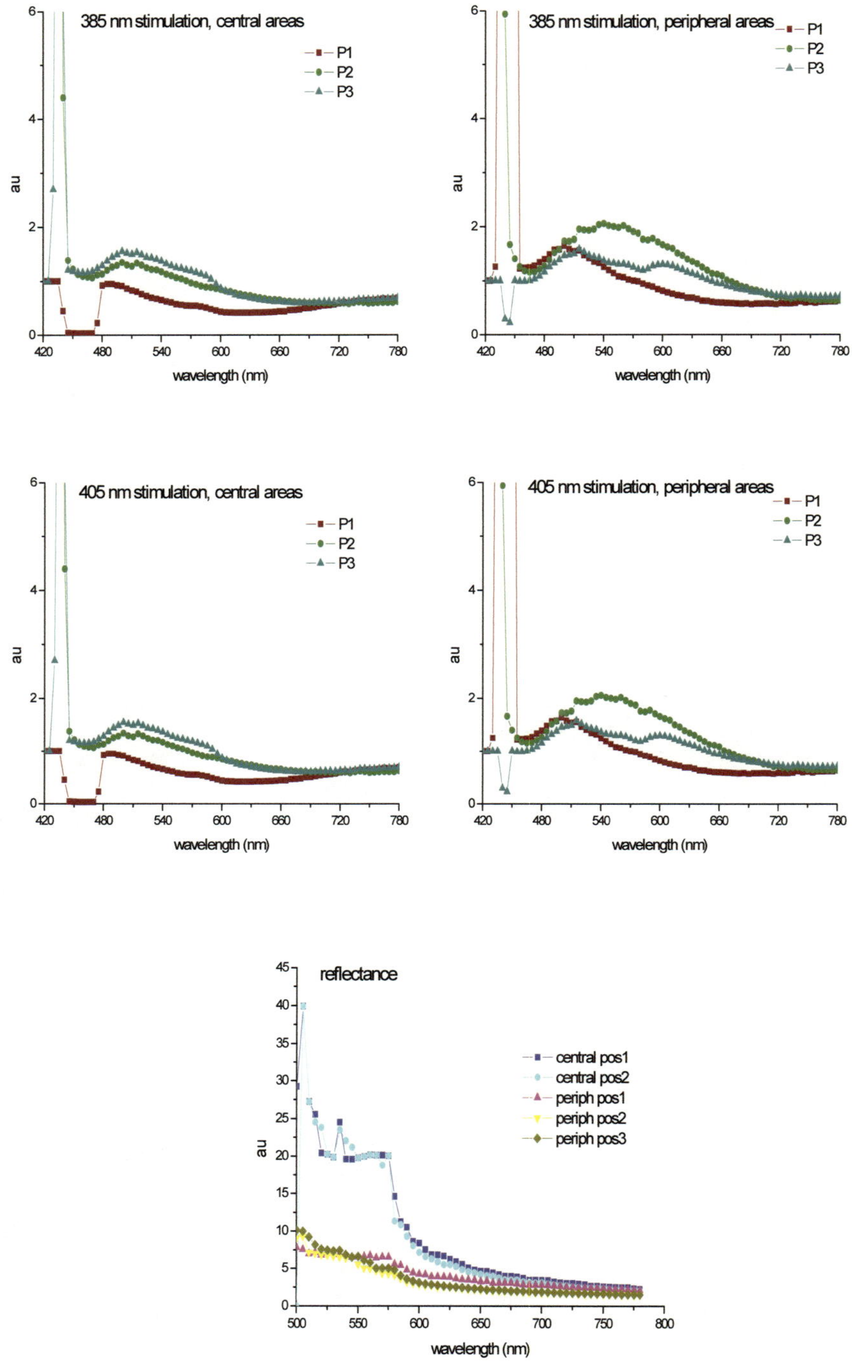

Fig. 6. Reflected and fluorescence spectra ratio of several points in dependence on the wavelength of stimulation for benign nevus diagnose.

4.2 Dysplastic nevus

Figure 7 illustrates the results of applying the techniques discussed to the image of a dysplastic nevus. The damaged area has clear outlined borders and could be easily extracted again by setting a threshold to the greyscale. The internal structure shows a low-density area concentrated into the centre of the lesion, and higher density near the borders. It could be assumed that the spectra would have different shape and intensity in dependence on the position of registering.

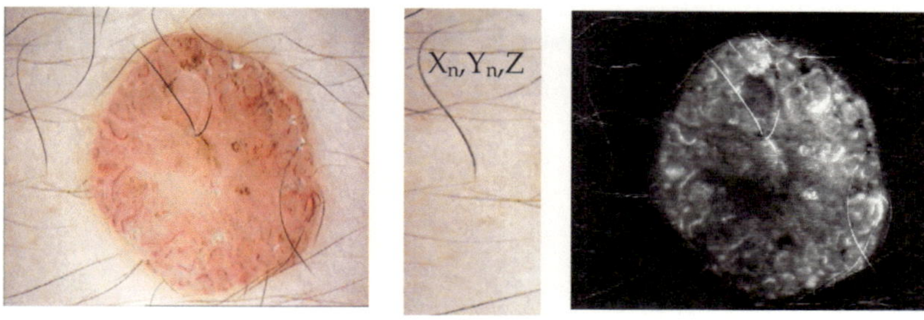

a b c

Fig. 7. Dysplastic nevus. Initial image - a, healthy area - b and the "chroma" image after processing – c.

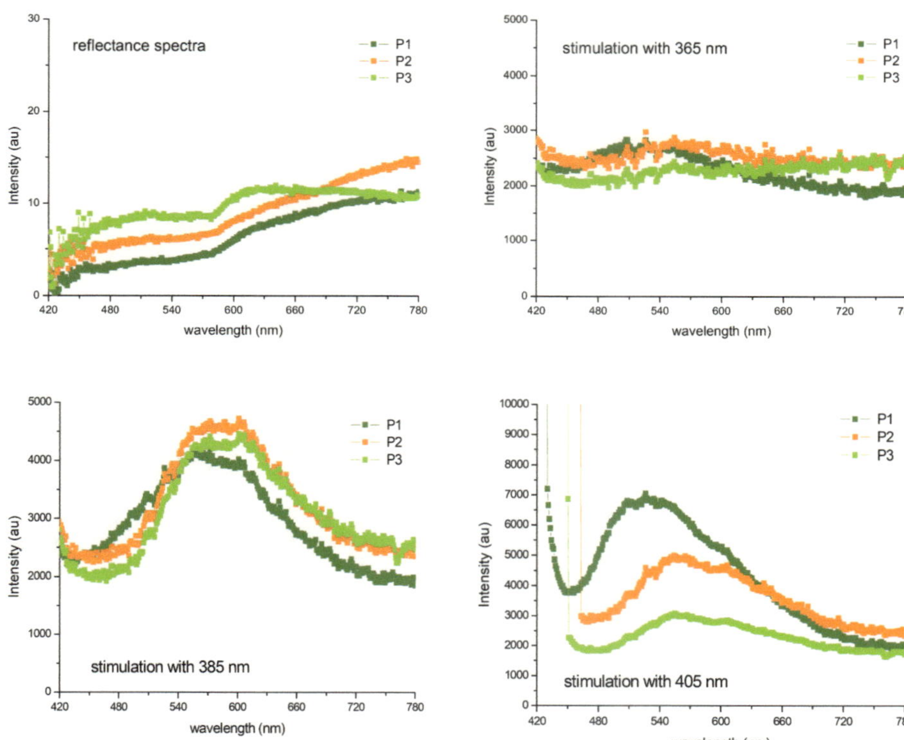

Fig. 8. Reflected and fluorescent spectra of the central area obtained from different patients in dependence on the wavelength of stimulation for dysplastic nevus diagnose.

Figure 8 shows reflected and fluorescent spectra of the central area obtained from three patients denoted again by P1, P2 and P3. The intensity of the reflected light is almost similar for the different patients, but the shape of the curves is different. Concerning the emitted spectra intensity, a higher level is seen again in case of stimulation at 385 nm. The next figure 9 also shows the reflected and fluorescent spectra of the central and peripheral areas and the spectra of the healthy areas. It could be seen that the shape of the fluorescent spectra does not depend on the position in all wavelengths stimulations tested. However, only the stimulation with 385 nm gives simultaneously a similarity between the spectra ratios and sufficient differences from the other spectra ratio (figure 10) in the cases of stimulations at 365 and 405 nm.

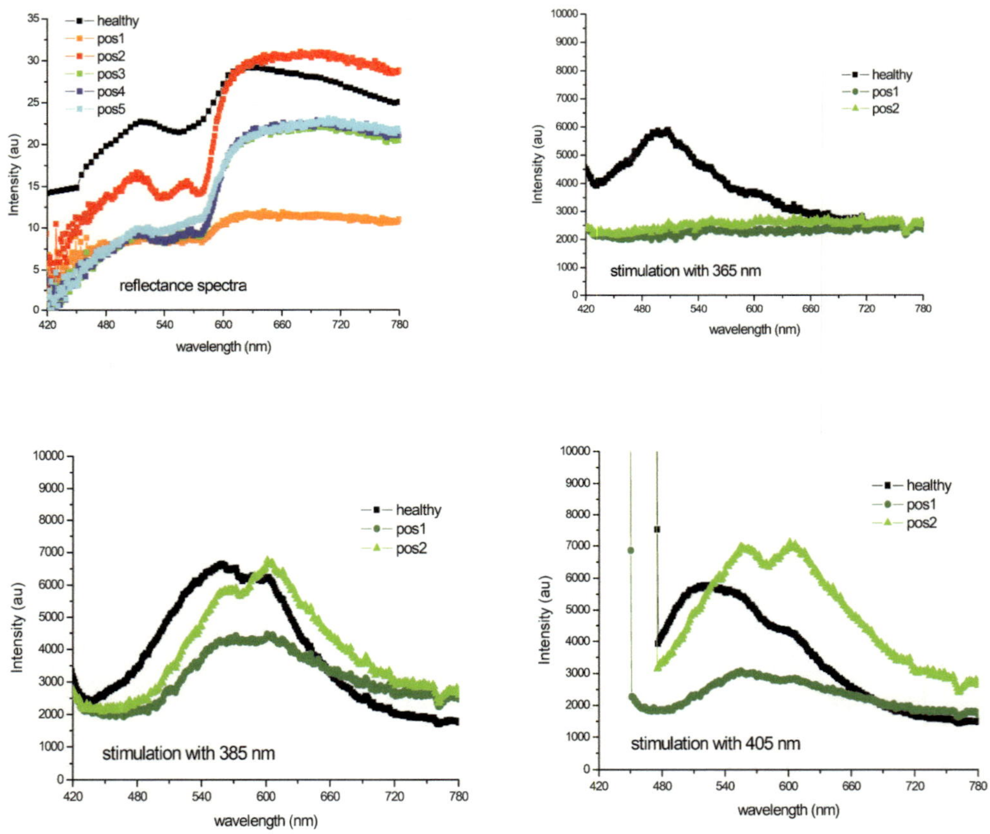

Fig. 9. Reflected and fluorescent spectra of several points in dependence on the wavelength of stimulation for dysplastic nevus diagnose.

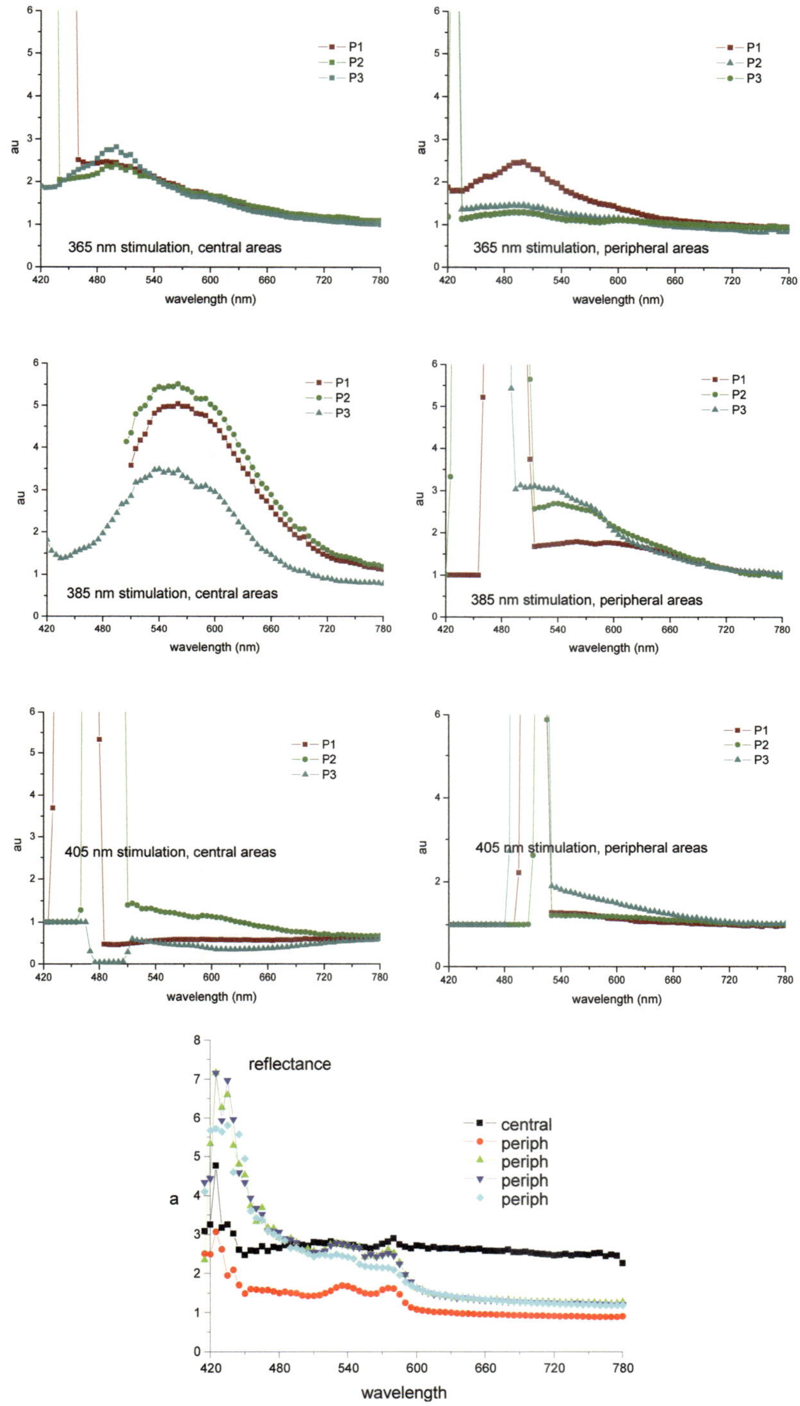

Fig. 10. Reflected and fluorescent spectra ratios of several points in dependence on the wavelength of stimulation for dysplastic nevus diagnose

4.3 Malignant melanoma

A malignant melanoma lesion is presented in fig. 11 by images resulting from two different processing: the one described above, the other using the program of MoleMax system. The latter uses ABCD criteria to set a diagnose by image analyses. The technique of greyscale „chroma" image shows better visibility of the differences inside the lesions than the method used in the MoleMax program. The density spreading implies the absence of a relation between the position (centred or near borders) and the shape and intensity of the spectrum.

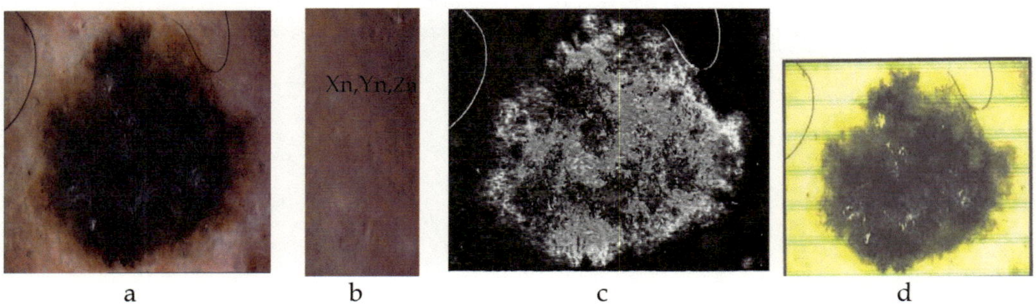

Fig. 11. Malignant melanoma: initial image-a, healthy area b, the "chroma" image –c, and image after MoleMax system processing-d.

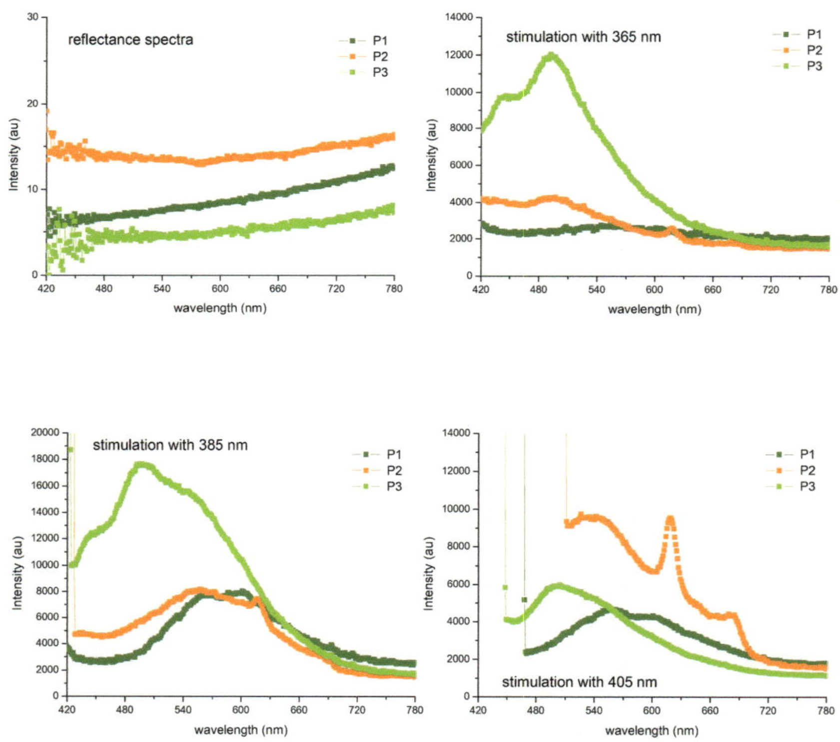

Fig. 12. Reflected and fluorescent spectra of the central area obtained from different patients in dependence on the wavelength of stimulation for malignant melanoma desease.

Figure 12 shows reflected and fluorescent spectra of the central area obtained from three patients denoted by P1, P2 and P3. The intensity of the reflected spectra varies from patient to patient. The same is valid for emitted spectra independently of the stimulation wavelength. The shapes of the spectra obtained from different areas of one patient are similar, but those of the spectra from different patients are different (figure 13). The spectra ratio given in figure 14 show different intensity, but the shape obtained by stimulation at 365 and 385 nm of peripheral areas are similar. The same applies to the reflected light spectra for.

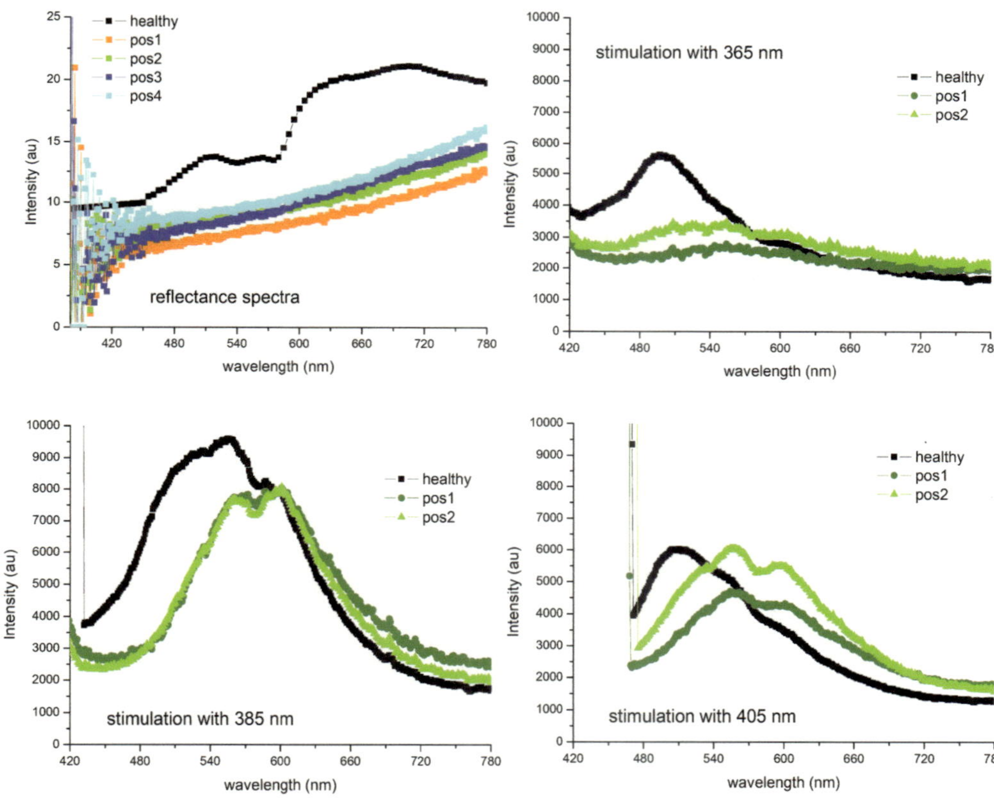

Fig. 13. Reflected and fluorescence spectra of several points in dependence on the wavelength of stimulation for malignant melanoma disease.

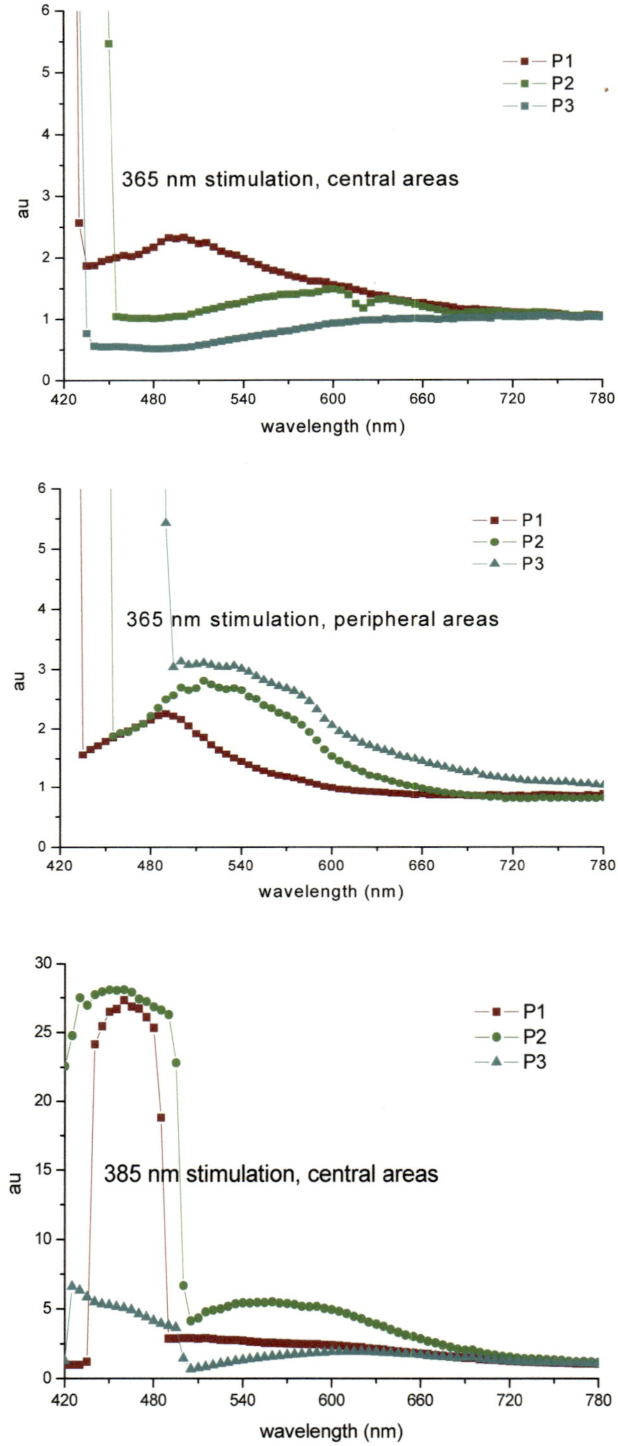
P1
P2
P3
365 nm stimulation, central areas
au
wavelength (nm)
P1
P2
P3
365 nm stimulation, peripheral areas
au
wavelength (nm)
P1
P2
P3
385 nm stimulation, central areas
au
wavelength (nm)

Fig. 14. (a)

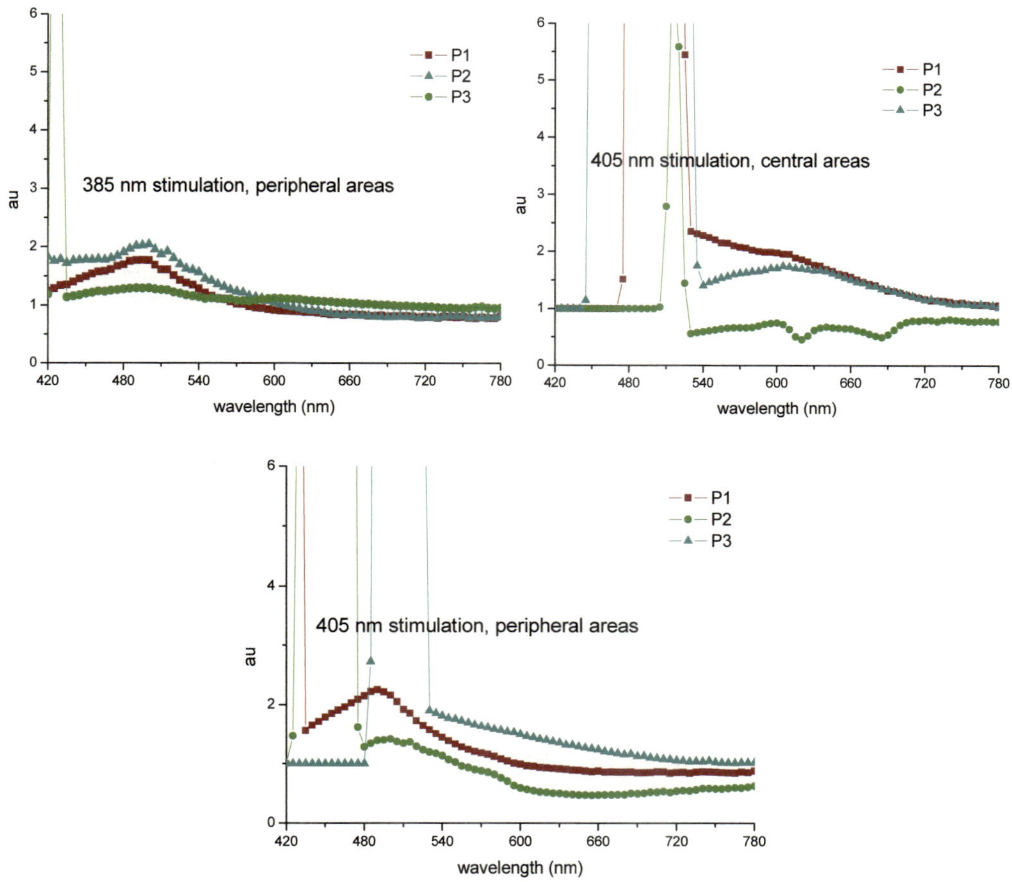

(b)

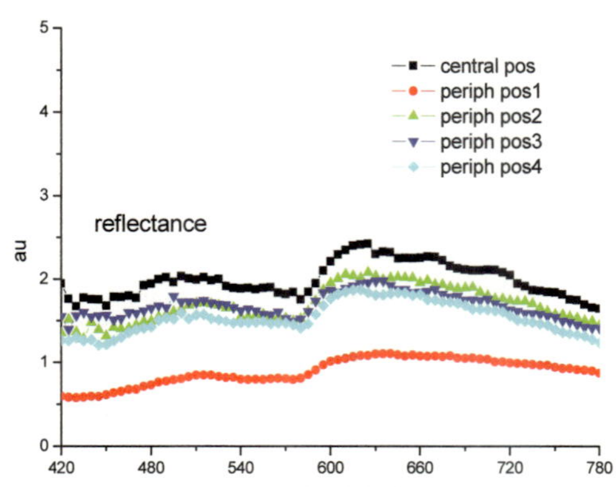

(c)

Fig. 14. Reflected and fluorescence spectra ratio of several points in dependence on the wavelength of stimulation for malignant melanoma desease.

Many technical advances and new optical methodologies for early detection of cancer have been recently developed, but there still exist considerable challenges concerning the precise diagnosis and differentiation of cutaneous malignant lesions. Most dermatologists still rely on their practical experience in visual evaluation of pigmented lesions. It is well known that the diagnostic accuracy depends on the clinical experience of the specialist (Morton and Mackie (1998)). In general practice, where such experience is low, diagnostic accuracy is quite bad (Bedlow 1995). In the early stages of the disease, the diagnosis is difficult even for experienced clinicians.

Within the wavelength range 400 - 800 nm, which we used in our observations, the stratum corneum, epidermis and dermis have relatively high scattering coefficients and lower absorption coefficients, particularly at longer wavelengths. Consequently, the spectrum of white light passing through such a tissue can be affected by the various components and thus become biased towards the longer wavelengths (Jones, 2000).

To benefit fully from optical spectroscopy's advantages, one needs to relate the spectral features with the morphology and biochemical composition of the tissue investigated. Account needs to be taken of various other skin tissue characteristics, such as melanin content in the epidermal layer, haemoglobin derivatives in the dermis and their influence on the detected spectra, so adding to the complexity of the conditions to be monitored.

Chromatic techniques have the potential for providing a means for quantifying the tissue spectral characteristics selectively under such conditions and for producing an assistive automated diagnosis means. When a combination of fluorescence, reflectance and chromatic techniques for analysis is applied, the diagnostic accuracy for malignant melanoma detection reaches 90 % (Borisova, 2008). In the situation when only one of these analytic techniques is applied, the diagnostic accuracies achieved are very similar for all three methods - about 70%.

Such an increase in diagnostic accuracy (by 20 %) demonstrates that applying chromatic techniques for monitoring biological tissues via the fluorescence, reflectance, absorption and scattering of polychromatic light could be extremely useful in tumour detection and evaluation. Therefore, unification of spectral and chromatic techniques in a common diagnostic tool is a very promising future step in the development of medical diagnostic systems, as it leads to increasing the diagnostic accuracy (ed. Jones, 2008, Borisova 2008) and allows one to develop computerized automatic systems for diagnostics decisions when one investigates cutaneous pathologies.

5. Conclusion

There are two common problems that impede one in obtaining optimal results.

- First, the greyscale "chroma" image resulting from the image processing depends on the healthy area; thus, any sparkles are able to produce incorrect chroma spreading inside the lesion. The problem could be avoided by controlling the image registration.
- The second problem is related to the wavelength interval of visibility of the stimulating laser pulse. In fact, the interval under 480 nm becomes useless.

Overcoming these problems is a task of data registration and do not have relation to the processing mentioned above.

Final greyscale images yield enough information about the density spreading inside one lesion. It makes it possible to control precisely the position of obtaining the spectrum.

Calculated spectra ratios emphasize the differences resulting from skin damages independently of the patients. A simple analysis shows that the data from emitted spectra after stimulation at 385 nm are suitable for setting a diagnose. For a benign nevus, the data

could be extracted from the any part of the lesion; for the dysplastic nevus, from the centre of the area; and from the peripheral area for the malignant melanoma.
The spectra ratios from reflectance calculated for a benign nevus could be distinguished from the spectra ratios for a dysplastic nevus, while the same spectra ratios for malignant melanoma clearly differ from the others.
Summarising the test results, we can conclude that the techniques described above form a good basis for the development a non-invasive method for estimating the type of skin damage.

6. Acknowledgements

This work was supported by the National Science Fund of Bulgarian Ministry of Education, Youth and Science under grant DO-02-112/2008 "National Centre of Biomedical Photonics".

7. References

Lademann, J.; Patzelt, A.; Worm M.; Richter, H.; Sterry, W. & Meinke, M. "Analysis of in vivo Penetration of Textile Dyes Causing Allergic Reactions," (2009) *Laser Phys. Lett.* 6, pp. 759–763

Chorvat, D.; Chorvatova, Jr. and A. "Multi-wavelength Fluorescence Lifetime Spectroscopy: A New Approach to the Study of Endogenous Fluorescence in Living Cells and Tissues," (2009) *Laser Phys. Lett.* 6, pp. 175–193

Vlasova, I. M.; Saletsky, A. M. "Raman Spectroscopy in Comparative Investigations of Mechanisms of Binding of Three Molecular Probes—Fluorescein, Eosin, and Erythrosin—to Human Serum Albumin," (2008) *Laser Phys. Lett.* A 5, pp. 834–839 .

Vaishakh, M. ; Murukeshan, V. M.; Sean L. K. "AnImage Fiber Based Fluorescent Probe with Associated Signal Processing Scheme for Biomedical Diagnostics," (2008) *Laser Phys. Lett.* 5, pp. 760–763.

Lemelle, B. ,Veksler, I.; Kozhevnikov, S. ; Akchurin, G. G. ; Piletsky, S. A.; Meglinski, I. "Application of Gold Nanoparticles as Contrast AGents in Confocal Laser Scanning Microscopy," (2009) *Laser Phys. Lett.* 6, pp. 71–75.

Lademann, J.; Patzelt, A.; Darvin, M. ; Richter, H.; Antoniou, C.; Sterry, W.; Koch, S. "Application of Optical Non-invasive Methods in Skin Physiology," (2008) *Laser Phys. Lett.* 5, pp. 335–346.

Vlasova, I. M.; Saletsky, A. M. "Raman Spectroscopy in Investigations of Mechanism of Binding of Human Serum Albumin to Molecular Probe Fluorescein," (2008) *Laser Phys. Lett.* 5, pp. 384–389.

Scheller, E. E.; Rohde, E.; Minet, O.; Muller, G.; Bindig, U. "Calculations Regarding Cell Metabolism Stimulation Using Photons in the Visible Wavelength Range," *Laser Phys. Lett.* (2008) 5, pp. 70–74 .

Borisova, E.; Troyanova, P.; Pavlova, P.; Avramov, L. "Pigmented Skin Tumors Diagnosis Based on Laser induced Autofluorescence and Diffuse Reflectance Spectroscopy," (2008) *Quantum Electron.* 38, pp. 597–605.

CIE, *Colorimetry*, 2nd ed., Publication CIE No.15.2 Central Bureau of the CIE, Vienna, Austria, (1986).

Pascale, D. RGB coordinates of the Macbeth ColorChecker (2006), Available from http://www.bablelcolor.com/download/

Pavlova, P. ; Borisova, E. ; Avramov, L. "Automation of the Skin Cancer Diagnostics on the Bases of Reflectance Spectroscopy," in *Proc. of the 9th Intern. Conf. On Biomedical Physics and Engineering* (Sofia, 2004), pp. 260–265.

Ed. by Jones, G.; Deakin, A. ; Spenser J.(2008) *Chromatic Monitoring of Complex Conditions,* CRC Press Taylor & Francis Group, ISBN 9781584889885, London, GB

Pavlova, P. ; Borisova, E. ; Avramov, L.; Petkova, El.; Troyanova P. "Investigation of Relations between Skin Cancer Lesions' Images and Their Fluorescent Spectra" Laser Phys. Lett. (2010) ,3, pp. 596–603.

Bigio I.; Mourant J. (1997) "Ultraviolet and visible spectroscopies for tissue diagnostics: fluorescence spectroscopy and elastic-scattering spectroscopy", *Phys Med Biol* 42, pp 803 - 814

Bachmann L; Zezell D.; da Costa Ribeiro A.; Gomes L.; Ito A. (2006) "Fluorescence spectroscopy of biological tissues - a review", *Appl Spectr Rev* 41, 575-590

Tuchin V., (2002) *Handbook of Biomedical Diagnostics*, (Bellingham: SPIE Press, 2002).

Wang L., Wu H.(2007), *Biomedical optics: principles and imaging* Hoboken: Wiley-Interscience,.

Sinichkin Yu.; Utz S.; Mavliutov A.; Pilipenko H.(1998) "In vivo fluorescence spectroscopy of the human skin: experiments and models", *J Biomed Opt* 3, pp 201- 211.

Borisova E.; Avramov L., (2000)"Laser System for Optical Biopsy and in vivo Study of the Human Skin", *Proc. SPIE*, 4397, pp. 405-409

Troyanova P.,; Borisova E.; Stoyanova V.; Avramov L., (2006) "Laser-induced autofluorescence spectroscopy of benign and dysplastic nevi and malignant melanoma", *Proc. SPIE* 6284, pp 62840K-1-8.

Mourant J.; Bigio I.,(2003) " Elastic-Scattering Spectroscopy and Diffuse Reflectance" in *Biomedical Photonics Handbook, ed. T. Vo-Dinh*, (CRC Press).

Borisova E.; Troyanova P.; Avramov L. (2006) "Optical biopsy of non-melanin pigmented cutaneous benign and malignant lesions", *Proc. SPIE* 6257, 62570U-1-8.

Jones G. R.; Russell P.C.; Vourdas A.; Cosgrave J.; Stergioulas L.; Haber R. (2000), "The Gabor Transform Basis of Chromatic Monitoring", *Meas. Sci. Tech.* 11, pp. 489-498.

Bedlow A. J. (1995) "Impact of skin cancer education on general practitioners' diagnostic skills", *Br. J. Dermatol* 133(suppl 45), pp 29-30.

Morton C A and R M.Mackie. (1998) "Clinical accuracy of the diagnosis of cutaneous malignant melanoma", *Br J Dermatol* 138, pp283-287.

Part 2

Immunology and the Association with Melanoma

7

Co-operation of Innate and Acquired Immunity for Controlling Tumor Cells

Hidemi Takahashi
Department of Microbiology and Immunology,
Nippon Medical School, Tokyo,
Japan

1. Introduction

The body is composed of various types of cells that unite in harmony to live in the natural environment. Viral infections, toxic products, and environmental stresses may affect the cells to initiate transformation for the development of tumors, an uncontrollable and unfavorable state of cells. Such a tumor state of cells is closely watched by the internal immune-surveillance system that generally controls or eliminates them to maintain the harmony of the body.

The internal immune-surveillance system is composed of two distinct parts; an innate immune system predominantly located on the surface areas of the body, such as the skin or mucosal compartments, and an acquired/adaptive immune system found mainly in systemic compartments, including circulating blood, lymph nodes, spleen, and various organs (Medzhitov and Janeway, 1997a) (Fig. 1). The cells of the innate immune system find and fight foreign bodies intruding from the outside, such as viruses and bacteria, through their pattern-recognition receptors (PRRs) (Medzhitov, 2007), such as Toll-like receptors (TLRs) (Akira et al., 2001) and C-type lectin receptors (CLRs) that recognize pathogen-associated molecular patterns (PAMPs) (Medzhitov and Janeway, 1997b), although they do not have any specific memories of foreign bodies. In contrast, the acquired immune system will respond to foreign elements only when competent cells of the acquired system recognize them specifically through their receptors established via gene-rearrangements (Palm and Medzhitov, 2009). Among these acquired receptors, a T-cell receptor (TCR) can specifically recognize foreign antigens as a specific structural component composed of protein-derived amino acids presented particularly by self-restricted antigen-presenting molecules, termed major histocompatibility complex (MHC) (Takahashi, 2003)

Although the precise mechanisms remain to be elucidated, such specific memories mediated through TCRs are instructed by innate cells, particularly dendritic cells (DCs), which are key cells to present antigenic information though their MHC together with co-stimulatory molecules that will promote memory formation via gene-rearrangements in acquired T cells. Therefore, innate DCs have the ability to capture tumor-derived antigens, processed them into antigenic fragments, and present the antigenic fragments in association with their MHC and co-stimulation molecules (Azuma et al., 1993; Chen et al., 1992), such as B7-1 (CD80), B7-2 (CD86), or CD40, to establish TCR-mediated antigen-specific memories in acquired immunity (Fig. 2).

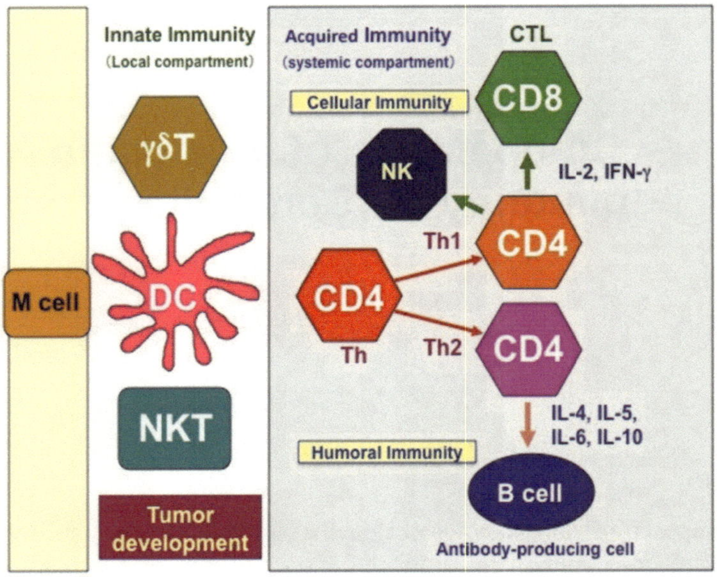

Fig. 1. Innate immunity and acquired immunity.

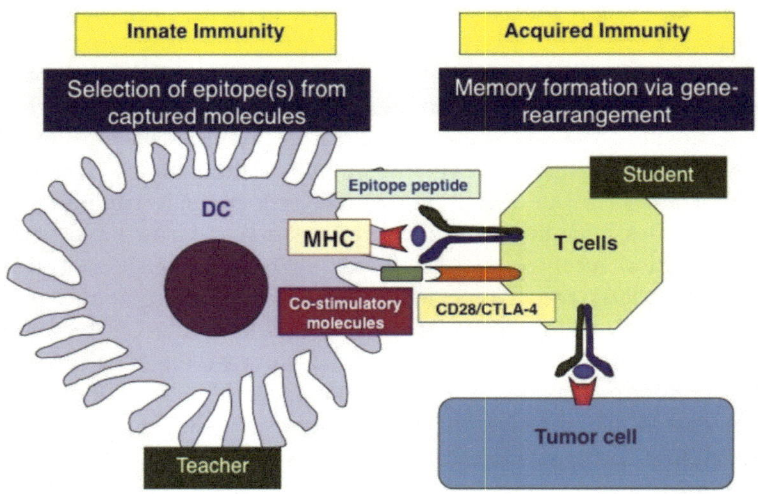

Fig. 2. Antigen selection and presentation by innate DCs to acquired T cells.

Two distinct MHC molecules are expressed on the surface of antigen-presenting cells, class I and class II MHC. In general, class I MHC molecules can present processed fragments of internally produced tumor-gene or virus-gene-derived antigens to $CD8^+$ T cells, whereas class II MHC present processed fragments of externally captured antigens to $CD4^+$ T cells (Takahashi, 1993) (Fig. 3).

Among TCR-mediated specific acquired immunity, class I MHC molecule-restricted tumor-peptide-specific immunity by $CD8^+$ cytotoxic T lymphocytes (CTLs) is particularly important in the elimination of tumor cells and both class I MHC molecule-associated antigenic stimulation and co-stimulatory signals on the same antigen-presenting cells (APCs) are required to elicit such CD8+ CTLs; however, in general, tumor cells that present tumor-derived antigenic peptides in association with their class I MHC do not express appropriate co-stimulation molecules and thus they cannot induce tumor-specific CD8+ CTLs.

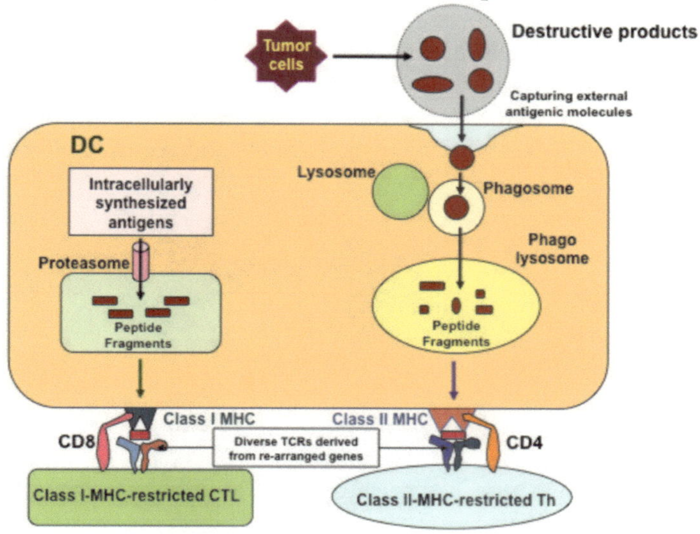

Fig. 3. Two distinct antigen presentation pathways mediated in DCs via class I and class II MHC molecules.

In addition, DCs will not usually become tumor cells and thus are unable to present tumor antigens in conjunction with their class I MHC, despite expressing suitable co-stimulation molecules for the elicitation of tumor-specific CD8+ CTLs.

On the basis of our recent findings (Moriya et al., 2010), this chapter propose a new direction for the establishment of tumor immunotherapy to generate tumor-derived epitope-specific class I MHC molecule-restricted acquired CD8+ CTLs against tumors by selective activation of DEC-205+ DCs that have the ability to process and cross-present antigenic fragments from externally captured tumor-derived products via class I MHC as well as innate effectors such as NKT cells and γδ T cells through their CD1 molecules (Takahashi, 2010).

2. Innate and acquired effectors against tumor cells

Tumor cells originate from normal functional cells, like melanoma from melanocytes, via several transformation steps, which can be classified into two types; early transformation steps initiated by stress-related substances and late transformation steps that generate mutated genes to gain uncontrollable proliferative capacity. The stress-associated products are expressed on the cell surface in association with MHC class I chain-related A (MICA) and MICB molecules, which are composed of a similar structural pattern of class I MHC. These MICA/MICB-associated compounds are recognized by NK group 2D (NKG2D) receptors of activated innate effectors, such as natural killer (NK) cells, natural killer T (NKT) cells, and γδT cells, bearing invariant receptors produced without gene-rearrangements (Higuchi et al., 2009). These innate effectors recognize early transformed tumors via NKG2D receptors and eliminate them. Also, MICA/MICB expressing tumor cells usually show down-modulation of class I MHC that will stimulate NK cells to eliminate them (Suarez-Alvarez et al., 2009).

In contrast, mature tumor cells with mutated genes and expressing tumor-gene-encoded antigenic peptides on their surface in association with class I MHC molecules can be specifically recognized and eliminated by acquired $CD8^+$ CTLs. Thus, stress-associated early transformed tumor cells appear to be regulated mainly by innate effectors, while mature tumor cells with specific structural mutations with high proliferative capacity can be specifically controlled by acquired $CD8^+$ CTLs in a class I MHC molecule-restricted manner. Taken together, internally transformed tumor cells gained uncontrollable proliferating capacity can be recognized and regulated by both innate and acquired effectors (Fig. 4).

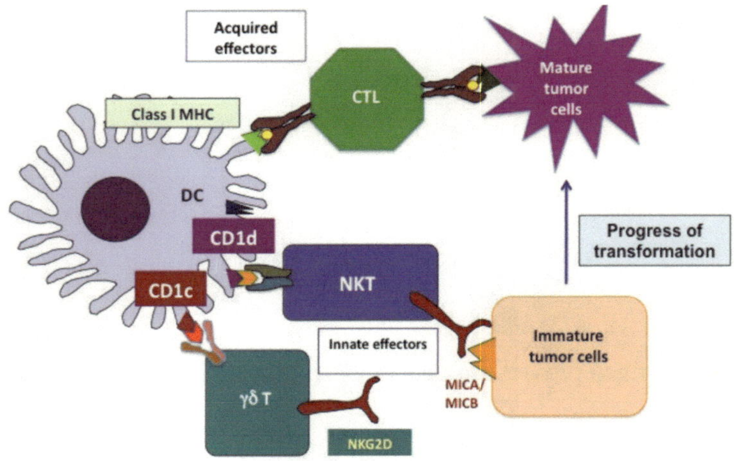

Fig. 4. Immune control of immature and mature tumor cells.

3. Antigen-presenting molecules on DCs

Induction of these innate and acquired effectors seems to be regulated by DCs via various antigen-presenting molecules. Innate immunity is chiefly regulated via species-restricted CD1 antigen-presenting molecules and acquired immunity is controlled via individually restricted MHC molecules on DCs. CD1 molecules are further divided into four classes, CD1a, CD1b, CD1c, and CD1d. These CD1s have been found to present lipid/glycolipid antigens to T cells bearing relatively invariant αβT-cell receptors (TCR), most of which are conserved among species (Barral and Brenner, 2007; Cohen et al., 2009). For example, highly conserved CD1d molecules present α-galactosyl ceramide (α-GalCer) to NKT cells of their own species (Saito et al., 2005). Indeed, human NKT cells generally express unique combinations of TCRs that consist of an invariant Vα24 chain preferentially paired with a Vβ11 (Dellabona et al., 1994), while murine α-GalCer-reactive CD1d-restricted NKT cells express invariant Vα14 paired with various Vβ combinations (Gui et al., 2001).

In contrast to species-restricted CD1 antigen-presenting molecules, both class I and class II MHC molecules are highly diverse among individuals as self-restricted elements presenting internally processed peptides as antigens, which can be recognized by the same MHC molecule-bearing αβTCR-expressing T cells with antigen-specificity established by intracellular gene rearrangements. Such gene rearrangements for the establishment of T cell-mediated acquired immunity can be initiated through the combination of antigen-loaded MHC molecules plus appropriate co-stimulatory signals on DCs, although the induction of CD1-associated T cells does not require such co-stimulatory signals. Thus, co-stimulatory signals appear to be required for the development of MHC molecule-restricted highly specific acquired immunity (Nakatsuka et al., 1999). Generally, CD8αβ-positive T cells recognize the processed epitope peptide from internally synthesized proteins presented by class I MHC molecules, whereas CD4-positive T cells recognize epitope peptide from externally captured proteins in association with class II MHC (Dustin, 2009). The structures of the two distinct groups of antigen-presenting molecules, CD1 and class I MHC, closely resemble each other, having three regions of α–chains (α1, α2, and α3) with non-covalently bound β2-microglobulin that may regulate the antigen-binding capacity of the presenting molecules (Kozlowski et al., 1991). However, although CD1-encoding genes are highly conserved and their structures are shared among species with limited polymorphism (Couedel et al., 1998), the class I MHC-encoding gene is highly diverse among individuals. So far, it has been reported that most innate NKT cells can be activated through CD1d and some γδT cells are activated through CD1c molecules on DCs (Cohen et al., 2009). Moreover, we have recently observed that live bacillus Calmette-Guerin (BCG)-activated DCs elicit innate effectors, such as NK cells, NKT cells, and γδT cells, to inhibit the growth of bladder carcinoma via IL-12 secretion (Higuchi et al., 2009). Collectively, DCs have the ability to manipulate innate effectors through CD1s and cytokines, as well as acquired effectors via MHC molecules to control internal tumors.

4. DC subset and "cross-presentation"

Recently, it has been demonstrated that two non-overlapping subsets of DCs are arranged to regulate internal immune responses *in vivo*; 33D1 (recognizing dendritic cell inhibitory receptor-2 (DCIR2))-positive and DEC-205-positive DCs (Dudziak et al., 2007). It has also been reported that *in vivo* targeting of DEC-205 with either poly(I:C) (Trumpfheller et al., 2008) or an antibody specific for DC-NK lectin group receptor-1 (DNGR-1) (Sancho et al., 2008) induced dominant Th1 immunity or potent CTL responses via cross-presentation, respectively. As indicated in Fig 5, it has turned out that the most suitable CTL epitope peptides within externally captured antigenic proteins are selected to present in association with class I MHC in DEC-205-positive DCs via cross-presentation (Moriya et al., 2010).
We have shown that such cross-presentation, the shift of the antigen-presentation pathway from the class II MHC to class I MHC processing route for externally captured antigenic proteins, can be achieved by a bark-derived saponin-associated adjuvant, such as ISCOMs (Takahashi et al., 1990), cholera toxin (CT) (Wakabayashi et al., 2008), and BCG (Higuchi et al., 2009). We have also demonstrated (Fujimoto et al., 2004) that TLR3-signaling of DCs, previously loaded antigenic proteins, by double-stranded RNA, polyriboinosinic polyribocytidylic acid (poly(I:C)), which reflects a natural genetic product from a variety of viruses, can generate the cross-presentation.
These results suggest that selective stimulation of DEC-205$^+$ DCs *in vivo* may elicit effective acquired CD8$^+$ CTL responses through Th1 dominancy by which protective immunity against tumors will be achieved even in the absence of externally added tumor antigens. We have recently established 33D1$^+$ DC-depleted C57BL/6 mice obtained by treatment with 33D1-specific monoclonal antibody (Moriya et al., 2010). As expected, 33D1$^+$ DC-depleted mice, implanted with syngeneic B16-F10 melanoma cells into the dermis, showed apparent inhibition of already established tumor growth *in vivo* when subcutaneously (sc) injected with LPS after tumor implantation, in which serum IL-12 secretion that may be mediated by the remaining DEC-205$^+$ DCs was markedly enhanced upon TLR4 signaling (Moriya et al., 2010). Unexpectedly, LPS-stimulated 33D1$^+$ DC-deleted tumor-bearing mice apparently produced H-2K^b-restricted epitope-specific CD8$^+$ CTLs among tumor infiltrating

lymphocytes (TILs) against already established syngeneic tumor cells (Moriya et al., 2010). These findings indicate the importance and effectiveness of selective targeting of a specific subset of DCs, such as DEC-205+ DCs, for the activation of tumor-specific class I MHC molecule-restricted CD8+ CTLs without externally added tumor antigen stimulation *in vivo*.

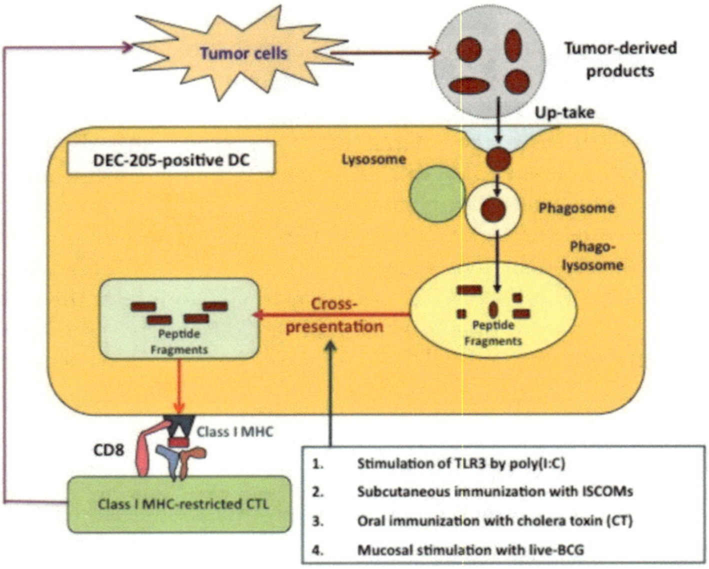

Fig. 5. New direction for tumor immuno-therapy.

5. Concluding remarks: A new direction for tumor immunotherapy

Because tumor epitope-specific CD8+ CTLs can be primed *in vivo* by immunization with epitope peptide-pulsed syngeneic DCs (Takahashi et al., 1993), most of the present works for the establishment of cancer immunotherapy have focused on identifying tumor-derived epitope peptides in each tumor; however, tumor-derived specific epitope peptides are generally very difficult to determine for most tumors because the structure of each epitope and its MHC cassette is highly diverse among individuals.

Here, we would like to propose a new, promising strategy for the development of cancer immunotherapy; selective activation of DEC-205+ DCs *in vivo*. It should be noted that innate DEC-205+ DCs do not have memories and thus, repetitive intermittent stimulation is required to carry out this procedure. By this method, selectively activated DEC-205+ DCs recognizing newly appeared tumor cells capture antigenic molecules and present their antigenic epitopes in association with class I MHC via cross-presentation, and the presented epitope will prime acquired tumor-specific class I MHC molecule-restricted CD8+ CTLs that specifically recognize tumor cells with mutated genes and attack them. As far as we have examined, ISCOMs, CT and BCG have the capacity to selectively stimulate DEC-205+ DCs *in vivo*. Indeed, repetitive immunization with adjuvant alone shows apparent inhibition in the growth of syngeneic implanted tumors (Wakabayashi, A., Nakagawa, Y., Date, T., Tomita, Y., Shimizu, M, and Takahashi, H.; manuscript in preparation).

In addition, as has been shown above, live BCG has the ability to activate innate effectors such as NK cells, NKT cells, and γδT cells to suppress the growth of early transformed tumors expressing MICA/MICB and stress-related substances via NKG2D (Higuchi et al.,

2009). These results strongly suggest that we can manipulate appropriate immunity to control tumor cells by repetitive stimulation of DEC-205+ DCs with a BCG-derived substance. Now we should recall the name of Chisato Maruyama (1901-1992), a professor of the Department of Dermatology as well as the past President of Nippon Medical School in Japan, who had noticed that there were a very low number of cancer patients suffered from tuberculosis and established special substance from *Mycobacterium tuberculosis* as a cancer vaccine, named the "Maruyama Vaccine (SSM; special substance of Maruyama)" in 1944. The SSM has been widely used, particularly for various cancer patients in Japan; however, the actual mechanism of the SSM has been unknown until now. Thus, although a number of cases with excellent effects on cancer regression by SSM have been reported, many doctors are still suspicious of the effect of SSM. Here, it is proposed that new adjuvant therapy should be considered, including BCG or SSM that will activate internal innate immunity, particularly DEC-205+ DCs.

6. References

Akira, S., Takeda, K., and Kaisho, T. (2001). Toll-like receptors: critical proteins linking innate and acquired immunity. *Nat Immunol,* 2, 675-680.

Azuma, M., Ito, D., Yagita, H., Okumura, K., Phillips, J.H., Lanier, L.L., and Somoza, C. (1993). B70 antigen is a second ligand for CTLA-4 and CD28. *Nature,* 366, 76-79.

Barral, D.C., and Brenner, M.B. (2007). CD1 antigen presentation: how it works. *Nat Rev Immunol,* 7, 929-941.

Chen, L., Ashe, S., Brady, W.A., Hellstrom, I., Hellstrom, K.E., Ledbetter, J.A., McGowan, P., and Linsley, P.S. (1992). Costimulation of antitumor immunity by the B7 counterreceptor for the T lymphocyte molecules CD28 and CTLA-4. *Cell,* 71, 1093-1102.

Cohen, N.R., Garg, S., and Brenner, M.B. (2009). Antigen Presentation by CD1 Lipids, T Cells, and NKT Cells in Microbial Immunity. *Adv Immunol,* 102, 1-94.

Couedel, C., Peyrat, M.A., Brossay, L., Koezuka, Y., Porcelli, S.A., Davodeau, F., and Bonneville, M. (1998). Diverse CD1d-restricted reactivity patterns of human T cells bearing "invariant" AV24BV11 TCR. *Eur J Immunol,* 28, 4391-4397.

Dellabona, P., Padovan, E., Casorati, G., Brockhaus, M., and Lanzavecchia, A. (1994). An invariant V alpha 24-J alpha Q/V beta 11 T cell receptor is expressed in all individuals by clonally expanded CD4-8- T cells. *J Exp Med,* 180, 1171-1176.

Dudziak, D., Kamphorst, A.O., Heidkamp, G.F., Buchholz, V.R., Trumpfheller, C., Yamazaki, S., Cheong, C., Liu, K., Lee, H.W., Park, C.G., *et al.* (2007). Differential antigen processing by dendritic cell subsets in vivo. *Science,* 315, 107-111.

Dustin, M.L. (2009). The cellular context of T cell signaling. *Immunity,* 30, 482-492.

Fujimoto, C., Nakagawa, Y., Ohara, K., and Takahashi, H. (2004). Polyriboinosinic polyribocytidylic acid [poly(I:C)]/TLR3 signaling allows class I processing of exogenous protein and induction of HIV-specific CD8+ cytotoxic T lymphocytes. *Int Immunol,* 16, 55-63.

Gui, M., Li, J., Wen, L.J., Hardy, R.R., and Hayakawa, K. (2001). TCR beta chain influences but does not solely control autoreactivity of V alpha 14J281T cells. *J Immunol,* 167, 6239-6246.

Higuchi, T., Shimizu, M., Owaki, A., Takahashi, M., Shinya, E., Nishimura, T., and Takahashi, H. (2009). A possible mechanism of intravesical BCG therapy for human bladder carcinoma: involvement of innate effector cells for the inhibition of tumor growth. *Cancer Immunol Immunother,* 58, 1245-1255.

Kozlowski, S., Takeshita, T., Boehncke, W.H., Takahashi, H., Boyd, L.F., Germain, R.N., Berzofsky, J.A., and Margulies, D.H. (1991). Excess beta 2 microglobulin promoting functional peptide association with purified soluble class I MHC molecules. *Nature,* 349, 74-77.

Medzhitov, R., and Janeway, C.A., Jr. (1997a). Innate immunity: impact on the adaptive immune response. *Curr Opin Immunol,* 9, 4-9.

Medzhitov, R., and Janeway, C.A., Jr. (1997b). Innate immunity: the virtues of a nonclonal system of recognition. *Cell,* 91, 295-298.

Medzhitov, R. (2007). Recognition of microorganisms and activation of the immune response. *Nature,* 449, 819-826.

Moriya, K., Wakabayashi, A., Shimizu, M., Tamura, H., Dan, K., and Takahashi, H. (2010) Induction of tumor-specific acquired immunity against already established tumors by selective stimulation of innate DEC-205(+) dendritic cells. *Cancer Immunol Immunother,* 59, 1083-1095.

Nakatsuka, K., Sugiyama, H., Nakagawa, Y., and Takahashi, H. (1999). Purification of antigenic peptide from murine hepatoma cells recognized by Class-I major histocompatibility complex molecule-restricted cytotoxic T-lymphocytes induced with B7-1-gene-transfected hepatoma cells. *J Hepatol,* 30, 1119-1129.

Palm, N.W., and Medzhitov, R. (2009). Pattern recognition receptors and control of adaptive immunity. *Immunol Rev,* 227, 221-233.

Saito, N., Takahashi, M., Akahata, W., Ido, E., Hidaka, C., Ibuki, K., Miura, T., Hayami, M., and Takahashi, H. (2005). Analysis of evolutionary conservation in CD1d molecules among primates. *Tissue Antigens,* 66, 674-682.

Sancho, D., Mourao-Sa, D., Joffre, O.P., Schulz, O., Rogers, N.C., Pennington, D.J., Carlyle, J.R., and Reis e Sousa, C. (2008). Tumor therapy in mice via antigen targeting to a novel, DC-restricted C-type lectin. *J Clin Invest,* 118, 2098-2110.

Suarez-Alvarez, B., Lopez-Vazquez, A., Baltar, J.M., Ortega, F., and Lopez-Larrea, C. (2009). Potential role of NKG2D and its ligands in organ transplantation: new target for immunointervention. *Am J Transplant,* 9, 251-257.

Takahashi, H., Takeshita, T., Morein, B., Putney, S., Germain, R.N., and Berzofsky, J.A. (1990). Induction of CD8+ cytotoxic T cells by immunization with purified HIV-1 envelope protein in ISCOMs. *Nature,* 344, 873-875.

Takahashi, H. (1993). Antigen processing and presentation. *Microbiol Immunol,* 37, 1-9.

Takahashi, H., Nakagawa, Y., Yokomuro, K., and Berzofsky, J.A. (1993). Induction of CD8+ cytotoxic T lymphocytes by immunization with syngeneic irradiated HIV-1 envelope derived peptide-pulsed dendritic cells. *Int Immunol,* 5, 849-857.

Takahashi, H. (2003). Antigen presentation in vaccine development. *Comp Immunol Microbiol Infect Dis,* 26, 309-328.

Takahashi, H. (2010) Species-specific CD1-restricted innate immunity for the development of HIV vaccine. *Vaccine,* 28(Suppl 2), B3-7.

Trumpfheller, C., Caskey, M., Nchinda, G., Longhi, M.P., Mizenina, O., Huang, Y., Schlesinger, S.J., Colonna, M., and Steinman, R.M. (2008). The microbial mimic poly IC induces durable and protective CD4+ T cell immunity together with a dendritic cell targeted vaccine. *Proc Natl Acad Sci U S A,* 105, 2574-2579.

Wakabayashi, A., Nakagawa, Y., Shimizu, M., Moriya, K., Nishiyama, Y., and Takahashi, H. (2008). Suppression of an already established tumor growing through activated mucosal CTLs induced by oral administration of tumor antigen with cholera toxin. *J Immunol,* 180, 4000-4010.

8

Adoptive T-Cell Therapy of Melanoma: Promises and Challenges

Patrick Schmidt and Hinrich Abken
Centre for Molecular Medicine Cologne and Clinic I for Internal Medicine, University of Cologne, Cologne Germany

1. Introduction

Adoptive immunotherapy for the treatment of melanoma has attracted growing interest in recent years. The trend reflects, at least in part, the disappointing results of conventional chemotherapy to induce lasting remission in advanced stages of the disease with multiple metastases and to cure patients even after initially complete response. The isolation of tumor infiltrating T cells from melanoma lesions, the identification of melanoma-associated antigens and the significant progress in our understanding in redirecting an immune response favored the development of novel strategies in adoptive immunotherapy of melanoma. Most recent advances in selectively eliminating melanoma cell subsets from tumor tissues together with the identification of so-called melanoma stem cells, however, imply to re-define the therapeutic target in melanoma. The review discusses current challenges and perspectives in the rational design of cellular immunotherapy of melanoma.

2. The need for novel options in the treatment of advanced stage melanoma

Despite of major improvements in the therapy of melanoma, the frequency of partial or complete responses after chemo- and radiotherapy has not significantly risen since years (Garbe et al. 2010). Disseminated melanoma is still an incurable disease and overall survival correlates with the stage of the disease at time of diagnosis. A 10-year-survival rate of 75-85% can be reached when the primary tumor was diagnosed in stage I or II, melanoma in stage III or IV, however, is commonly associated with poor survival (Garbe et al. 2010). The situation is mainly caused by two major drawbacks due to the particular biology of melanoma cells. Firstly, melanoma early disseminates into distant organs including the brain by forming micro-metastases which are small in cancer cell numbers and beyond the detection limit of current tomographic procedures (Denninghoff et al. 2004; Bedikian et al. 2010). Micro-metastases can persist for long time without any change in size in a "dormant" stage (Leiter et al. 2010). Secondly, many melanoma cells are notoriously resistant against chemo- and radiation therapy (Bradbury & Middleton 2004; Pak et al. 2001; Pak et al. 2004). Both drawbacks result in the unsatisfactory situation that surgical removing of tumor lesions in early stages is the only curative option to fight melanoma. In more progressed stages of the disease recruitment of the cellular immune defense is thought to be an option. In this context immune-modulatory adjuvants, including interferon α-2b, exhibit some effect although are not curative (Kirkwood et al. 2000; Kirkwood et al. 1996) and still a matter of debate. These efforts, however, indicate that activation of the patient's immune response can be effective in fighting melanoma; a more tumor-specific way of immune cell activation needs to be explored. We here summarize evidence for the potency of adoptive immune cell therapy in melanoma and discuss premises and future treatment options.

3. Adoptively transferred T cells are capable to fight melanoma

Based on early evidences that the concerted action of the immune system is capable to fight cancer efforts were focused to redirect cytolytic effector cells towards autologous cancer cells. First experiments following the strategy were performed by the Rosenberg group in 1984 by treating transplanted tumors in mice by adoptive transfer of syngeneic lymphocytes in combination with IL-2 (Rosenberg 1984; Grimm et al. 1982). In addition to promote activation and proliferation of both cytolytic and helper T cells, IL-2 also activates natural killer (NK) cells as well as macrophages (Waldmann & Tagaya 1999) which provided the rationale to administer IL-2 as immune adjuvant in cancer patients. Between 1985 and 1993 overall 270 melanoma patients were treated with IL-2 in the context of eight clinical trials with an objective response rate of 16%, comprising 6% complete and 10% partial responses (Atkins et al. 1999). While IL-2 doubtless induced an immune cell anti-tumor response, the immune cell activation was not specifically redirected towards melanoma.

The elucidation of so-called "tumor antigens" preferentially expressed on melanoma cells led to the concept to immunize patients with defined T cell antigens in order to activate by natural selection melanoma specific T cells in a more specific fashion. Two antigens were primarily considered as promising candidates, namely Melan-A/MART 1 and gp100 (Rivoltini et al. 1996; Rivoltini et al. 1995). By using different strategies of vaccination including injection of antigen or application of antigen-pulsed dendritic cells melanoma reactive T cells could be amplified in the cancer patient (Kawakami & Rosenberg 1997). Until today a variety of clinical studies using dendritic cells loaded with T cell recognition peptides were performed with various therapeutic effects. A meta-analysis in 2008 comprising 38 trials with overall 626 patients revealed that 3% of the patients responded to treatment with complete and 6% with partial remission, 21% achieved stable disease (Engell-Noerregaard et al. 2009). These results were irrespective of both the antigen used for loading and the type of DCs. The route of injection and the administration of adjuvant had no impact on clinical outcome. In conclusion no therapeutic advantage could be documented for patients treated with vaccines compared to treatment with immune stimulatory cytokines.

As a consequence further developments in the immunotherapy of melanoma were thereon focused on the adoptive transfer of immune effector cells itself. The development was further strengthened by the success in isolating tumor infiltrating lymphocytes (TILs) which are found in substantial numbers in a variety of melanoma lesions. First described in 1969 (Clark et al. 1969) TILs particularly from melanoma gained interest in during the last years since these cells are believed to recognize melanoma-associated antigens and thereby specifically accumulate in melanoma lesions. Freshly isolated from melanoma lesions TILs are mainly of T cell origin consisting of both effector and helper T cell subsets. While the prevalence of TILs in primary melanoma lesions and metastases is not a prognostic factor itself, high numbers of infiltrating lymphocytes, however, correlate with better clinical outcome (Clemente et al. 1996; Burton et al. 2011), moreover providing a rationale to use these lymphocytes as effector cells in the treatment of melanoma. Protocols according to GMP standards were developed to isolate TILs and to amplify them ex vivo to numbers suitable for re-infusion (Figure 1). To expand preferentially highly melanoma reactive T cells first lymphocyte expansion protocols were based on cultures in presence of IL-2 on feeder layer cells expressing melanoma antigens (Vignard et al. 2005). While the concept perfectly worked in mouse models, the application in patients turned out to need further improvements. Upon adoptive TIL infusions regression of metastases could be observed in the majority of patients, only few, however, remained in complete remission (Besser et al. 2010). In most cases a partial shrinkage of the tumor mass followed by stable disease was observed. The disappointing results despite the high numbers of infused TILs is thought to be due to the fact that the cells were extensively amplified over weeks ex vivo and have entered anergy unable to be properly rescued for an anti-melanoma attack after infusion (Chhabra 2010). More recent expansion protocols therefore aim to select so-called "young TILs" which underwent minimal culture times and which were not selected for melanoma reactivity prior re-infusion. A first phase I trial showed improved response with increased frequencies in partial and complete remission (Besser et al. 2009). All trials were performed under myeloablative conditions and IL-2 administration based on the rationale to provide space and stimuli for homeostatic expansion of adoptively transferred T cells. Other cytokines like IL-7 and/or IL-15 are worth to be explored since they do not activate regulatory T cells.

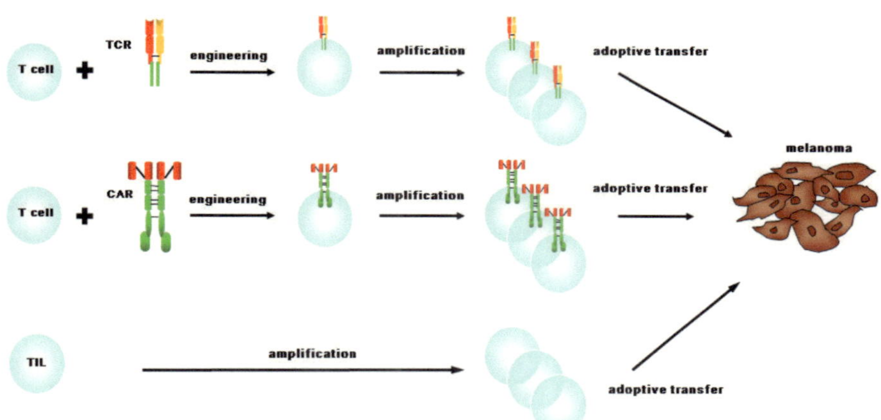

Fig. 1. Strategies in the adoptive immunotherapy of melanoma.

Tumor infiltrating lymphocytes (TIL) are isolated from a melanoma lesion, amplified ex vivo and re-administered without further modification. Alternatively, T cells from the peripheral blood of the melanoma patient are engineered ex vivo to express either a chimeric antigen receptor (CAR), which forms a homo-dimer, or a recombinant T cell receptor (TCR), which is composed of the α and β chain, with specificity for a melanoma associated antigen, amplified and re-administered in therapeutic doses to the patient.

4. Redirecting T cells with pre-defined specificity towards melanoma

While adoptive transfer of TILs is showing promising efficacy in first trials, attempts are made to redirect blood T cells with pre-defined specificity toward melanoma. The rationale for using effector T cells from the peripheral blood is provided by the frequent inability to isolate TILs in sufficient amounts from a given melanoma lesion and the more progressed proliferative stage of TILs compared to blood T cells.

To redirect peripheral blood T cells specifically towards melanoma antibodies were combined in a bi-specific antibody format which targets T cells with by an anti-CD3 antibody as one arm and the melanoma cell with the other arm. Upon application it is assumed that bi-specific antibodies build a bridge between T cells and melanoma cells thereby forcing peripheral blood cytolytic effectors towards their target. Bi-specific antibodies were directed against melanoma p97, gp100 (Cochlovius et al. 1999), and melanoma chondroitin sulfate proteoglycan (MCSP, also called high molecular weight-melanoma associated antigen HMW-MAA) (Grosse-Hovest et al. 1999). Therapeutic potency was demonstrated by long-term survival in pre-clinical models resulting, the efficacy, however, critically depends on the number of recruitable effector cells at the tumor site. Bi-specific constructs triggering CD28 costimulation of T cells furthermore increased tumor-cell killing predominantly by recruiting cytolytic cells without targeted specificity (Grosse-Hovest et al. 1999; Grosse-Hovest et al. 2003).

While first generation bi-specific reagents were conventional hetero-dimeric antibodies, second generation antibodies are constituted of two single polypeptide chain antibodies covalently joined by a linker domain (Grosse-Hovest et al. 1999; Bluemel et al. 2010a). Those so-called bi-specific T cell engager (BiTE) antibodies targeting CD3 on T cells and a tumor-associated antigen on malignant cells of solid tumors showed efficacy even in nano-molar concentrations in a clinical trial (Bargou et al. 2008). The size of antigen as well as the targeted epitope impacts the efficacy in T cell activation since a BiTE antibody targeting the membrane proximal domain of HMW-MAA on melanoma cells showed more potent than those binding to more distal domains (Bluemel et al. 2010b). The same observations were made when targeting EpCAM indicating that there is obviously a correlation between epitope positioning relative to the cell membrane and the potency in T cell activation.

Technical advances in genetically engineering blood T cells ex vivo fueled efforts to design T cells with pre-defined specificity for redirected targeting melanoma cells. Recombinant DNA technology and the structural elucidation of the T cell receptor (TCR) complex together with recent developments in vector design made the genetic T cell modification with a recombinant TCR feasible. The melanoma gp100 specific TCR was one of the first be cloned from T cells accumulating at the tumor site. TCR α and β chains were introduced ex vivo by retroviral gene transfer into naïve, fresh T cells which gained specificity as indicated by redirected cytotoxicity towards primary melanoma and established melanoma cell lines and by increased secretion of pro-inflammatory cytokines including IFN-γ (Schaft et al. 2003; Morgan et al. 2003). TCR modified T cells were amplified ex vivo and re-infused in therapeutic doses to the patient (Figure 1). Similarly, recombinant TCRs with specificity for MART1/Melan-A or MAGE-A1 could be transferred into naïve T cells (Hughes et al. 2005; Willemsen et al. 2005).

In 2006 the Rosenberg group published the first clinical trial using T cells with engineered specificity for melanoma. Adoptive transfer of those T cells caused a strong response against metastases in distant organs. Engineered T cells persisted in circulation of most patients for nearly 2 months. The therapeutic efficacy, however, was disappointingly low with 2 out of 17 patients showing objective regression of metastases resulting in complete response. In those patients, interestingly, engineered T cells were detected in the blood for a year after treatment implying that therapeutic efficacy may correlate with long-term anti-melanoma immunity (Morgan et al. 2006; Coccoris et al. 2008). In a very recent trial, similarly TCR engineered T cells showed efficacy towards brain metastases of melanoma indicating that this procedure may be useful to treat otherwise incurable metastatic sites (Hong et al. 2010). Although these and other trials showed technical feasibility in engineering TCR modified T cells and clinical practicability in the adoptive transfer of those cells, the unexpected low clinical response raised concerns with respect to clonal variability of the targeted melanoma lesion.

Melanoma like other malignant diseases displays clonal evolution during tumor progression which enables the tumor to evade T cell recognition. Common mechanisms are the down-regulation of MHC complex expression (Seliger 2008), point mutations in the β_2 microglobulin chain (Sigalotti et al. 2004), and deregulation of various components of the antigen processing machinery (Seliger 2008; Vitale et al. 2005). As a consequence TCR engineered T cells are no longer able to recognize and destroy those melanoma cells with mutant or lack of MHC-peptide complexes.

Limitations in the expression of a recombinant TCR in T cells additionally dampened enthusiasm in the strategy. Co-expression of a recombinant TCR together with the physiological TCR in T cells turned out to create new but unpredictable specificities which may result in severe auto-reactivity. The molecular basis is the similarity of the recombinant α and β TCR chains to the respective chains of the physiological TCR which leads to the formation of hetero-dimers loosing the specificity of the recombinant TCR (Coccoris et al. 2010). In mouse models hetero-dimer formation resulted in severe auto-immunity (Bendle et al. 2010). Tremendous efforts were undertaken to solve the problem including replacement of TCR constant domains by homologous murine domains (Cohen et al. 2006) and introducing cysteine bridges (Kuball et al. 2007) to enforce αβ-pairing of the recombinant TCR chains.

Advances in the engineering of recombinant signaling molecules facilitated the development of a "one-chain-receptor" molecule for redirected T cell activation. Zelig Eshhar pioneered the strategy in generating a chimeric antigen receptor (CAR) molecule composed of an extracellular single chain antibody for binding and an intracellular TCR signaling domain (Eshhar et al. 1993). The CAR, also named immunoreceptor or nick-named "T-body", thereby combines the MHC-independent recognition of antigen by an antibody with the T cell activating machinery of the TCR. Naïve T cells from the peripheral blood of melanoma patients are engineered ex vivo to express the CAR, amplified and administered to the patient (Figure 1). Due to the modular design a nearly unlimited variety of antigens can be targeted as long as an antibody is available, including non-classical T cell antigens like carbohydrates as HMW-MAA, also called MCSP (Reinhold et al. 1999). Different CARs were reported to target melanoma antigens, including HMW-MAA (Reinhold et al. 1999), melanotransferrin (Schmidt et al. 2011), GD2 (Yvon et al. 2009) and GD3 (Lo et al. 2010). The modular composition of CARs moreover allowed combining primary signaling moieties with costimulatory signals in order to modulate the T cell response in a predicted fashion (Hombach & Abken 2007). Along with multiple other modifications the stability of expression and antigen binding has been substantially improved during the last years (Bridgeman et al. 2010). Although CARs use the TCR signaling machinery, the strategy is obviously not restricted to redirect T cells; monocytes, macrophages as well as NK cells can be specifically redirected by CARs as well (Pegram et al. 2008; Kruschinski et al. 2008). Appropriate models and, finally, trials need to address whether redirected non-T cells have a benefit in tumor elimination in general and in melanoma therapy in particular.

Some TCRs and CARs specific to melanoma associated antigens are already applied in phase I clinical trials, and several others are in an advanced phase of preparation (Table 1). Only a few of these studies have been published; other information is derived from registries and from personal communications.

A clinical trial by the Brenner group, Baylor College of Medicine, (Pule et al. 2008) has shown a correlation between the persistence of adoptively transferred, modified T cells and the clinical outcome. Epstein-Barr virus specific cytotoxic T cells were engineered to express a CAR directed to the diasialoganglioside GD2, an antigen expressed by human neuroblastoma cells, aiming that redirected T cells would receive optimal costimulation after engagement of their EBV-specific TCR, enhancing survival and anti-tumor activity mediated through their CAR (Savoldo et al. 2007). When administered to tumor patients the EBV-specific T cells engineered with a GD2-specific CAR indeed survived longer than T cells with the same CAR but lacking virus specificity. Infusion of these genetically modified T cells was associated with tumor regression or necrosis in half of the patients. Results show the safety, feasibility, and potential anti-tumor activity of adoptive therapy with CAR modified T cells; clinical application, however, has to take into account some particular aspects as recently summarized (Büning et al. 2010) and briefly discussed below.

5. Advantages, premises and challenges of engineered T cells in their attack against melanoma

There are potential balances to advantages of the CAR or the TCR strategy in the adoptive T cell therapy of melanoma which need careful consideration. Melanoma cells frequently down-regulate proteins associated with antigen processing and presentation (Seliger et al. 1997) which effectively renders the tumor cell invisible to a physiological T cell attack. Consequently, the MHC-independent targeting of cell surface molecules through a CAR makes those melanoma cells vulnerable to T cell attack while remaining invisible for TCR engineered T cells. The CAR strategy moreover has the advantage that immune cells with defined specificity for a variety of cell surface molecules can be produced. Powerful selection systems, such as phage display provide a plethora of binding domains to target virtually any cell surface molecule. Melanoma cells which do not express the targeted antigen, however, are not attacked by CAR redirected T cells making antigen-loss cell variants a source of potential tumour relapse after initially successful treatment. TCR redirected T cells, on the other hand, may recognize even those melanoma cells when they cross-present the targeted antigen. Most recently, TCR-like single chain antibodies were generated and used as targeting domain in a CAR, thereby combining the MHC-restricted recognition of antigen with the CAR strategy. T cells with TCR-like CAR were redirected towards NY-ESO-1 and MAGE-A1, respectively (Stewart-Jones et al. 2009; Willemsen et al. 2001). The advantage of these MHC restricted CARs over the use of recombinant TCRs remains unclear aside from the fact that the CAR consists of a single expressed protein while the TCR approach requires co-expression of both α and β TCR chains.

The high complexity of the recognition and signaling process in the T cell and the variety of antigen structures on the melanoma cell imply that the optimized configuration of a CAR universal for each antigen may not exist. In contrast the TCR recognition and activation process through MHC presented antigen is much more standardized. The antibody-derived binding domain of a CAR moreover displays extraordinary high affinity compared to a TCR. By mutagenesis the affinity of a given antibody binding domain can be increased or reduced (Stewart-Jones et al. 2009; Chmielewski et al. 2004). Increase in affinity, however, does not necessarily improve CAR redirected T cell activation which is assumed for TCR mediated T cell activation as well. CD28 costimulation, moreover, does not impact the activation threshold of CAR redirected T cells (Chmielewski et al. 2011).

Critical to the success of therapy will moreover be the choice of targeted antigen and the membrane topography of the targeted epitope. In vitro data suggest that an optimal T cell-to-target cell spacing distance is required for T cell activation. For instance, binding the more membrane distal epitope of the targeted antigen showed less T cell activation than binding of the membrane proximal epitope (Hombach et al. 2007). The rigidity of the antigen itself as well as the antigen mobility in the cell membrane will moreover impact redirected T cell activation. Carbohydrate antigens like HMW-MAA are thought to act differently than polypeptide antigens like melanotransferin, both expressed on the same melanoma cell. As such, empirical testing may be required to identify the best targeted epitope for the particular antigen for redirected T cell activation.

The TCR or CAR binding avidity impacts recruitment of engineered T cells to tumor sites. Strong binding to target antigen may cause the T cells to be locally trapped while low avidity interactions may not provide sufficiently long T cell – melanoma cell contact to execute the cytolytic attack. On the other hand, the amount of antigen on the melanoma cell surface is also important. In essence, low affinity binding directs the activity of engineered T cells preferentially against targets with abundant antigen levels; high affinity binding is thought to be also effective against low antigen levels on target cells. The optimized affinity which sustains selective T cell trafficking to the tumor, however, is still unclear. Homing and migration of engineered T cells may also be manipulated through co-expression of chemokine receptors alongside with CARs (Cheadle et al. 2007). Alternatively, isolated T cell subpopulations which express or lack certain chemokine receptors may be used, in particular when targeting melanoma lesions in the periphery. Studies investigating these issues in animal models are now gaining momentum and are likely to improve the anti-tumor efficacy. Once entered the tumor lesion engineered T cells are assumed to efficiently re-cycle lytic capacity and to kill multiple targets. While this is suggested by in vitro evidences formal in vivo confirmation is still lacking.

A beneficial effector cell-to-target cell ratio at the tumor site is likely to be required for efficient target cell lysis. Higher numbers of engineered T cells applied per dose are likely to increase clinical efficacy, an estimation based on clinical data, however, is not yet available. Current trials are applying up to 10^{10} cells per dose. These and higher numbers of engineered T cells can be generated by current expansion protocols; cells with the optimal phenotype for adoptive transfer, however, may not be generated under these conditions. Short term amplification protocols are therefore discussed for both TILs from melanoma lesions and for engineered T cells.

Auto-immunity may result from off-target T cell activation against healthy tissues which physiologically express low levels of the targeted antigen. A number of so-called "tumor-associated antigens" are also expressed on healthy tissues, although frequently at lower levels, e.g., MART-1 on melanocytes. When targeting those antigens, vitiligo and deafness (Offringa 2009; Johnson et al. 2009a) to a certain degree is frequently observed; uveitis and inner ear toxicity were observed upon adoptive therapy with TCR engineered T cells (Johnson et al. 2009b). Since nearly all tumor-associated antigens are self-antigens, strategies need to be adopted to ensure off-target toxicities are kept to a minimum although toxicity may be a surrogate for clinical efficacy. In the adoptive therapy of melanoma, indeed, off-target toxicities generally predict for anti-tumour responses (Overwijk et al. 2003). It is currently under investigation whether T cells with low-avidity TCR are less prone to induce such unwanted side effects. Toxicity, however, can be controlled using steroids to deplete modified T cells locally (Johnson et al. 2009b) or systemically as has been the case in CAR targeting carboanhydrase IX (G250), a renal cell carcinoma antigen also expressed at low levels on bile duct epithelia (Lamers et al. 2006a; Lamers et al. 2006b).

One of the major hurdles of redirected immunotherapy of melanoma is the heterogeneity of antigen expression within the malignant lesions which negatively affects the long-term therapeutic efficacy of the approach. Whereas melanotransferin-positive or HMW-MAA-positive melanoma cells may be successfully eliminated by redirected T cells engineered with the respective CAR, antigen-negative tumor cells, however, will not be recognized by those T cells. The limitation may be overcome by utilizing mixed T cell populations modified with different CARs recognizing different antigens of the same tumor. On the other hand, activation of pro-inflammatory immune cells in the tumor microenvironment led to the speculation whether IL-2, secreted in high concentrations by activated T cells, may attract a second wave of non-antigen restricted effector cells which eradicate antigen-negative tumor cells. Experiments with antibody-cytokine fusion proteins indicate that at least in an animal model antigen-negative melanoma cells are indeed eliminated when co-inoculated with antigen-positive melanoma cells and that the T cell mediated immune response is followed by a long-lived transferable protective immunity (Becker et al. 1996).

As far as safety concerns, insertional mutagenesis by retro- or lentiviral gene transfer of the TCR or CAR encoding transgene also needs to be addressed. While more than 100 patients have been treated so far, malignant transformation of blood T cells has not been observed in any case which is in contrast to genetic modification of hematopoietic stem cells. Retrovirally modified, mature polyclonal T cells seem not to produce clonal amplification upon adoptive transfer (Newrzela et al. 2008). Apart from that, the search for a safer vector system using non-integrating vectors (Perro et al. 2010), RNA transfer (Zhao et al. 2010), or targeted recombination (Carroll 2008) into safe sites is still ongoing. Once adoptively transferred, controlling the engineered T cell in vivo represents an important option. Novel gene suicide systems using tagged receptor molecules which can be targeted by T cell depleting antibodies in vivo (Kieback et al. 2008) and inducible caspase-based suicide systems (de Witte et al. 2008) have recently been developed to permit specific depletion of the engineered T cells rather than total T cell depletion by steroids.

6. Targeting the heart of melanoma: do cancer stem cells play a role?

Current therapeutic strategies in oncology aim to eliminate all cancer cells within a tumor lesion. The histology, however, teaches us that a variety of different cancer cells make up most tumor tissues in addition to non-malignant cells which form the so-called stroma. Transplantation of individual cancer cell subsets from melanoma under limiting dilution conditions revealed that a subset of cancer cells is capable to induce tumors of the same histological phenotype as the parental tumor (Al-Hajj et al. 2003; Schatton et al. 2008; Zabierowski & Herlyn 2008). Transplantation assays moreover revealed that a low number of sorted cells, most rigorously one cancer cell, is capable to induce tumors when transplanted under appropriate conditions (Quintana et al. 2008). The conclusion drawn from these experiments was that melanoma is organized in a hierarchical manner following an initiator cell or so-called cancer stem cell (CSC). The same observation was drawn from other tumor entities (Ailles & Weissman 2007; Clevers 2011). Low abundance, induction of tumors, self-renewal and differentiation into heterogeneous phenotypes of cancer cells are properties postulated for CSCs. While established as early as 1968 (Fiala 1968), the CSC paradigm experienced revival when Bonnet and Dick (1997) showed that most subtypes of acute myeloid leukemia can be established in their broad diversity by transplantation of a defined and rare subset of malignant $CD34^+$ cells fully recapitulating the leukemic phenotype (Bonnet & Dick 1997). A variety of cancer stem cells were subsequently identified in solid tumors including mammary, prostate, pancreatic and colon carcinoma as well as glioma (Al-Hajj et al. 2003; Dalerba et al. 2007; Singh et al. 2003; Ricci-Vitiani et al. 2007; Li et al. 2007). In melanoma, however, the identity of CSCs, their frequency and more even their existence in a given lesion is still controversially debated (Marotta & Polyak 2009; Rosen & Jordan 2009; Hill 2006; Shackleton et al. 2009; Shackleton & Quintana 2010). A first study using the limiting dilution transplantation assay identified a melanoma cell subset which exhibits stem-like capacities and expresses CD20 (Fang et al. 2005). Under more strict assay conditions other groups isolated tumor initiating cells which express either the transporter protein ABCB5 (Schatton et al. 2008) or the nerve growth factor receptor CD271 (Boiko et al. 2010). A recent study from Weissman and colleagues calculated the frequency of tumorigenic cells in melanoma of about 1/2000 cells (Boiko et al. 2010). Investigations by Quintana et al. (Quintana et al. 2010; Quintana et al. 2008) questioned the existence of any melanoma stem cell. Transplantation under more rigorous conditions revealed that nearly every forth randomly chosen melanoma cell (1/2 - 1/15) is capable to induce melanoma in the appropriate host and that the potential of melanoma induction is not associated with any surface marker tested so far. This demonstrates that the number of potential CSCs in melanoma may not be necessarily low and that the melanoma inducing capacity is not associated with a fixed phenotype of melanoma cells while these cells reconstitute the exact marker pattern of the parental tumor irrespective of marker positivity or negativity. The observations imply that reversible transformation of the melanoma cell is crucial for the initiation of a new melanoma after xeno-transplantation and that a substantial number of melanoma cells are capable to undergo this transformation process. The melanoma cell may express a variety of different markers at the time of isolation from an established lesion, after transplantation, however, the cell re-programs to the tumor initiating phenotype.

Another so far not appropriately recognized consequence of the CSC paradigm is that a hierarchy of cancer cells is preserved in an established tumor lesion. If the hypothesis is fulfilled for melanoma, some melanoma cells maintain tumor progression whereas the bulk of tumor cells does not. Consequently, specific ablation of the properly rare melanoma sustaining cells, which may but must not be identical to CSCs identified by the transplantation assay, from the established tumor tissue must inevitably lead to a decay of the tumor lesion independently of targeting the cancer cell mass. A most recent study addressed whether specific elimination of defined melanoma cells from an established lesion causes tumor regression (Schmidt et al. 2011). By adoptive transfer of engineered T cells with a CD20 specific CAR established xeno-transplanted tumors could be completely eradicated whereas targeted elimination of any random melanoma cell population did not. The frequency of $CD20^+$ melanoma cells in the tumor tissues was about 1 - 2% irrespective of the melanoma subtype; in about 20% of melanoma samples no $CD20^+$ melanoma cells could be detected. In those tumors, consequently, adoptive transfer of CD20 redirected T cells did not induce tumor regression. Re-expression of CD20 in those tumor cells, moreover, did not reconstitute the capacity to maintain melanoma progression indicating that CD20 per se does not induce the capacity. CD20 expression, however, indicates melanoma cells in an established lesion with such tumor maintaining properties. The observations have substantial impact on the future design of melanoma therapy.

First, eradication of hierarchically organized melanoma needs to eliminate those cancer cells which maintain melanoma progression. Elimination of any other cancer cell populations will de-bulk the tumor lesion and induce rapid tumor regression but the tumor will inevitably relapse due to surviving melanoma sustaining cells. The prediction reflects the clinical observation of frequent melanoma relapse after chemotherapy and radiation.

Second, melanoma maintaining cells are rare and unlikely to be eliminated by random targeting as provided by most therapeutic agents. Specific targeting by cytotoxic T cells redirected towards CD20 or by CD20-specific therapeutic antibodies like Rituxan™ (rituximab) or Arzerra™ (ofatumumab) will be required.

Third, melanoma maintaining cells like other CSCs will less replicate than the majority of cancer cells making anti-proliferative drugs less efficient. Moreover, melanoma CSCs express transporter molecules like ABCB5 (Schatton et al. 2008) which efficiently counteract chemotherapy. Both properties together contribute to CSC resistance towards a variety of physiological and pharmaceutical signals which is frequently described as "dormancy". The dormant state, however, re-activates under so far unknown conditions resulting in melanoma relapse.

Forth, the prevalence of $CD20^+$ melanoma maintaining cells in a tumor lesion may correlate with prognosis. It is unresolved, however, whether those cells accumulate during tumor progression and metastasis.

Fifth, functional and phenotypic plasticity of melanoma maintaining cells may require continuous presence of therapeutic agents specifically targeting those cells which freshly gained melanoma initiating capacities. Clonal evolution of genetic and epigenetic modifications may moreover contribute to cancer cell heterogeneity. In their therapeutic approach, Schmidt and colleagues (2011) used engineered T cells which are known to penetrate tissues, scan for targets and persist for long-term acting as an antigen-specific guardian. This is a major advantage of cellular therapy in comparison to other drugs which need to be present in therapeutic levels over long times which in the case of melanoma may be years. It will therefore be of benefit to de-bulk the tumor mass by conventional therapy in advance to eliminating melanoma initiating cells by specific agents.

7. Thoughts on future developments

Current trials using melanoma TILs show first promising results, the efficacy in long-term needs to be confirmed. Using artificially redirected T cells previous and ongoing phase I studies demonstrate the feasibility in generating suitable numbers of gene-modified T cells for adoptive transfer. Each trial is being performed with CARs and TCRs which have been empirically optimised and possess subtle but significant differences suggesting that the direct comparison between clinical trial outcomes may not be possible. While lymphodepletion prior T cell therapy is widely accepted, substitution of IL-2 in high, medium or low doses is still a matter of debate. As such, it is likely that some basic formulations will need to be determined before the field moves on towards larger, multi-centre clinical testing of modified T cells.

There are currently clear limitations in adoptive immunotherapy of melanoma and of other malignant diseases. Adoptive immunotherapy uses "drugs" which need to be individually generated for each patient. Whilst T cells can be produced for early phase trials, the ability to generate sufficient cells to perform large scale trials is currently beyond the capabilities of any production centre. With clinical success the biotechnological issues need to be investigated.

therapeutic agent	targeted antigen	modification	clinical phase	principal investigator	clinicaltrials.gov or reference
TIL	unknown	none	II	Jacob Schachter, Sheba Medical Center, Tel Hashomer, Israel	NCT00287131
TIL	DMF5	none	I/II	Steven A. Rosenberg, NIH, Bethesda, USA	NCT00924001
TIL	unknown	none	I/II	Brigitte Dreno, CHU de Nantes, Nantes, France	NCT01082887
TIL	unknown	none	I	Cassian Yee, Fred Hutchinson Cancer Center, Seattle, USA	NCT00045149
TIL	MART-1	none	I	Marcus Butler, Dana Farber Cancer Institute, Boston, USA	NCT00512889
TIL	unknown	IL-12	I/II	Steven A. Rosenberg, NIH, Bethesda, USA	NCT01236573
young TIL	unknown	none	II	Steven A. Rosenberg, NIH, Bethesda, USA	NCT01118091
young TIL	unknown	none	II	Steven A. Rosenberg, NIH, Bethesda, USA	NCT00513604
T cells	MART-1	TCR	I/II	Brigitte Dreno, CHU de Nantes, Nantes, France	NCT00720031
T cells	MART-1	TCR	I	Steven A. Rosenberg, NIH, Bethesda, USA	(Morgan et al. 2006)
T cells	MART-1	TCR	II	Antoni Ribas, UCLA, Los Angeles, USA	NCT00910650
$CD8^+$ T cells	NY-Eso-1	TCR	I/II	Aude Chapuis, Fred Hutchinson Cancer Center, Seattle, USA	NCT00871481
$CD8^+$ T cells	VEGFR2	CAR	I/II	Steven A. Rosenberg, NIH, Bethesda, USA	NCT01218867

Table 1. Clinical trials in the adoptive immunotherapy of melanoma.

As a system eminent limitation the TIL approach is limited by the lack of knowledge of melanoma specificity and the failure to isolate TILs in sufficient numbers from all tumor lesions. The CAR approach, on the other hand, is limited to targets on the cell surface while intracellular antigens cannot be targeted; the TCR approach is limited to proper MHC expression and antigen presentation. While novel strategies are currently explored by combining the advantages and eliminating the limitations, the key aspect for adoptive immunotherapy is that the effector cells need to get to the tumor site and infiltrate the solid tumor tissue. In the tumor tissue infiltrating T cells experience the counter-attack by the immune suppressive environment provided by suppressive cytokines and regulatory cells. Different T cell subsets may be more effective than others in resisting repression, eliminating regulatory T cells by lymphodepletion favours therapeutic efficacy of adoptively transferred T cells.

Taken together, strong arguments support the development of cellular immunotherapy of melanoma. Since the initial descriptions of the approach, most of the early technological hurdles in generating melanoma-specific effector cells have been largely overcome and an increasing focus is upon understanding the clinically relevant mechanisms of T cell directed therapies and how to make the methodology more economic and widely applicable. Adoptive cell therapy in melanoma has moved at a pace and the current clinical and pre-clinical activities will furthermore determine whether adoptive immunotherapy with redirected T cells can control melanoma in long-term.

8. Acknowledgements

Work in the author's laboratory was funded by a grant from the Deutsche Krebshilfe, Bonn, Germany.

9. References

Ailles, L.E. & Weissman, I.L., 2007. Cancer stem cells in solid tumors. *Current Opinion in Biotechnology*, 18(5), pp.460-466.

Al-Hajj, M. et al., 2003. Prospective identification of tumorigenic breast cancer cells. *Proceedings of the National Academy of Sciences of the United States of America*, 100(7), pp.3983-3988.

Atkins, M.B. et al., 1999. High-dose recombinant interleukin 2 therapy for patients with metastatic melanoma: analysis of 270 patients treated between 1985 and 1993. *Journal of Clinical Oncology: Official Journal of the American Society of Clinical Oncology*, 17(7), pp.2105-2116.

Bargou, R. et al., 2008. Tumor regression in cancer patients by very low doses of a T cell-engaging antibody. *Science (New York, N.Y.)*, 321(5891), pp.974-977.

Becker, J.C. et al., 1996. An antibody-interleukin 2 fusion protein overcomes tumor heterogeneity by induction of a cellular immune response. *Proceedings of the National Academy of Sciences of the United States of America*, 93(15), pp.7826-7831.

Bedikian, A.Y. et al., 2010. Predictive Factors for the Development of Brain Metastasis in Advanced Unresectable Metastatic Melanoma. *American Journal of Clinical Oncology*. Available at: http://www.ncbi.nlm.nih.gov/pubmed/21150567 [Accessed March 9, 2011].

Bendle, G.M. et al., 2010. Lethal graft-versus-host disease in mouse models of T cell receptor gene therapy. *Nature Medicine*, 16(5), pp.565-570, 1p following 570.

Besser, M.J. et al., 2010. Clinical responses in a phase II study using adoptive transfer of short-term cultured tumor infiltration lymphocytes in metastatic melanoma patients. *Clinical Cancer Research: An Official Journal of the American Association for Cancer Research*, 16(9), pp.2646-2655.

Besser, M.J. et al., 2009. Minimally cultured or selected autologous tumor-infiltrating lymphocytes after a lympho-depleting chemotherapy regimen in metastatic melanoma patients. *Journal of Immunotherapy (Hagerstown, Md.: 1997)*, 32(4), pp.415-423.

Bluemel, C. et al., 2010a. Epitope distance to the target cell membrane and antigen size determine the potency of T cell-mediated lysis by BiTE antibodies specific for a large melanoma surface antigen. *Cancer Immunology, Immunotherapy: CII*, 59(8), pp.1197-1209.

Bluemel, C. et al., 2010b. Epitope distance to the target cell membrane and antigen size determine the potency of T cell-mediated lysis by BiTE antibodies specific for a large melanoma surface antigen. *Cancer Immunology, Immunotherapy: CII*, 59(8), pp.1197-1209.

Boiko, A.D. et al., 2010. Human melanoma-initiating cells express neural crest nerve growth factor receptor CD271. *Nature*, 466(7302), pp.133-137.

Bonnet, D. & Dick, J.E., 1997. Human acute myeloid leukemia is organized as a hierarchy that originates from a primitive hematopoietic cell. *Nature Medicine*, 3(7), pp.730-737.

Bradbury, P.A. & Middleton, M.R., 2004. DNA repair pathways in drug resistance in melanoma. *Anti-Cancer Drugs*, 15(5), pp.421-426.

Bridgeman, J.S. et al., 2010. Building better chimeric antigen receptors for adoptive T cell therapy. *Current Gene Therapy*, 10(2), pp.77-90.

Büning, H. et al., 2010. Do CARs need a driver's license? Adoptive cell therapy with chimeric antigen receptor-redirected T cells has caused serious adverse events. *Human Gene Therapy*, 21(9), pp.1039-1042.

Burton, A.L. et al., 2011. Prognostic significance of tumor infiltrating lymphocytes in melanoma. *The American Surgeon*, 77(2), pp.188-192.

Carroll, D., 2008. Progress and prospects: zinc-finger nucleases as gene therapy agents. *Gene Therapy*, 15(22), pp.1463-1468.

Cheadle, E.J. et al., 2007. Eotaxin-2 and colorectal cancer: a potential target for immune therapy. *Clinical Cancer Research: An Official Journal of the American Association for Cancer Research*, 13(19), pp.5719-5728.

Chhabra, A., 2010. Mitochondria-centric activation induced cell death of cytolytic T lymphocytes and its implications for cancer immunotherapy. *Vaccine*, 28(29), pp.4566-4572.

Chmielewski, M., Hombach, A.A. & Abken, H., 2011. CD28 cosignalling does not affect the activation threshold in a chimeric antigen receptor-redirected T-cell attack. *Gene Therapy*, 18(1), pp.62-72.

Chmielewski, M. et al., 2004. T cell activation by antibody-like immunoreceptors: increase in affinity of the single-chain fragment domain above threshold does not increase T cell activation against antigen-positive target cells but decreases selectivity. *Journal of Immunology (Baltimore, Md.: 1950)*, 173(12), pp.7647-7653.

Clark, W.H. et al., 1969. The histogenesis and biologic behavior of primary human malignant melanomas of the skin. *Cancer Research*, 29(3), pp.705-727.

Clemente, C.G. et al., 1996. Prognostic value of tumor infiltrating lymphocytes in the vertical growth phase of primary cutaneous melanoma. *Cancer*, 77(7), pp.1303-1310.

Clevers, H., 2011. The cancer stem cell: premises, promises and challenges. *Nature Medicine*, 17(3), pp.313-319.

Coccoris, M. et al., 2010. T cell receptor (TCR) gene therapy to treat melanoma: lessons from clinical and preclinical studies. *Expert Opinion on Biological Therapy*, 10(4), pp.547-562.

Coccoris, M. et al., 2008. Long-term functionality of TCR-transduced T cells in vivo. *Journal of Immunology (Baltimore, Md.: 1950)*, 180(10), pp.6536-6543.

Cochlovius, B. et al., 1999. Human melanoma therapy in the SCID mouse: in vivo targeting and reactivation of melanoma-specific cytotoxic T cells by bi-specific antibody fragments. *International Journal of Cancer. Journal International Du Cancer*, 81(3), pp.486-493.

Cohen, C.J. et al., 2006. Enhanced antitumor activity of murine-human hybrid T-cell receptor (TCR) in human lymphocytes is associated with improved pairing and TCR/CD3 stability. *Cancer Research*, 66(17), pp.8878-8886.

Dalerba, P. et al., 2007. Phenotypic characterization of human colorectal cancer stem cells. *Proceedings of the National Academy of Sciences of the United States of America*, 104(24), pp.10158-10163.

Denninghoff, V.C. et al., 2004. Sentinel lymph node: detection of micrometastases of melanoma in a molecular study. *Molecular Diagnosis: A Journal Devoted to the Understanding of Human Disease Through the Clinical Application of Molecular Biology*, 8(4), pp.253-258.

Engell-Noerregaard, L. et al., 2009. Review of clinical studies on dendritic cell-based vaccination of patients with malignant melanoma: assessment of correlation between clinical response and vaccine parameters. *Cancer Immunology, Immunotherapy: CII*, 58(1), pp.1-14.

Eshhar, Z. et al., 1993. Specific activation and targeting of cytotoxic lymphocytes through chimeric single chains consisting of antibody-binding domains and the gamma or zeta subunits of the immunoglobulin and T-cell receptors. *Proceedings of the National Academy of Sciences of the United States of America*, 90(2), pp.720-724.

Fang, D. et al., 2005. A tumorigenic subpopulation with stem cell properties in melanomas. *Cancer Research*, 65(20), pp.9328-9337.

Fiala, S., 1968. The cancer cell as a stem cell unable to differentiate. A theory of carcinogenesis. *Neoplasma*, 15(6), pp.607-622.

Garbe, C. et al., 2010. Diagnosis and treatment of melanoma: European consensus-based interdisciplinary guideline. *European Journal of Cancer*, 46(2), pp.270-283.

Grimm, E.A. et al., 1982. Lymphokine-activated killer cell phenomenon. Lysis of natural killer-resistant fresh solid tumor cells by interleukin 2-activated autologous human peripheral blood lymphocytes. *The Journal of Experimental Medicine*, 155(6), pp.1823-1841.

Grosse-Hovest, L. et al., 1999. Tumor-growth inhibition with bispecific antibody fragments in a syngeneic mouse melanoma model: the role of targeted T-cell co-stimulation via CD28. *International Journal of Cancer. Journal International Du Cancer*, 80(1), pp.138-144.

Grosse-Hovest, L. et al., 2003. A recombinant bispecific single-chain antibody induces targeted, supra-agonistic CD28-stimulation and tumor cell killing. *European Journal of Immunology*, 33(5), pp.1334-1340.

Hill, R.P., 2006. Identifying cancer stem cells in solid tumors: case not proven. *Cancer Research*, 66(4), pp.1891-1895; discussion 1890.

Hombach, A. & Abken, H., 2007. Costimulation tunes tumor-specific activation of redirected T cells in adoptive immunotherapy. *Cancer Immunology, Immunotherapy: CII*, 56(5), pp.731-737.

Hombach, A.A. et al., 2007. T cell activation by antibody-like immunoreceptors: the position of the binding epitope within the target molecule determines the efficiency of activation of redirected T cells. *Journal of Immunology (Baltimore, Md.: 1950)*, 178(7), pp.4650-4657.

Hong, J.J. et al., 2010. Successful treatment of melanoma brain metastases with adoptive cell therapy. *Clinical Cancer Research: An Official Journal of the American Association for Cancer Research*, 16(19), pp.4892-4898.

Hughes, M.S. et al., 2005. Transfer of a TCR gene derived from a patient with a marked antitumor response conveys highly active T-cell effector functions. *Human Gene Therapy*, 16(4), pp.457-472.

Johnson, L.A. et al., 2009a. Gene therapy with human and mouse T-cell receptors mediates cancer regression and targets normal tissues expressing cognate antigen. *Blood*, 114(3), pp.535-546.

Johnson, L.A. et al., 2009b. Gene therapy with human and mouse T-cell receptors mediates cancer regression and targets normal tissues expressing cognate antigen. *Blood*, 114(3), pp.535-546.

Kawakami, Y. & Rosenberg, S.A., 1997. Immunobiology of human melanoma antigens MART-1 and gp100 and their use for immuno-gene therapy. *International Reviews of Immunology*, 14(2-3), pp.173-192.

Kieback, E. et al., 2008. A safeguard eliminates T cell receptor gene-modified autoreactive T cells after adoptive transfer. *Proceedings of the National Academy of Sciences of the United States of America*, 105(2), pp.623-628.

Kirkwood, J.M. et al., 2000. High- and low-dose interferon alfa-2b in high-risk melanoma: first analysis of intergroup trial E1690/S9111/C9190. *Journal of Clinical Oncology: Official Journal of the American Society of Clinical Oncology*, 18(12), pp.2444-2458.

Kirkwood, J.M. et al., 1996. Interferon alfa-2b adjuvant therapy of high-risk resected cutaneous melanoma: the Eastern Cooperative Oncology Group Trial EST 1684. *Journal of Clinical Oncology: Official Journal of the American Society of Clinical Oncology*, 14(1), pp.7-17.

Kruschinski, A. et al., 2008. Engineering antigen-specific primary human NK cells against HER-2 positive carcinomas. *Proceedings of the National Academy of Sciences of the United States of America*, 105(45), pp.17481-17486.

Kuball, J. et al., 2007. Facilitating matched pairing and expression of TCR chains introduced into human T cells. *Blood*, 109(6), pp.2331-2338.

Lamers, C.H.J. et al., 2006. Process validation and clinical evaluation of a protocol to generate gene-modified T lymphocytes for imunogene therapy for metastatic renal cell carcinoma: GMP-controlled transduction and expansion of patient's T lymphocytes using a carboxy anhydrase IX-specific scFv transgene. *Cytotherapy*, 8(6), pp.542-553.

Lamers, C.H.J. et al., 2006. Treatment of metastatic renal cell carcinoma with autologous T-lymphocytes genetically retargeted against carbonic anhydrase IX: first clinical experience. *Journal of Clinical Oncology: Official Journal of the American Society of Clinical Oncology*, 24(13), pp.e20-22.

Leiter, U. et al., 2010. Excision guidelines and follow-up strategies in cutaneous melanoma: Facts and controversies. *Clinics in Dermatology*, 28(3), pp.311-315.

Li, C. et al., 2007. Identification of pancreatic cancer stem cells. *Cancer Research*, 67(3), pp.1030-1037.

Lo, A.S.Y. et al., 2010. Anti-GD3 chimeric sFv-CD28/T-cell receptor zeta designer T cells for treatment of metastatic melanoma and other neuroectodermal tumors. *Clinical Cancer Research: An Official Journal of the American Association for Cancer Research*, 16(10), pp.2769-2780.

Marotta, L.L.C. & Polyak, K., 2009. Cancer stem cells: a model in the making. *Current Opinion in Genetics & Development*, 19(1), pp.44-50.

Morgan, R.A. et al., 2003. High efficiency TCR gene transfer into primary human lymphocytes affords avid recognition of melanoma tumor antigen glycoprotein 100 and does not alter the recognition of autologous melanoma antigens. *Journal of Immunology (Baltimore, Md.: 1950)*, 171(6), pp.3287-3295.

Morgan, R.A. et al., 2006. Cancer Regression in Patients After Transfer of Genetically Engineered Lymphocytes. *Science*, 314(5796), pp.126 -129.

Newrzela, S. et al., 2008. Resistance of mature T cells to oncogene transformation. *Blood*, 112(6), pp.2278-2286.

Offringa, R., 2009. Antigen choice in adoptive T-cell therapy of cancer. *Current Opinion in Immunology*, 21(2), pp.190-199.

Overwijk, W.W. et al., 2003. Tumor regression and autoimmunity after reversal of a functionally tolerant state of self-reactive CD8+ T cells. *The Journal of Experimental Medicine*, 198(4), pp.569-580.

Pak, B.J. et al., 2001. Lineage-specific mechanism of drug and radiation resistance in melanoma mediated by tyrosinase-related protein 2. *Cancer Metastasis Reviews*, 20(1-2), pp.27-32.

Pak, B.J. et al., 2004. Radiation resistance of human melanoma analysed by retroviral insertional mutagenesis reveals a possible role for dopachrome tautomerase. *Oncogene*, 23(1), pp.30-38.

Pegram, H.J. et al., 2008. Adoptive transfer of gene-modified primary NK cells can specifically inhibit tumor progression in vivo. *Journal of Immunology (Baltimore, Md.: 1950)*, 181(5), pp.3449-3455.

Perro, M. et al., 2010. Generation of multi-functional antigen-specific human T-cells by lentiviral TCR gene transfer. *Gene Therapy*, 17(6), pp.721-732.

Pule, M.A. et al., 2008. Virus-specific T cells engineered to coexpress tumor-specific receptors: persistence and antitumor activity in individuals with neuroblastoma. *Nature Medicine*, 14(11), pp.1264-1270.

Quintana, E. et al., 2010. Phenotypic Heterogeneity among Tumorigenic Melanoma Cells from Patients that Is Reversible and Not Hierarchically Organized. *Cancer Cell*, 18(5), pp.510-523.

Quintana, E. et al., 2008. Efficient tumour formation by single human melanoma cells. *Nature*, 456(7222), pp.593-598.

Reinhold, U. et al., 1999. Specific lysis of melanoma cells by receptor grafted T cells is enhanced by anti-idiotypic monoclonal antibodies directed to the scFv domain of the receptor. *The Journal of Investigative Dermatology*, 112(5), pp.744-750.

Ricci-Vitiani, L. et al., 2007. Identification and expansion of human colon-cancer-initiating cells. *Nature*, 445(7123), pp.111-115.

Rivoltini, L. et al., 1995. Induction of tumor-reactive CTL from peripheral blood and tumor-infiltrating lymphocytes of melanoma patients by in vitro stimulation with an immunodominant peptide of the human melanoma antigen MART-1. *Journal of Immunology (Baltimore, Md.: 1950)*, 154(5), pp.2257-2265.

Rivoltini, L. et al., 1996. Binding and presentation of peptides derived from melanoma antigens MART-1 and glycoprotein-100 by HLA-A2 subtypes. Implications for peptide-based immunotherapy. *Journal of Immunology (Baltimore, Md.: 1950)*, 156(10), pp.3882-3891.

Rosen, J.M. & Jordan, C.T., 2009. The increasing complexity of the cancer stem cell paradigm. *Science (New York, N.Y.)*, 324(5935), pp.1670-1673.

Rosenberg, S.A., 1984. Immunotherapy of cancer by systemic administration of lymphoid cells plus interleukin-2. *Journal of Biological Response Modifiers*, 3(5), pp.501-511.

Savoldo, B. et al., 2007. Epstein Barr virus specific cytotoxic T lymphocytes expressing the anti-CD30zeta artificial chimeric T-cell receptor for immunotherapy of Hodgkin disease. *Blood*, 110(7), pp.2620-2630.

Schaft, N. et al., 2003. Peptide fine specificity of anti-glycoprotein 100 CTL is preserved following transfer of engineered TCR alpha beta genes into primary human T lymphocytes. *Journal of Immunology (Baltimore, Md.: 1950)*, 170(4), pp.2186-2194.

Schatton, T. et al., 2008. Identification of cells initiating human melanomas. *Nature*, 451(7176), pp.345-349.

Schmidt, P. et al., 2011. Eradication of melanomas by targeted elimination of a minor subset of tumor cells. *Proceedings of the National Academy of Sciences of the United States of America*, 108(6), pp.2474-2479.

Seliger, B., Maeurer, M.J. & Ferrone, S., 1997. TAP off--tumors on. *Immunology Today*, 18(6), pp.292-299.

Seliger, B., 2008. Molecular mechanisms of MHC class I abnormalities and APM components in human tumors. *Cancer Immunology, Immunotherapy: CII*, 57(11), pp.1719-1726.

Shackleton, M. & Quintana, E., 2010. Progress in understanding melanoma propagation. *Molecular Oncology*, 4(5), pp.451-457.

Shackleton, M. et al., 2009. Heterogeneity in Cancer: Cancer Stem Cells versus Clonal Evolution. *Cell*, 138(5), pp.822-829.

Sigalotti, L. et al., 2004. Intratumor heterogeneity of cancer/testis antigens expression in human cutaneous melanoma is methylation-regulated and functionally reverted by 5-aza-2'-deoxycytidine. *Cancer Research*, 64(24), pp.9167-9171.

Singh, S.K. et al., 2003. Identification of a cancer stem cell in human brain tumors. *Cancer Research*, 63(18), pp.5821-5828.

Stewart-Jones, G. et al., 2009. Rational development of high-affinity T-cell receptor-like antibodies. *Proceedings of the National Academy of Sciences of the United States of America*, 106(14), pp.5784-5788.

Vignard, V. et al., 2005. Adoptive transfer of tumor-reactive Melan-A-specific CTL clones in melanoma patients is followed by increased frequencies of additional Melan-A-specific T cells. *Journal of Immunology (Baltimore, Md.: 1950)*, 175(7), pp.4797-4805.

Vitale, M. et al., 2005. HLA class I antigen down-regulation in primary ovary carcinoma lesions: association with disease stage. *Clinical Cancer Research: An Official Journal of the American Association for Cancer Research*, 11(1), pp.67-72.

Waldmann, T.A. & Tagaya, Y., 1999. The multifaceted regulation of interleukin-15 expression and the role of this cytokine in NK cell differentiation and host response to intracellular pathogens. *Annual Review of Immunology*, 17, pp.19-49.

Willemsen, R. et al., 2005. Redirecting human CD4+ T lymphocytes to the MHC class I-restricted melanoma antigen MAGE-A1 by TCR alphabeta gene transfer requires CD8alpha. *Gene Therapy*, 12(2), pp.140-146.

Willemsen, R.A. et al., 2001. A phage display selected fab fragment with MHC class I-restricted specificity for MAGE-A1 allows for retargeting of primary human T lymphocytes. *Gene Therapy*, 8(21), pp.1601-1608.

de Witte, M.A. et al., 2008. An inducible caspase 9 safety switch can halt cell therapy-induced autoimmune disease. *Journal of Immunology (Baltimore, Md.: 1950)*, 180(9), pp.6365-6373.

Yvon, E. et al., 2009. Immunotherapy of metastatic melanoma using genetically engineered GD2-specific T cells. *Clinical Cancer Research: An Official Journal of the American Association for Cancer Research*, 15(18), pp.5852-5860.

Zabierowski, S.E. & Herlyn, M., 2008. Melanoma stem cells: the dark seed of melanoma. *Journal of Clinical Oncology: Official Journal of the American Society of Clinical Oncology*, 26(17), pp.2890-2894.

Zhao, Y. et al., 2010. Multiple injections of electroporated autologous T cells expressing a chimeric antigen receptor mediate regression of human disseminated tumor. *Cancer Research*, 70(22), pp.9053-9061.

9

Current Perspectives on Immunomodulation of NK Cells in Melanoma

Tadepally Lakshmikanth and Maria H. Johansson
Department of Microbiology, Tumor and Cell Biology, Karolinska Institutet, Stockholm, Sweden

1. Introduction

Malignant Melanoma is a highly aggressive, deadly, chemoresistant and difficult-to-treat form of skin cancer (Flaherty and Gadgeel, 2002), which develops as a consequence of multifactorial perturbations from a series of architectural and phenotypically distinct stages, finally culminating into metastasis. It continues to increase in most western countries amongst the white population, the incidence has been increasing yearly by 5-7% and the prognosis for this metastatic disease remains poor (Greenlee et al., 2001). Melanoma incidence is influenced by pigmentation of the population as well as geographical parameters such as latitude and altitude (Armstrong and Kricker, 2001). According to epidemiological and experimental studies, the major risk factor of melanoma is ultraviolet radiation, which is associated with intermittent burning doses, especially during childhood (Whiteman et al., 2001). Melanoma is usually diagnosed at an early stage and is amenable to primary surgical treatment. However, it is sometimes characterized by an aggressive disease course with widespread metastasis and poor prognosis, which does not respond to standard therapy. Melanoma is largely refractory to current adjuvant therapies including chemotherapy, radiation therapy and/or immunotherapy (Chin et al., 2006) and therefore remains as a significant cause of mortality in Caucasians.

Immune responses are believed to have an important function in the natural history of melanoma since tumor infiltrating lymphocytes (TILs) are commonly found in melanoma, often associated with spontaneous regression and considered a favorable prognostic factor in primary melanoma (Mackensen et al., 1994). Hence, melanoma is the most studied tumor model in the field of human tumor immunology. NK cells represent a critical first line of defense against malignant transformation. NK cells were identified in melanoma in the 80s by Kornstein (Kornstein et al., 1987). Tumor immune surveillance allows recognition and destruction of cancer (host-protective) but may also shape cancer immunogenicity (tumor-promoting) through a 'cancer immunoediting process' due to selective pressure from the immune system. We have shown evidence for an immunoediting process enabling melanoma cells to escape from NK cell recognition (Lakshmikanth et al., 2009). In this chapter, we have taken into consideration the work accomplished by many investigators in trying to understand the immunology of melanoma and to identify various treatment strategies. The immune system basically has two main possibilities for dealing with malignant tissue which are Antigen (Ag)-specific CTLs and Ag-non-specific immune response by NK cells. We here put forth current perspectives on therapeutical strategies used against melanoma with specific focus on NK cells and provide insights into new opportunities for NK cell-based immunotherapy of melanoma disease.

2. NK cells and their role in melanoma

NK cells comprise approximately 10-15% of peripheral blood lymphocytes in human and are known to kill transformed cells and produce cytokines critical to the innate immune response (Cooper et al., 2001). NK cells are found in peripheral tissues, including the liver, peritoneal cavity and placenta. Resting NK cells circulate in the blood, but following activation by cytokines, they are capable of extravasation and infiltration into most tissues that contain pathogen-infected or malignant cells (Morris and Ley, 2004). NK cells were originally described based on their ability to lyse certain tumors in the absence of prior stimulation (Herberman et al., 1975; Kiessling et al., 1975a). NK cells may play a role in antitumor surveillance (Kiessling et al., 1975b), in vivo rejection of tumor cells (Porgador et al., 1995) and prevention of tumor metastases (Taniguchi et al., 1985). Much knowledge has been acquired with respect to origin, differentiation, receptor repertoire and effector functions of NK cells, as well as to their ability to shape adaptive immune responses (Colucci et al., 2003). NK cells induce target cell lysis and apoptosis in a cell-contact-dependent manner through release of cytotoxic granules containing perforin and granzymes (Trapani et al., 2000), and/or ligands engaging death receptors on the target cell, such as Fas or TRAIL-R (Lieberman, 2003). In addition, NK cells can secrete a number of effector cytokines such as interferon-γ (IFN-γ) which play critical roles in antiviral defense as well as in tumor surveillance (Biron et al., 1999; Street et al., 2001), tumor necrosis factor-α (TNF-α), granulocyte-macrophage colony stimulating factor (GM-CSF), Interleukin (IL)-5, IL-10 and IL-13, all of which influence adaptive immune responses (Loza et al., 2002). NK cells respond to a variety of cytokines, such as IL-2 (Talmadge et al., 1987), IL-12 (Trinchieri, 1998), IL-15 and Type I IFNs (α and β) (Santoni et al., 1985), which increase their cytolytic, secretory, proliferative and antitumor functions. NK cells express a variety of adhesion molecules like integrins, selectins (Morris and Ley, 2004), and immunoglobulin (Ig) superfamily molecules like DNAM-1 (CD226) (Shibuya et al., 1996), aiding migration to peripheral tissues (Colucci et al., 2003), and infiltration of tumors (Fogler et al., 1996).

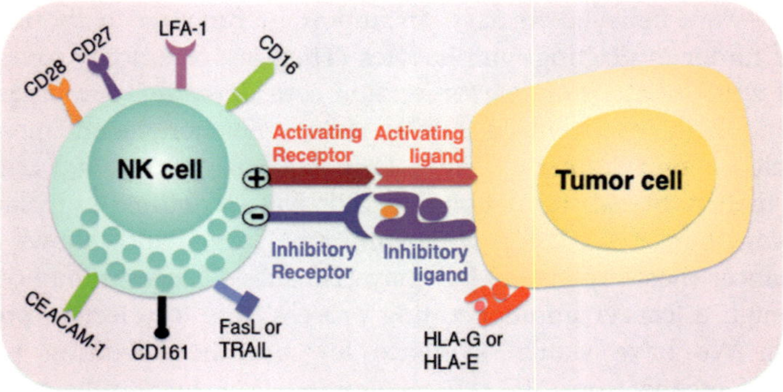

Fig. 1. A schematic figure showing interaction of a human NK cell with a tumor target by ligation of NK cell activating receptors and inhibitory receptors with corresponding ligands on the targets. Activating receptors include NCRs, NKG2D or DNAM-1. Inhibitory receptors are KIRs and CD94/NKG2A.

2.1 NK cell recognition

NK cells utilize several parallel recognition mechanisms to distinguish and eliminate aberrant cells (Karre, 1991; Lanier, 2005). Recognition is based on an array of activating and inhibitory receptors. Activating receptors often bind to cognate ligands that are up-regulated on 'stressed' cells (e.g. tumor or virus-infected cells), while the major inhibitory receptors bind to MHC class I molecules which may be down-regulated on tumors and virus-infected cells, referred to as 'missing-self' recognition (Fig 1) (Ljunggren and Karre, 1990).

Activating NK receptors mainly involved in tumor cell lysis are represented by the Fcγ-receptor, CD16 (Lanier, 2005), the NKp46, NKp30, and NKp44 (collectively called natural cytotoxicity receptors; NCRs), all belonging to the Ig superfamily (Moretta et al., 2001). There is limited information on the ligands for NCRs with the exception of B7-H6 ligand recognized by NKp30 (Pogge von Strandmann et al., 2007). In addition, C-type lectin-like receptors like NKG2D are expressed by NK cells as well as CTLs. NKG2D recognizes the stress inducible MICA/B and ULBP proteins (Lanier, 2005). DNAM-1 is expressed by NK cells, partially expressed by T lymphocytes and monocytes and recognizes PVR (CD155) and Nectin-2 (CD112) (Bottino et al., 2003). The activating receptors have a short cytoplasmic tail without signaling motifs and associate with adaptor proteins via charged amino acids in their transmembrane domains. Adaptor proteins contain the immune receptor tyrosine-based activation motifs (ITAMs), which get phosphorylated upon receptor engagement and recruit tyrosine kinases, leading to activation of lymphocytes. Synergy between different activating receptors is important in activation of naive NK cells by target cells. Engagement of specific combinations of receptors govern the degree of activity but also dictates qualitatively distinct events, such as target cell adhesion, granule polarization and NK cell degranulation (Bryceson et al., 2005). A large number of adhesion and costimulatory molecules such as CD2, CD7, CD161, CD59, NTB-A, CD62L, NKp80, and LFA-1 also play an important role in fine tuning the NK cell activity (Lanier, 2005).

Inhibitory NK receptors ligate major histocompatibility (MHC) molecules to modulate the immune response. Human NK cell inhibitory receptors that recognize antigens encoded by the HLA-A, -B, -C loci are members of the Ig superfamily and termed Killer immunoglobulin-like receptors (KIRs) (Long, 1999). Other receptor families include natural killer group 2 (NKG2) which are C-type lectins that heterodimerize with CD94 and recognize non-classical HLA-E molecules. Engagement of inhibitory receptors can turn an NK cell off via intracellular signaling mediated through phosphorylation of immunoreceptor tyrosine-based inhibitory motifs (ITIMs) in their cytoplasmic tail (Lanier, 2005). In contrast, the absence or incomplete expression of host MHC class I molecules will result in lack of inhibition and render a cell susceptible to NK cell attack (Ljunggren and Karre, 1990).

NK cell response thus depends on the net effect of activating and inhibitory receptors and is regulated through a balance between positive and negative signals. NK-mediated killing can occur if the target cell expresses appropriate activating ligands and/or lacks inhibitory ligands (Lanier, 2005). Stimulation is initiated through a combination of signals from multiple receptor/ligand interactions, which initiates several signaling cascades, resulting in cytokine secretion and release of cytolytic granules (Davis and Dustin, 2004).

2.2 NK cells in melanoma

Melanoma is the most studied tumor model in tumor immunology since it responds to various immunotherapeutic approaches and displays spontaneous regressions (Lotze et al.,

1992). Immunotherapy treatment-related skin depigmentation is considered a favorable prognostic sign during melanoma intervention. NK cells were identified as important effectors in the host defense against melanoma in the 80s (Trinchieri and Perussia, 1984). Experiments demonstrated that loss of HLA-I expression in melanoma cell lines, accompanied by escape from autologous CTLs, sensitized targets for NK cell attack (Pandolfi et al., 1991). NK cells, being present in the skin and able to sense stress-induced ligands on premalignant cells, may be important early before clinically detectable malignancy arises (Luci et al., 2009). NK cells could thus orchestrate a response in the microenvironment before overt tumor transformation (Strid et al., 2008). Some studies have reported that NK cells were less represented in TILs (Lakshmikanth et al., 2009; Vetter et al., 2002) while others have reported frequent NK cells in malignant melanoma specimens (Becker et al., 2000; Kornstein et al., 1987). NK cells play a critical role in tumor immunosurveillance (Smyth et al., 2002). A role for NK cells in the control of hematogenous dissemination and growth of melanoma metastases was observed by Kornstein (Kornstein et al., 1987). Animal models have demonstrated a critical role in preventing the establishment of metastatic disease dependent on IFN-γ and perforin (Kim et al., 2011; Markovic and Murasko, 1991). The involvement of NK cells in antitumor immunity in vivo was demonstrated in several mouse tumor models using NK cell-depleting antibodies and genetically modified mutant mice (Diefenbach et al., 2001; Shankaran et al., 2001; Smyth et al., 2002). Using the B16 murine melanoma model, NK cells were shown to be major mediators of the natural control of both spontaneous and experimental metastatic dissemination (Markovic and Murasko, 1990). Defects in NK activity in patients with metastatic disease have been described (Muller et al., 1989), however, there is no correlation between NK activity and prognosis in melanoma patients (Hersey et al., 1980). Some studies have shown a decrease in NK cell activity of all melanoma patients, associated with advancing stage of melanoma disease (Sibbitt et al., 1984) and due to IL-10 and TGF-β (Jovic et al., 2001).

To date, little substantial information exists on the ability of autologous NK cells to kill melanoma tumors. One study shows efficient autologous NK-mediated lysis of HLA class I negative melanoma cells in patients undergoing specific T cell-therapy (Porgador et al., 1997). The susceptibility of melanoma cells obtained from patients to autologous NK cells and the role of activating/inhibitory receptors were comprehensively analyzed in one study (Carrega et al., 2009). However, there are no reports on autologous NK lines as a potential tool for treatment of melanoma patients. As loss of MHC class I expression renders tumor cells more sensitive to NK cell killing, it may be associated with improved prognosis in melanoma (Porgador et al., 1997). There is evidence for susceptibility of melanoma cells to NK-mediated lysis due to insufficient amounts of HLA class I molecules (Pende et al., 1998).

Some of our recent work points towards strategies for NK cell-based immunotherapy. These will be explained more in detail in a later section. First, in the B16-F10 mouse melanoma model, blockade of mouse NK cell inhibitory NK receptors (Ly49), mimicking a 'missing self' phenotype, in combination with IL-2 treatment significantly delayed outgrowth of established sub-cutaneous tumors in an NK cell-dependent manner (Vahlne et al., 2010). Second, syngeneic mouse NK cells, autologous human NK cells, and allogeneic NK cells from healthy donors were shown to have the intrinsic capacity to recognize and target melanoma cells. Further, autologous and allogeneic NK cells preferentially targeted lymph node (LN) melanoma metastases over metastases from skin, pleura and liver. The NCRs and DNAM-1 emerged as key receptors in directing the NK anti-melanoma cytotoxicity

(Lakshmikanth et al., 2009). These results have implications in patients with melanoma for the design of immunotherapeutic strategies.

A major part of melanoma patients are of old age. It is therefore important to consider age-dependent changes in the immune system in relation to immunotherapy of melanoma. With increasing age, the number of NK cells seems to increase. However, the killing activity of naive NK cells was decreased in some studies, but could sometimes be fully restored by IL-2 activation (Le Garff-Tavernier et al., 2010). NK cells from older donors may, however, require higher concentrations of IFN-α for activation (Burns and Leventhal, 2000).

3. Receptor-ligand interactions involved in NK cell recognition of melanoma

Lack of inhibition and recognition of activating structures on target cells are the key events to prime NK cell-mediated cytotoxicity and cytokine production (Bryceson et al., 2006). Therefore, integration of signals derived from multiple activating and inhibitory receptors regulates the NK recognition of tumors but the relative importance of different receptors varies between different cancerous situations (Farag and Caligiuri, 2006). The main activating NK cell receptors as described in section 2.1 are NCRs, NKG2D and DNAM-1. Signaling through these receptors has been shown to be important in NK recognition of melanoma that expresses ligands for these activating receptors (Lakshmikanth et al., 2009; Solana et al., 2007). The importance of ligands for the NCRs has been demonstrated by use of blocking monoclonal antibodies in vitro in several studies (Pende et al., 1999). Results from blockade of two or more NCRs indicate that multiple NCRs are involved in NK recognition of melanoma (Lakshmikanth et al., 2009; Pende et al., 1999). The importance of NCR in disease progression in vivo has been demonstrated in NKp46-deficient mice, which developed more lung colonies than wild type mice, when melanoma cells were transferred intravenously (Lakshmikanth et al., 2009). NK cells along with $CD8^+$ and $\gamma\delta$T cells express NKG2D (Hayakawa and Smyth, 2006). The role of NKG2D in NK recognition of melanoma cells has been demonstrated, as well as a correlation between NKG2D function and expression of ligands on melanoma cells (Pende et al., 2002). Recent observations show that the ligands, MICA/B, may be downregulated in metastatic lesions (Vetter et al., 2002), but there are contrasting data (Markel et al., 2009), as well as data showing heterogeneity in NKG2D ligand expression (Lakshmikanth et al., 2009). It is therefore important to understand if NKG2D ligand expression changes with disease progression. The DNAM-1 receptor is important in recognition of freshly isolated cells from melanoma by NK cells. In vivo interference of DNAM-1 by antibody-mediated blockade or genetic ablation compromises rejection of melanoma cells in transplanted mice (Gilfillan et al., 2008; Lakshmikanth et al., 2009). PVR and Nectin-2 ligands were recently shown to bind also to T cell immunoglobulin and ITIM domain (TIGIT), a recently identified inhibitory receptor that counteracts the activating effects of DNAM-1 (Yu et al., 2009). Potential modulation of DNAM-1 ligands during melanoma disease progression requires further investigation. The relative roles of NCRs, NKG2D or DNAM-1 in NK cell recognition will vary depending on the expression of relevant ligands on tumors. Effective lysis is often seen when DNAM-1 is triggered in concert with other activation receptors, typically NCRs and/or NKG2D (Bryceson et al., 2006; Pende et al., 2001). Synergistic effects between different receptors have been demonstrated in melanoma (Carrega et al., 2009; Casado et al., 2009; Lakshmikanth et al., 2009) showing that in the absence of ligands for a particular receptor, other receptors would synergize for the complete eradication of the tumor. Similar findings were reported for suppression of poorly immunogenic melanoma metastases (Chan et al., 2010).

Melanoma cells also express death receptors that bind to ligands belonging to the Tumor necrosis factor (TNF) family: TNF-α, FAS ligand (FASL), TNF-related apoptosis-inducing ligand (TRAIL) and TNF-weak inducer of apoptosis (TWEAK) expressed on lymphocytes. Interaction with ligands on lymphocytes results in activation of the caspase pathway and apoptosis. This kind of ligand-receptor mechanism has been shown to be important in tumor recognition in vivo (Smyth et al., 2002).

4. Immunosurveillance of melanoma and cancer metastasis

Most patients with solid tumors die due to metastatic spread of the disease. Metastatic cells have a highly unstable phenotype and can rapidly adapt to selective pressure, allowing the cells to survive even under the most unfavorable circumstances (Meier et al., 1998). We have recently shown that melanoma metastases obtained from different anatomical sites of human melanoma patients display differential susceptibilities to NK cell lysis in relation to their phenotypic expression profile. Tumor metastasis of cutaneous melanoma is a stepwise process; where the tumor cells first colonize the lymph nodes, then enter the systemic circulation and reach remote tissues like skin, brain, lungs or liver. During the local invasion and metastatic spread of melanoma, invasive characteristics appear. Tumor cells then dissociate from the primary lesion, migrate through the surrounding stroma, and invade blood vessels and lymphatics (Haass et al., 2005). Most cancers spread early through the lymphatic vessels to lymph nodes, which can be a source of further metastases through the blood stream to the viscera, where development of secondary tumors can affect vital functions and cause death (Cochran et al., 2006). Tumors may even influence immune cells in adjacent lymph nodes. Significant differences were shown in lymphocyte subpopulations between different lymph nodes of patients with melanoma, with a marked decrease in the number of CD4+ T helper (T_H) and an increase in the number of CD56+ NK cells, which correlated with the clinical stage of melanoma, distance of the node from the primary tumor and the tumor status of the node (Farzad et al., 1990). There are also reports on reduced lymphocyte activity as well as immune inhibitory activity from cells in lymph nodes close to tumors (Wen et al., 1989). This may facilitate the establishment and expansive growth of metastatic tumors in lymph nodes (Cochran et al., 2001).

4.1 Mechanisms of tumor escape from Immune surveillance

Downregulation of MHC class I molecules to escape CTL recognition is a process well known to occur in solid tumors during metastatic progression (Marincola et al., 2000). This can remarkably sensitize tumor cells to NK-mediated lysis (Ferrone and Marincola, 1995). However, owing to the selective pressure posed by NK cells, tumors have evolved various mechanisms by which they can evade NK cell attack. These mechanisms include interference with NK cell activation or adhesion, induced inhibition as well as modulation of NK cell function.

Modulation of recognition via activating receptors

The MICA/B proteins are recognized by the activating receptor, NKG2D. Loss of MICA/B proteins during uveal melanoma tumor progression has been shown to occur, suggesting an immune selection of MIC-negative tumor variants with reduced NK sensitivity (Vetter et al., 2004). There is evidence for strong immunoediting of tumors by NK cells. The phenomenon has been well studied in receptor knock out mice for NKG2D (Guerra et al., 2008; Smyth et al., 2005) or DNAM-1 (Iguchi-Manaka et al., 2008) or NKp46 (Elboim et al., 2010). We have recently shown evidence for this phenomenon in human melanoma patients (Lakshmikanth et al., 2009). Several studies have also reported various alterations in expression of activating receptors on NK cells from melanoma patients. Decreased expression of receptors like CD161, NKG2D, CD16, NKp30 and NKp46 has been reported (Konjevic et al., 2007). There are also reports on NK cell activity changes between stage I and II melanoma in lymph nodes (Farzad et al., 1990; Hersey et al., 1980), suggesting the involvement of NK cells in the early phase of melanoma development. Sustained exposure of NK cells to NKG2D ligands on the target cell can strongly downregulate the NKG2D receptor as shown in vitro (Benitez et al., 2011) and in vivo using ligand over-expressing transgenic mice (Oppenheim et al., 2005; Wiemann et al., 2005). Furthermore, soluble forms of MICA/B can bind to NKG2D, leading to receptor internalization and escape from NK cell recognition (Groh et al., 2002). A similar phenomenon can occur when tumors overexpress PVR and release it as soluble factor (Baury et al., 2003), which will bind to DNAM-1 and prevent its immune recognition. This could be an effective immune escape mechanism for tumor cells to evade from NK cell surveillance or cytokine-based immunotherapies.

Modulation of inhibition via NK cell receptors

NK cells and subsets of CTLs express inhibitory receptors specific for non-classical HLA class Ib molecules with a restricted tissue distribution. Upregulation of HLA-G has been reported in many types of cancer including melanoma, this negatively regulated NK cells and conveyed evasion of NK recognition (Paul et al., 1998). CEACAM-1 (CD66a), a member of the carcinoembryonic antigen family is a cell adhesion molecule, mediating homophilic and heterophilic interations and which can act as an inhibitory NK cell receptor (Markel et al., 2002). CD66a expression in primary tumors of melanoma patients is associated with and can be an independent predictor for risk of metastasis (Thies et al., 2002). Melanoma cells can evade attack from NK cells through CD66a interactions (Markel et al., 2002).

Modulation of costimulation, adhesion or susceptibility to apoptosis

A lack of expression of costimulatory molecules such as B7-1 (CD80), B7-2 (CD86), CD40 and CD70 by tumors hinders an optimal NK activation via CD28 and CD27 costimulatory pathways (Carbone et al., 1997; Galea-Lauri et al., 1999) and may lead to T cell anergy (Schwartz, 1990). The interaction between LFA-1 on NK cells and ICAM-1 (CD54) on tumor cells is important for cell adhesion and killing. Surprisingly, low expression of ICAM-1 by melanoma cells following immunotherapy lead to longer overall survival of patients (Quereux et al., 2007). Shedding of ICAM-1 from melanoma cells has also been described which results in masking of LFA-1 on effector cells (Haass et al., 2005). Melanoma cells can sometimes evade immune recognition from CD8+ T cells and NK cells by developing resistance to TRAIL- and granzyme-B-induced death pathways. In addition, lymphocytes from advanced melanoma patients demonstrated lower expression of TRAIL (Nguyen et al., 2000). Studies of melanoma patients have shown that there is a range of abnormalities that have been selected to inhibit TRAIL-mediated apoptosis (Hersey and Zhang, 2001).

Modulation of NK cell function

Tumors can influence the nature and efficacy of the immune responses of the host in order to escape immune surveillance. For example, induction of regulatory T cells (Tregs) or myeloid suppressor cells and/or production of several immunosuppressive factors including arginase-1, NOS-2, IDO, or TGF-β by tumor cells or components of the tumor microenvironment may result in functional subversion of tumor infiltrating immunocompetent cells (Zitvogel et al., 2006). A recent study showed that tumor cells can induce granzyme B expression in Tregs, which then utilizes this protease to induce the death of NK and CD8+ T cells in a perforin-dependent fashion (Cao et al., 2007). Release of prostaglandin E2 (PGE_2) by fibroblasts isolated from metastatic melanoma patients have been shown to interfere with induction of NK cell effector functions (Balsamo et al., 2009).

Immune surveillance of uveal melanoma

Uveal melanoma metastases were shown to frequently lose MHC class I molecules. However, in contrast to cutaneous melanoma where MHC class I loss correlated with worse survival, loss of MHC class I molecules in uveal melanoma lesions was associated with an improved prognosis. This difference may be explained by that uveal melanoma spreads hematogenously, and thereby immune surveillance may be mainly based on NK cells. In contrast, cutaneous melanoma is first spread via lymph nodes resulting in predominant exposure to T cells (Hanna, 1982; Jager et al., 2002). As noted above, uveal melanoma metastases may escape NK cells via downmodulation of MICA/B proteins. In vitro and in vivo studies of murine melanoma show evidence for NK cell killing of metastatic uveal melanoma in the liver in an IL-2- and TGF-β-dependent manner (Ma and Niederkorn, 1995). More details on uveal melanoma are discussed in other chapters of this book.

5. Immunomodulatory agents used to enhance NK cell activity against tumors

A convergence of information from the fields of molecular biology and cellular immunology has opened new opportunities for immunomodulating agents to be tested in the clinic. We here list some of the immunomodulating agents used to enhance NK cell activity against cancer, tested in vitro and in vivo using cell lines and preclinical mouse models, and some of which are in clinical trials (Fig 2). Other immunotherapeutic agents used against melanoma have been reviewed in the next section.

5.1 Cytokines

Many different cytokines are being tested to enhance NK cell activity against tumors. The role of IL-2, IFNs, IL-12, IL-15, IL-18 and IL-21 discretely or in combination with each other or with other modulators has been tested in cancer immunotherapy. Combinations of cytokines have been proposed to enhance NK cytolytic activity (Carson et al., 1994).

IL-2 comprises a cornerstone of systemic therapeutic modalities in disseminated melanoma (Tsao et al., 2004). IL-2 has been used to generate in vitro Lymphokine Activated Killer (LAK) cells, consisting of activated NK cells and T cells. Adoptive infusion of LAK cells is reviewed in section 6.1. Clinical trials have assessed effects of low-dose IL-2 administration on activation of NK cells in cancer patients. Whereas IL-2 significantly expanded the circulating NK cells in vivo, cytotoxicity was increased to some extent, as determined by in vitro assays (Miller et al., 1997). Infusion of IL-2-activated NK cell-enriched populations or intravenous IL-2 infusions combined with subcutaneous IL-2 augmented in vivo NK cell function but without consistent efficacy when compared with matched control cohorts (L. J. Burns et al., 2003). Objective clinical benefits were observed only in 20% of patients treated with IL-2, occasionally patients were cured. Immunocomplexing of cytokine and anti-cytokine monoclonal antibody (mAb) prolongs half-life and can increase or modify cytokine activities in vivo. Treatment with IL-2 immunocomplexes, lead to suppression of B16 tumor metastases in the lung (Jin et al., 2008). Hence, IL-2 immunocomplex treatment offers a novel therapeutic strategy to enhance NK cell activities also in humans. However, there are dose-limiting toxicities associated with IL-2, which have compromised its clinical use and other cytokines with an improved therapeutic index are therefore needed.

IFNs are a group of cytokines mainly known for their antiviral effect. They have a wide range of activities in modulating the immune system and have been reported effective in mice against spontaneous as well as experimental metastases (IFN-α) (Brunda et al., 1984). IFN-α enhances innate immune antitumor activity by inducing NK cell proliferation and cytotoxicity (Konjevic et al., 2007) and induces a favorable Th1-response (Bremers and Parmiani, 2000). IFN-α induces cytokines, perforin and FasL and mediates antitumor activity via interferon response factor-1 (IRF-1) (Kroger et al., 2002). It also promotes an increase in NKG2D and CD161 expression on NK cells in melanoma patients (Konjevic et al., 2010). IFN-α is currently approved as adjuvant therapy in high-risk melanoma patients, to eradicate micrometastases after surgical removal of the primary tumor and has demonstrated improved disease free survival but with conflicting results regarding overall survival (Ascierto and Kirkwood, 2008). Combination treatment with IFN-α and IL-2 induced expression of activating receptors on NK cells and was found to be clinically beneficial in melanoma patients (Konjevic et al., 2010). Upregulation of MHC class I expression is a major effect of IFN-γ, which may induce resistance to NK cells. Data on the effects of IFN-γ on tumor cell killing by NK cells have however been conflicting (Routes, 1992). The current notion on IFN-γ is that it can be pro-tumorigenic and anti-tumorigenic, depending on the context, intensity and durability of the IFN-γ signal (Zaidi et al., 2011). The IFN 'survival signature' is one of the mechanisms to evade immunosurveillance. Therefore IFN-γ/IFN-γ-R or their downstream pathway members represent potential prognostic markers in melanoma.

IL-12 acts as an NK cell and T cell growth factor (Perussia et al., 1992), enhances cytolytic activity of NK and LAK cells (Naume et al., 1992), and augments cytolytic T cell responses (Gately et al., 1992). IL-12 has direct effects on lymphocytes and NK cells by enhancing IFN-γ production (Lamont and Adorini, 1996). In a mouse melanoma model, intratumoral treatment with IL-12-encoding DNA resulted in NK cell-mediated significant regression in melanoma tumor development (Heinzerling et al., 2002). NK cells co-injected with IL-2 and IL-12 into SCID mice showed favorable antitumor effects (Hill et al., 1994). The interaction between IL-2 and IL-12 was found to enhance NK cell spontaneous cytotoxicity against tumor cells (Chehimi et al., 1992). In addition it stimulates NK cell cytokine production that may induce antitumor activity from macrophages and neutrophils (Perussia et al., 1992). The combination of IL-12 and Trastuzumab (Herceptin) in a mouse model led to tumor regression mediated through NK cell IFN-γ production (Jaime-Ramirez et al., 2011). HER2 is the target structure for the mAb Trastuzumab and its overexpression is associated with a poor prognosis (Ross and Fletcher, 1998). IL-12 in combination with stimulation of the TNF receptor superfamily member 4-1BB has been suggested to stimulate CD8+ T-cell responses in a mouse melanoma model. Hence a synergy between IL-12 and anti-4-1BB induced regression of established melanoma via NK and CD8+ T cells (Xu et al., 2004). Adenovirus-vector-mediated delivery of IL-12 was shown to improve efficacy of adenovirus-vector-mediated immunization with a melanoma antigen in a mouse B16 melanoma metastasis model. The effects of this combined therapy depended on both T cell-mediated immunity and NK cell-mediated cytotoxicity (Hirschowitz and Crystal, 1999).

IL-15 is involved in development and maintenance of NK cells and binds partly to the same receptor as IL-2 (Fehniger and Caligiuri, 2001). IL-15 overexpression in transgenic mice enhanced antitumor immunity (Yajima et al., 2002). A pronounced synergy between IL-15 and IL-12 that exceeds the IL-2 and IL-15 combination has been reported (Seidel et al., 1998). IL-15 is as efficacious as IL-2 but may have a superior therapeutic index (Munger et al., 1995). Clinical trials of IL-15 are expected soon (Fewkes and Mackall, 2010).

IL-18 is similar to IL-12 in inducing IFN-γ secretion from NK and T cells and augments NK cytolytic activity (Okamura et al., 1995). Although IL-18 and IL-12 synergize in IFN-γ production, their receptors and signal-transduction pathways appear to be different (Kohno et al., 1997). Evaluation of IL-18+IL-12 in a mouse melanoma model showed synergistic antitumor effects that associated with markedly elevated IFN-γ production but also had side effects. The IL-18 effect was mediated by NK cells and CD4+ T cells, independent of IFN-γ and IL-12 (Osaki et al., 1998). A phase II study of IL-18 in patients with metastatic melanoma has confirmed its safety but suggested limited efficacy of IL-18 monotherapy in this setting. IL-18 may be of better use in combination with other immunostimulatory cytokines, vaccines, or monoclonal antibodies (Srivastava et al., 2010).

IL-21 is produced by CD4+ T cells, have sequence homology to IL-2, IL-4, and IL-15 and stimulate T and NK cells. Synergy between IL-21, FLT3 ligand and IL-15, promotes expansion and differentiation of NK cells from the bone marrow and enhances their lytic function against B16 melanoma targets in vitro (Parrish-Novak et al., 2000). Administration of plasmid DNA encoding murine IL-21 significantly induced tumor killing by NK cells in vivo without obvious toxicity and prolonged survival of s.c tumor bearing mice (G. Wang et al., 2003). Clinical trials have been initiated, showing that IL-21 is well tolerated and possesses antitumor effects when administered as a single agent to patients with malignant melanoma and renal cell carcinoma. Future studies may combine IL-21 with vaccines and adoptive cell therapies (Fewkes and Mackall, 2010).

5.2 Chemotherapeutic agents

This section will focus on chemotherapeutic agents with immunomodulatory function on NK cells. The epidermal growth factor receptor (EGFR) pathway inhibitors, erlotinib and gefitinib, induce NKG2D ligands on cancer cells and sensitize them to NK cell-mediated killing as demonstrated in lung cancer (Kim et al., 2011). The small molecule multiple protein kinase inhibitors, sorafenib and sunitinib, have been approved for treatment of renal cell carcinoma. Sorafenib and sunitinib upregulate NKG2D ligands as observed on nasopharyngeal carcinoma (Huang et al., 2011). Sorafenib also inhibits the shedding of MICA on hepatocellular carcinoma (Kohga et al., 2010). The ubiquitin-proteasome pathway inhibitor bortezomib was shown to sensitize tumors to autologous NK cytotoxicity and this effect was enhanced upon depletion of Tregs (Lundqvist et al., 2009), as will be further discussed in section 7. Therapeutic compounds like thalidomide (Davies et al., 2001) in multiple myeloma and imatinib in gastrointestinal stromal tumors (Borg et al., 2004) might indirectly enhance NK cell functions, survival and proliferation (Fig 2). MICA and MICB proteins may be induced on hepatoma cells with an increase in NK cell-mediated lysis, using the histone deacetylase (HDAC) inhibitor, Valproic acid (Armeanu et al., 2005).

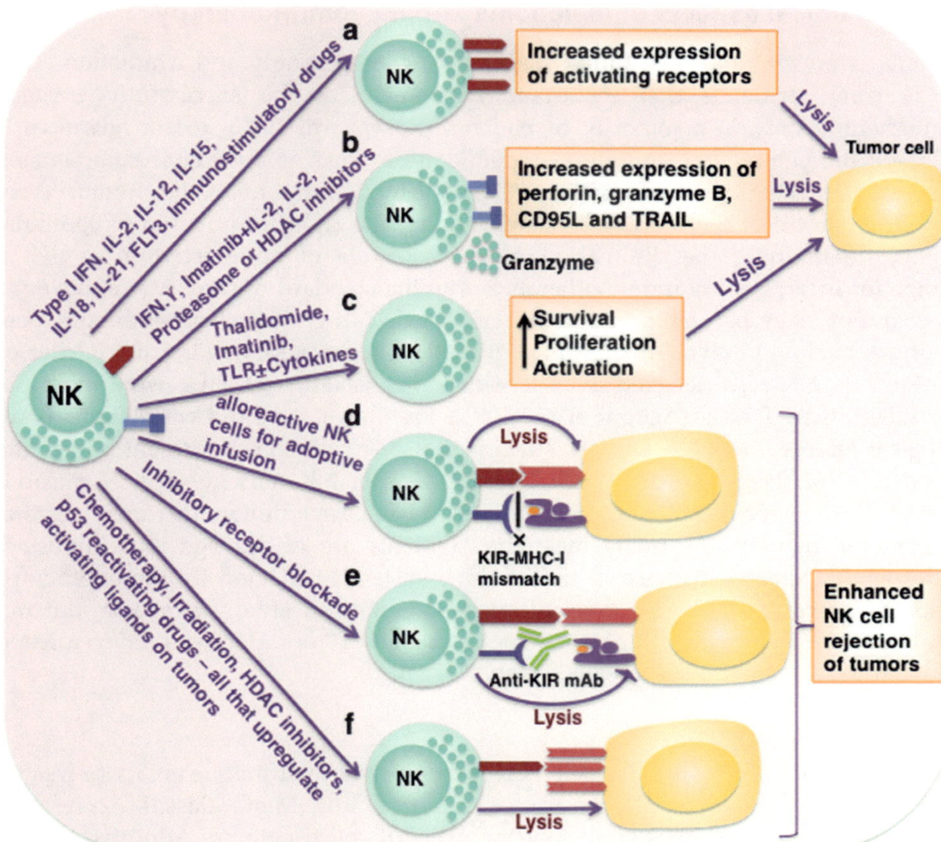

Fig. 2. Immunomodulatory strategies to harness NK cells in melanoma.

5.3 Blockade of inhibitory NK cell receptors

NK cell missing-self-reactivity (as alluded to in section 2.2) can be mimicked by blocking interaction between inhibitory receptors on NK cells and cognate MHC class I ligands. Blocking of inhibitory receptors using $F(ab')_2$ fragments enhanced anti-tumor activity both in vitro and in vivo and inhibited growth of syngeneic leukemia cells in an NK cell-dependent manner (Koh et al., 2001). However, it was not clear whether the in vivo effect occurred through direct induction of NK cell rejection or long-term influence on the NK cell population. Using a mouse model, we investigated this further using $F(ab')_2$ fragments to block Ly49C/I NK cell inhibitory receptors on mouse NK cells. When used alone, inhibitory receptor blockade lead to enhanced rejection of RMA lymphoma cells. In combination with high-dose IL-2 it further boosted the anti-lymphoma activity of NK cells. Combination therapy even delayed growth of B16 melanoma tumors established s.c (Vahlne et al., 2010) (Fig 2). Recently, Romagne et al have generated and characterized a fully human anti-KIR therapeutic candidate mAb, 1-7F9, which is currently in clinical development with the overall aim to increase antitumor responses of endogenous NK cells in patients with hematological malignancies without transplantation (Romagne et al., 2009), this therapy was not tested with solid tumors yet.

6. Immunological aspects of melanoma and its immunotherapy

Melanoma is an immunogenic tumor resistant to chemotherapy and irradiation. Though there is some evidence that metastatic melanoma can be successfully treated by immunotherapy only in a minority of patients (Rosenberg, 1997), recent advances have highlighted the potential of immunotherapeutic approaches as a valuable complement for cancer therapy (Dudley et al., 2002). While chemotherapy treats the tumor directly, immunotherapy treats the immune system. Finding the right formulation of combination therapies, determining the optimal dose and schedule of administration is the main challenge for incorporating immunotherapies into the standard of care. As tumors evade T cell recognition, they become prone to NK cell attack. NK cell numbers in tumors increase following activation in vivo (Albertsson et al., 2003) or after adoptive transfer (Geller et al., 2011). Further, NK cells detected in melanomas after isolation of TILs, were more potent tumor killers than T cells (Azogui et al., 1991). Previously reported correlations between histological features and NK activity suggest that NK cells may represent an additional prognostic factor (Hersey et al., 1982). The detection of NK cells in stage IV melanomas (Fregni et al., 2011) further encourages us to design NK-based immunotherapeutic strategies for melanoma patients. As many melanoma patients are of old age it is important to consider age-dependent changes in the immune system in relation to immunotherapy of melanoma. Information on responses to immunotherapy in elderly is sparse, but in one study, high dose IL-2 treatment of tumor patients, aged 70 or older, resulted in a response rate similar to that in younger patients (Quan et al., 2005).

6.1 Adoptive NK cell therapy

NK cells are attractive for adoptive cell therapy because of their unique ability to lyse target cells without any priming. Moreover, the reported low MHC class I expression on melanoma metastases (Algarra et al., 1997) allows NK cell triggering. Adoptive transfer of immune cells to patients with cancer was pioneered in the mid-1980s by Rosenberg and collaborators who infused autologous LAK cells together with high-doses of IL-2 to patients with advanced metastatic melanoma and renal cell carcinoma (Rosenberg et al., 1985). The FDA approved this treatment for patients with melanoma metastases (Rosenberg et al., 1987) with 20% of patients responding to the LAK cell infusion containing autologous NK cells. In follow up studies there was a response rate of 13-17% of the patients. The limited success may be explained by that high doses of IL-2 expand regulatory T cells, inhibiting NK cell activity via TGF-β (Ghiringhelli et al., 2005). The modest results of LAK cell/IL-2 therapy were further limited by serious side effects. A new era in the exploitation of NK cells in cancer immunotherapy started with Ruggeri et al who demonstrated that in bone marrow transplanted patients with a donor-KIR/host-KIR-ligand mismatch, alloreactive donor-derived NK cells were protective against acute myeloid leukemia (AML) relapse (Ruggeri et al., 2002). This study has been reproduced in AML patients by Giebel S et al (Giebel et al., 2003). Furthermore, alloreactive KIR-incompatible NK cells effectively eliminate melanoma and renal cancer cells in vitro (Igarashi et al., 2004). These data would suggest that allogeneic NK cells may have potent antitumor effects but this strategy remains to be tested in melanoma patients. A potential problem with adoptive transfer of NK cells is to direct the NK cells to the site of the tumor. Even if adoptively transferred NK cells produce cytokines like IFN-γ and TNF-α that may be able to function systemically, these cells need to be in close contact with the tumor for recognition and complete elimination of tumor targets. Activation of NK cells with IL-2 ex vivo increased their migration to the tumor site, and in vivo cytokine treatment may improve this further (Yang et al., 2003).

6.2 Combinatorial therapies

Immunological and biological agents convey their antitumor effect by potentiating cytotoxic and anti-proliferative effects of chemotherapy by modulating antitumor reactions mediated primarily by cell subpopulations of the innate immunity. The range of therapeutic options against melanoma encompasses chemotherapeutic, immune, anti-angiogenic and hormonal strategies. The sequence of these therapies used should correlate with the therapeutic activity. One study demonstrated that a subcutaneous metastasis obtained after two rounds of therapy with fotemustine, IFN-α and IL-2 showed strong expression of MICA/B on tumor cells and NKG2D on the infiltrating immune cells, while metastases from the same patient prior to therapy lacked these molecules. So chemotherapy may offer a great alternative in the induction of activating ligands on tumors (Vetter et al., 2004).

7. Strategies and current opportunities for NK cell-based immunotherapy of melanoma

The challenges faced by clinicians and the scientific community working with melanoma are formidable and it is required that we translate the growing body of scientific information clinically to be useful in targeting melanoma in patients and prolonging their survival. T cell-based immunotherapies have shown limited success so far (Fang et al., 2008). The main obstacle in using adoptive cell therapy with T cells is MHC class I-negative tumor variants that are insensitive to T cells (R. F. Wang and Rosenberg, 1996). Further, a cancer vaccine based solely on T cell therapy might drive development of class I-negative melanoma variants and/or variants that have lost the immunodominant target antigen (Yee et al., 2002). Therefore, new strategies are required. Reduced MHC class I expression opens up opportunities for NK cell-based immunotherapy at early stages of the disease when ligands for NK receptors are first expressed. Based on findings obtained on immunomodulation of NK cells we put forth our opinion on promising strategies and opportunities that can be explored for NK cell-based immunotherapy of melanoma.

Over the past years, there have been several reports on the importance of NK cells in immunotherapy (Fernandez et al., 1999). As the knowledge on NK cells has been growing over the last two decades, successful NK-based therapeutic breakthroughs have however not been accomplished. One potential reason for failure of adoptively transferred autologous NK cells or LAKs to mediate objective rejection of metastatic solid tumors is that autologous NK cells are subject to inhibition via KIR-ligands on tumor cells (Law et al., 1995). In addition, autologous NK cells in melanoma often have decreased expression of stimulating NK cell receptors. KIR/KIR-ligand mismatched NK cells have shown enhanced efficacy against melanoma and renal cell carcinoma in vitro (Igarashi et al., 2004). Thus, allogeneic NK cells may have a greater anti-tumor effect than autologous ones in adoptive transfer (Ljunggren and Malmberg, 2007; Terme et al., 2008). In a promising study by Miller et al, human allogeneic NK cells derived from haploidentical related donors were adoptively transferred along with IL-2 in the presence of high-dose cyclophosphamide and fludarabine immunosuppression. NK cells expanded and persisted in vivo accompanied by a rise in endogenous IL-15 levels (Miller et al., 2005). This lead to an enhanced antitumor effect, which was prevalent when KIR/KIR-ligand mismatch existed between donor and recipient, reminiscent of results in AML patients receiving haploidentical hematopoietic transplantation. Further, 'unlicensed' or 'hyporesponsive' NK cells, i.e. NK cells expressing no inhibitory receptors for self-HLA class I, lysed melanoma cells in vitro (Carrega et al., 2009). Appropriate activation may enable these NK cells to kill autologous melanomas. These cells can act independently of HLA class I expression in melanoma cells, but more studies are needed to understand their functional properties and trafficking patterns to utilize them successfully in cancer immunotherapeutic approaches. Clinical trials using adoptive transfer of NK cells are currently ongoing (Velardi et al., 2009).

Recently, a new strategy was proposed by Markel et al to augment anticancer activity by NK cells based on matching of activating NK cell receptors and their ligands. Increased killing was observed against melanomas in vitro in matched effector-target combinations (Markel et al., 2009). Matching of activating receptors/ligands as well as ex vivo testing of tumor susceptibility to lysis by NK cells (Carlsten et al., 2007) may improve adoptive cell therapy protocols.

Most clinical studies exploiting allogeneic NK cells for adoptive immunotherapy have been performed with NK cells selected from leukapheresis products by immunomagnetic bead selection protocol (Iyengar et al., 2003; Meyer-Monard et al., 2009). Ex vivo expansions of NK cells will facilitate infusion of higher numbers of activated NK cells (Carlens et al., 2001). Several approaches are being tested. Large-scale expansion of functional human NK cells from hematopoietic progenitor and stem cells without use of animal products and feeder cells (cytokine-based method) generated 100% pure and activated NK cells at a high log-scale magnitude which were able to lyse AMLs and solid tumors like melanoma (Spanholtz et al., 2010). This method may hold a great promise for ex vivo generation of clinical grade NK cell products for cellular immunotherapy against melanoma.

Tumors can be sensitized to NK cell killing via death receptors. Bortezomib treatment of B16 melanoma has been shown to augment their susceptibility to syngeneic NK cells in mice by increasing TRAIL receptors on tumor cells, as growth of Bortezomib treated human melanomas was delayed in SCID mice adoptively transferred with human NK cells (Lundqvist et al., 2009). Hence, NK cell activity against cancer can be substantially bolstered by combining adoptive NK infusions with bortezomib treatment (Lundqvist et al., 2006). Other therapeutic approaches used to activate the TRAIL-system are reviewed by Hersey (Hersey and Zhang, 2001).

As elucidated in the previous sections, we have recently demonstrated that NK cells have the intrinsic capacity to recognize and target malignant melanoma cells. Tumor metastases in the lymph nodes were more susceptible to peripheral blood NK cells. NCRs and DNAM-1, but not NKG2D, emerged as key receptors in NK cell-melanoma cytotoxicity, indicating that NK subsets expressing these receptors might be good candidates for adoptive transfer in melanoma patients. Furthermore, using a xenogeneic model of cell therapy we have shown that allogeneic NK cells potently eliminated LN metastases expressing ligands for NCRs and DNAM-1, but did not affect metastases from skin, ascites, or pleura (Lakshmikanth et al., 2009). The use of allogeneic NK cells in therapy of melanoma patients needs to be further tested (Fig 3) but the results suggest enhanced potency of KIR-mismatched allogeneic NK cells against melanoma cells (Igarashi et al., 2004) and provides important implications for the use of NK cell immunotherapy in melanoma. Based on the findings obtained in our study, we have presented our perspectives as two non-exclusive approaches that include augmentation of endogenous NK cell activation/migration pathways and intervention with allogeneic NK cell therapy. We have also raised a number of unanswered questions whose knowledge will help better in designing the most effective therapy for melanoma (Burke et al., 2010). It is understood that once the melanoma tumor spreads beyond the skin and regional lymph nodes, it is frequently incurable by available chemotherapeutic agents. Since tumor metastases from lymph nodes were more susceptible to NK cells it may be crucial to recruit NK cells and elicit response in that site to prevent hematogenous tumor dissemination and further metastasis development. Autologous peripheral blood NK cells could be redirected to the LN by administration of TLR ligands as shown in a mouse model (Martin-Fontecha et al., 2004). It is of note that most of the TLR ligands can serve as excellent adjuvants in classical T cell vaccines. It has been shown that only a small proportion of advanced melanoma patients respond to IL-2. However, it is still one of the few cytokine therapies with demonstrable clinical activities. Recent data from a mouse model suggest that NK-tumor cell interaction via DNAM-1 or NKG2D receptors was important for the efficacy of IL-2, -12 or -21 therapy (Chan et al., 2010). Hence assessment of ligand expression on tumors may be a predictive marker for the efficacy of cytokine therapy (Fig 3). Further, in light of our results, augmenting DNAM-1–mediated recognition of melanoma appears as an attractive approach. Recently, Santoni and coworkers found that melphalan, doxorubicin and bortezomib increase DNAM-1 ligands on multiple myeloma cell surface, similar immuno-chemotherapy could optimize melanoma patients' treatment leading to a more effective autologous NK cell anti-melanoma cytotoxicity (Soriani et al., 2009). Furthermore, genotoxic chemotherapeutic agents have been shown to upregulate NK activating ligands for NKG2D like MICA/B on tumor cells by mechanisms that activate the Hsp70 promoter (Liu et al., 1996). This is of particular interest as it would link chemotherapy and immunotherapy and explains the synergistic effects of these different therapeutic approaches observed clinically. Similarly, chemotherapeutic agents that activate p53 can also induce NK specific activating ligands on tumors and augment NK cell-mediated killing of melanomas and other tumor cell types as shown by us in a more recent study (Li et al., manuscript submitted, 2011). Thus, re-establishing NK cell immunosurveillance by strategically forcing the expression of NK activating ligands on tumor cells by appropriate chemotherapeutic antiblastic drugs can be an interesting approach for melanoma therapy (Fig 3).

As mentioned in previous sections, we have recently shown that NK cell missing-self-reactivity can be mimicked by blocking self-specific inhibitory receptors on NK cells using $F(ab')_2$ fragments which in combination with IL-2 lead to delayed outgrowth of melanoma tumor cells (Vahlne et al., 2010). Further, Romagne et al have characterized a fully human anti-KIR therapeutic candidate mAb, which is currently in clinical development, with the overall aim to boost antitumor responses of endogenous NK cells from patients with hematological malignancies without transplantation (Romagne et al., 2009). This needs to be tested in solid tumors like melanoma as they do express a certain level of MHC class I molecules on their cell surface during the initial stages of their metastatic spread. Hence, NK-based therapeutic strategies in combination with each other, as well as with established treatments, could form the basis for future therapy developments in melanoma.

8. Conclusion

As advances made in tumor immunology are enabling fast-paced discovery and translation of results into potential clinical tools, there is clearly a dire need to improve response rates and overall survival of melanoma patients. Despite limitations in the NK cell field, a great interest has grown recently in exploiting the potential of NK cell-based immunotherapy

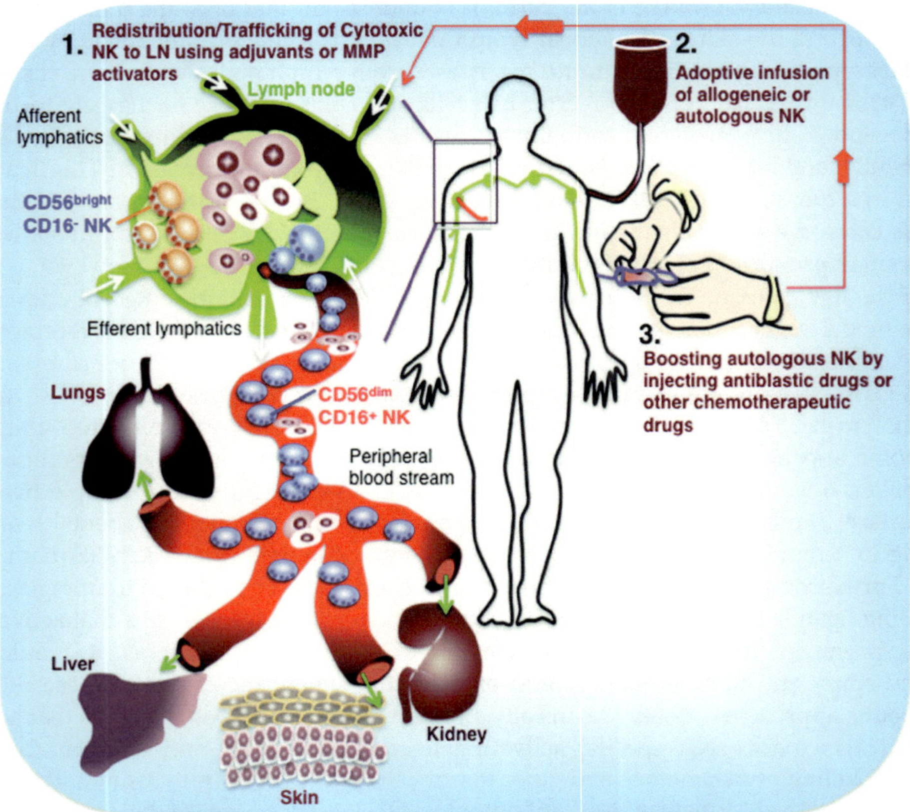

Fig. 3. Strategies to manipulate NK cells in targeting melanoma. 1). The subset of NK cells residing in the blood are $CD56^{dim}$ CD16+, a more cytotoxic subset unlike the $CD56^{bright}$ CD16- subset that resides in the lymph node which has a more cytokine secreting profile. Peripheral blood NK cells can be redistributed or trafficked into the LN by using TLR adjuvants or matrix metalloprotease (MMP) activators; 2) Adoptive transfer of higher numbers of autologous NK or allogeneic NK cells from healthy donors that can target metastases in LN which prevent further hematogenous spread of tumors into the viscera; 3) Boosting autologous NK cells by injecting antiblastic drugs like doxorubicin, bortezomib or melphalan, that might upregulate ligands for NKG2D or DNAM-1 on tumors.

(Long et al., 2001) as shown by in vitro studies (Igarashi et al., 2004), murine studies (Lundqvist et al., 2007), retrospective data from allogeneic transplant trials (Giebel et al., 2003; Ruggeri et al., 2007), and clinical trials evaluating adoptive allogeneic NK cell infusions in cancer patients (Miller et al., 2005). Clearly, many questions have to be answered before designing optimal NK-based therapy. Great achievements have been made at the bench and in the clinic over the last decade that will gain cancer patients in the coming future. Several prognostic markers have also been determined. Furthermore, by the use of comprehensive genomic, genetic and phenotypic analysis of human samples and with refined mouse models, molecular insights into the mechanisms of resistance of melanoma tumors to various immune-based therapies or chemotherapeutic drugs will be understood well. It is reasonable to anticipate that alternative therapeutics to resistant tumors and various combination strategies will emerge in the coming future. Development of effective therapeutic regimens against advanced melanoma will require more sustained effort and the hope is that the developments in understanding of melanoma tumor biology will translate into a significant benefit for patients.

9. Acknowledgement

We would like to thank Klas Kärre for critical reading of the manuscript and for providing thoughtful comments. This work was supported by grants from Karolinska Institutet, the Åke Wiberg foundation, the Magnus Bergwall foundation, the Royal Swedish Academy of Sciences, the Swedish National Board of Health and Welfare, 'Syskonen Svensssons fond' and Novo Nordisk A/S to M.H.J; Postdoctoral Research grants from Karolinska Institutet and The Swedish Research Council (524-2009-846) to T.L.K.

10. References

Albertsson, P.A., Basse, P.H., Hokland, M., Goldfarb, R.H., Nagelkerke, J.F., Nannmark, U., and Kuppen, P.J. (2003). NK cells and the tumour microenvironment: implications for NK-cell function and anti-tumour activity. *Trends Immunol*, 24, 11, 603-609.

Algarra, I., Collado, A., and Garrido, F. (1997). Altered MHC class I antigens in tumors. *Int J Clin Lab Res*, 27, 2, 95-102.

Armeanu, S., Bitzer, M., Lauer, U.M., Venturelli, S., Pathil, A., Krusch, M., Kaiser, S., Jobst, J., Smirnow, I., Wagner, A., Steinle, A., and Salih, H.R. (2005). Natural killer cell-mediated lysis of hepatoma cells via specific induction of NKG2D ligands by the histone deacetylase inhibitor sodium valproate. *Cancer Res*, 65, 14, 6321-6329.

Armstrong, B.K., and Kricker, A. (2001). The epidemiology of UV induced skin cancer. *J Photochem Photobiol B*, 63, 1-3, 8-18.

Ascierto, P.A., and Kirkwood, J.M. (2008). Adjuvant therapy of melanoma with interferon: lessons of the past decade. *J Transl Med*, 6, 62.

Azogui, O., Avril, M.F., Margulis, A., Guillard, M., Caillou, B., and Prade, M. (1991). Tumor-infiltrating CD3- NK cells are more effective than CD3+ T cells in killing autologous melanoma cells. *J Invest Dermatol*, 97, 3, 425-429.

Balsamo, M., Scordamaglia, F., Pietra, G., Manzini, C., Cantoni, C., Boitano, M., Queirolo, P., Vermi, W., Facchetti, F., Moretta, A., Moretta, L., Mingari, M.C., and Vitale, M. (2009). Melanoma-associated fibroblasts modulate NK cell phenotype and antitumor cytotoxicity. *Proc Natl Acad Sci U S A*, 106, 49, 20847-20852.

Baury, B., Masson, D., McDermott, B.M., Jr., Jarry, A., Blottiere, H.M., Blanchardie, P., Laboisse, C.L., Lustenberger, P., Racaniello, V.R., and Denis, M.G. (2003). Identification of secreted CD155 isoforms. *Biochem Biophys Res Commun*, 309, 1, 175-182.

Becker, J.C., Vetter, C.S., Schrama, D., Brocker, E.B., and thor Straten, P. (2000). Differential expression of CD28 and CD94/NKG2 on T cells with identical TCR beta variable regions in primary melanoma and sentinel lymph node. *Eur J Immunol*, 30, 12, 3699-3706.

Benitez, A.C., Dai, Z., Mann, H.H., Reeves, R.S., Margineantu, D.H., Gooley, T.A., Groh, V., and Spies, T. (2011). Expression, signaling proficiency, and stimulatory function of the NKG2D lymphocyte receptor in human cancer cells. *Proc Natl Acad Sci U S A*, 108, 10, 4081-4086.

Biron, C.A., Nguyen, K.B., Pien, G.C., Cousens, L.P., and Salazar-Mather, T.P. (1999). Natural killer cells in antiviral defense: function and regulation by innate cytokines. *Annu Rev Immunol*, 17, 189-220.

Borg, C., Terme, M., Taieb, J., Menard, C., Flament, C., Robert, C., Maruyama, K., Wakasugi, H., Angevin, E., Thielemans, K., Le Cesne, A., Chung-Scott, V., Lazar, V., Tchou, I., Crepineau, F., Lemoine, F., Bernard, J., Fletcher, J.A., Turhan, A., Blay, J.Y., Spatz, A., Emile, J.F., Heinrich, M.C., Mecheri, S., Tursz, T., and Zitvogel, L. (2004). Novel mode of action of c-kit tyrosine kinase inhibitors leading to NK cell-dependent antitumor effects. *J Clin Invest*, 114, 3, 379-388.

Bottino, C., Castriconi, R., Pende, D., Rivera, P., Nanni, M., Carnemolla, B., Cantoni, C., Grassi, J., Marcenaro, S., Reymond, N., Vitale, M., Moretta, L., Lopez, M., and Moretta, A. (2003). Identification of PVR (CD155) and Nectin-2 (CD112) as cell surface ligands for the human DNAM-1 (CD226) activating molecule. *J Exp Med*, 198, 4, 557-567.

Bremers, A.J., and Parmiani, G. (2000). Immunology and immunotherapy of human cancer: present concepts and clinical developments. *Crit Rev Oncol Hematol*, 34, 1, 1-25.

Brunda, M.J., Rosenbaum, D., and Stern, L. (1984). Inhibition of experimentally-induced murine metastases by recombinant alpha interferon: correlation between the modulatory effect of interferon treatment on natural killer cell activity and inhibition of metastases. *Int J Cancer*, 34, 3, 421-426.

Bryceson, Y.T., March, M.E., Barber, D.F., Ljunggren, H.G., and Long, E.O. (2005). Cytolytic granule polarization and degranulation controlled by different receptors in resting NK cells. *J Exp Med*, 202, 7, 1001-1012.

Bryceson, Y.T., March, M.E., Ljunggren, H.G., and Long, E.O. (2006). Activation, coactivation, and costimulation of resting human natural killer cells. *Immunol Rev*, 214, 73-91.

Burke, S., Lakshmikanth, T., Colucci, F., and Carbone, E. (2010). New views on natural killer cell-based immunotherapy for melanoma treatment. *Trends Immunol*, 31, 9, 339-345.

Burns, E.A., and Leventhal, E.A. (2000). Aging, immunity, and cancer. *Cancer Control*, 7, 6, 513-522.

Burns, L.J., Weisdorf, D.J., DeFor, T.E., Vesole, D.H., Repka, T.L., Blazar, B.R., Burger, S.R., Panoskaltsis-Mortari, A., Keever-Taylor, C.A., Zhang, M.J., and Miller, J.S. (2003). IL-2-based immunotherapy after autologous transplantation for lymphoma and breast cancer induces immune activation and cytokine release: a phase I/II trial. *Bone Marrow Transplant*, 32, 2, 177-186.

Cao, X., Cai, S.F., Fehniger, T.A., Song, J., Collins, L.I., Piwnica-Worms, D.R., and Ley, T.J. (2007). Granzyme B and perforin are important for regulatory T cell-mediated suppression of tumor clearance. *Immunity*, 27, 4, 635-646.

Carbone, E., Ruggiero, G., Terrazzano, G., Palomba, C., Manzo, C., Fontana, S., Spits, H., Karre, K., and Zappacosta, S. (1997). A new mechanism of NK cell cytotoxicity activation: the CD40-CD40 ligand interaction. *J Exp Med*, 185, 12, 2053-2060.

Carlens, S., Gilljam, M., Chambers, B.J., Aschan, J., Guven, H., Ljunggren, H.G., Christensson, B., and Dilber, M.S. (2001). A new method for in vitro expansion of cytotoxic human CD3-CD56+ natural killer cells. *Hum Immunol*, 62, 10, 1092-1098.

Carlsten, M., Bjorkstrom, N.K., Norell, H., Bryceson, Y., van Hall, T., Baumann, B.C., Hanson, M., Schedvins, K., Kiessling, R., Ljunggren, H.G., and Malmberg, K.J. (2007). DNAX accessory molecule-1 mediated recognition of freshly isolated ovarian carcinoma by resting natural killer cells. *Cancer Res*, 67, 3, 1317-1325.

Carrega, P., Pezzino, G., Queirolo, P., Bonaccorsi, I., Falco, M., Vita, G., Pende, D., Misefari, A., Moretta, A., Mingari, M.C., Moretta, L., and Ferlazzo, G. (2009). Susceptibility of human melanoma cells to autologous natural killer (NK) cell killing: HLA-related effector mechanisms and role of unlicensed NK cells. *PLoS One*, 4, 12, e8132.

Carson, W.E., Giri, J.G., Lindemann, M.J., Linett, M.L., Ahdieh, M., Paxton, R., Anderson, D., Eisenmann, J., Grabstein, K., and Caligiuri, M.A. (1994). Interleukin (IL) 15 is a novel cytokine that activates human natural killer cells via components of the IL-2 receptor. *J Exp Med*, 180, 4, 1395-1403.

Casado, J.G., Pawelec, G., Morgado, S., Sanchez-Correa, B., Delgado, E., Gayoso, I., Duran, E., Solana, R., and Tarazona, R. (2009). Expression of adhesion molecules and ligands for activating and costimulatory receptors involved in cell-mediated cytotoxicity in a large panel of human melanoma cell lines. *Cancer Immunol Immunother*, 58, 9, 1517-1526.

Chan, C.J., Andrews, D.M., McLaughlin, N.M., Yagita, H., Gilfillan, S., Colonna, M., and Smyth, M.J. (2010). DNAM-1/CD155 interactions promote cytokine and NK cell-mediated suppression of poorly immunogenic melanoma metastases. *J Immunol*, 184, 2, 902-911.

Chehimi, J., Starr, S.E., Frank, I., Rengaraju, M., Jackson, S.J., Llanes, C., Kobayashi, M., Perussia, B., Young, D., Nickbarg, E., and et al. (1992). Natural killer (NK) cell stimulatory factor increases the cytotoxic activity of NK cells from both healthy donors and human immunodeficiency virus-infected patients. *J Exp Med*, 175, 3, 789-796.

Chin, L., Garraway, L.A., and Fisher, D.E. (2006). Malignant melanoma: genetics and therapeutics in the genomic era. *Genes Dev*, 20, 16, 2149-2182.

Cochran, A.J., Huang, R.R., Lee, J., Itakura, E., Leong, S.P., and Essner, R. (2006). Tumour-induced immune modulation of sentinel lymph nodes. *Nat Rev Immunol*, 6, 9, 659-670.

Cochran, A.J., Morton, D.L., Stern, S., Lana, A.M., Essner, R., and Wen, D.R. (2001). Sentinel lymph nodes show profound downregulation of antigen-presenting cells of the paracortex: implications for tumor biology and treatment. *Mod Pathol*, 14, 6, 604-608.

Colucci, F., Caligiuri, M.A., and Di Santo, J.P. (2003). What does it take to make a natural killer? *Nat Rev Immunol*, 3, 5, 413-425.

Cooper, M.A., Fehniger, T.A., and Caligiuri, M.A. (2001). The biology of human natural killer-cell subsets. *Trends Immunol*, 22, 11, 633-640.

Davies, F.E., Raje, N., Hideshima, T., Lentzsch, S., Young, G., Tai, Y.T., Lin, B., Podar, K., Gupta, D., Chauhan, D., Treon, S.P., Richardson, P.G., Schlossman, R.L., Morgan, G.J., Muller, G.W., Stirling, D.I., and Anderson, K.C. (2001). Thalidomide and immunomodulatory derivatives augment natural killer cell cytotoxicity in multiple myeloma. *Blood*, 98, 1, 210-216.

Davis, D.M., and Dustin, M.L. (2004). What is the importance of the immunological synapse? *Trends Immunol*, 25, 6, 323-327.

Diefenbach, A., Jensen, E.R., Jamieson, A.M., and Raulet, D.H. (2001). Rae1 and H60 ligands of the NKG2D receptor stimulate tumour immunity. *Nature*, 413, 6852, 165-171.

Dudley, M.E., Wunderlich, J.R., Robbins, P.F., Yang, J.C., Hwu, P., Schwartzentruber, D.J., Topalian, S.L., Sherry, R., Restifo, N.P., Hubicki, A.M., Robinson, M.R., Raffeld, M., Duray, P., Seipp, C.A., Rogers-Freezer, L., Morton, K.E., Mavroukakis, S.A., White, D.E., and Rosenberg, S.A. (2002). Cancer regression and autoimmunity in patients after clonal repopulation with antitumor lymphocytes. *Science*, 298, 5594, 850-854.

Elboim, M., Gazit, R., Gur, C., Ghadially, H., Betser-Cohen, G., and Mandelboim, O. (2010). Tumor immunoediting by NKp46. *J Immunol*, 184, 10, 5637-5644.

Fang, L., Lonsdorf, A.S., and Hwang, S.T. (2008). Immunotherapy for advanced melanoma. *J Invest Dermatol*, 128, 11, 2596-2605.

Farag, S.S., and Caligiuri, M.A. (2006). Human natural killer cell development and biology. *Blood Rev*, 20, 3, 123-137.

Farzad, Z., Cochran, A.J., McBride, W.H., Gray, J.D., Wong, V., and Morton, D.L. (1990). Lymphocyte subset alterations in nodes regional to human melanoma. *Cancer Res*, 50, 12, 3585-3588.

Fehniger, T.A., and Caligiuri, M.A. (2001). Interleukin 15: biology and relevance to human disease. *Blood*, 97, 1, 14-32.

Fernandez, N.C., Lozier, A., Flament, C., Ricciardi-Castagnoli, P., Bellet, D., Suter, M., Perricaudet, M., Tursz, T., Maraskovsky, E., and Zitvogel, L. (1999). Dendritic cells directly trigger NK cell functions: cross-talk relevant in innate anti-tumor immune responses in vivo. *Nat Med*, 5, 4, 405-411.

Ferrone, S., and Marincola, F.M. (1995). Loss of HLA class I antigens by melanoma cells: molecular mechanisms, functional significance and clinical relevance. *Immunol Today*, 16, 10, 487-494.

Fewkes, N.M., and Mackall, C.L. (2010). Novel gamma-chain cytokines as candidate immune modulators in immune therapies for cancer. *Cancer J*, 16, 4, 392-398.

Flaherty, L.E., and Gadgeel, S.M. (2002). Biochemotherapy of melanoma. *Semin Oncol*, 29, 5, 446-455.

Fogler, W.E., Volker, K., McCormick, K.L., Watanabe, M., Ortaldo, J.R., and Wiltrout, R.H. (1996). NK cell infiltration into lung, liver, and subcutaneous B16 melanoma is mediated by VCAM-1/VLA-4 interaction. *J Immunol*, 156, 12, 4707-4714.

Fregni, G., Perier, A., Pittari, G., Jacobelli, S., Sastre, X., Gervois, N.I., Allard, M., Bercovici, N., Avril, M.F., and Caignard, A. (2011). Unique functional status of Natural Killer cells in metastatic stage IV melanoma patients and its modulation by chemotherapy. *Clin Cancer Res*,

Galea-Lauri, J., Darling, D., Gan, S.U., Krivochtchapov, L., Kuiper, M., Gaken, J., Souberbielle, B., and Farzaneh, F. (1999). Expression of a variant of CD28 on a subpopulation of human NK cells: implications for B7-mediated stimulation of NK cells. *J Immunol*, 163, 1, 62-70.

Gately, M.K., Wolitzky, A.G., Quinn, P.M., and Chizzonite, R. (1992). Regulation of human cytolytic lymphocyte responses by interleukin-12. *Cell Immunol*, 143, 1, 127-142.

Geller, M.A., Cooley, S., Judson, P.L., Ghebre, R., Carson, L.F., Argenta, P.A., Jonson, A.L., Panoskaltsis-Mortari, A., Curtsinger, J., McKenna, D., Dusenbery, K., Bliss, R., Downs, L.S., and Miller, J.S. (2011). A phase II study of allogeneic natural killer cell therapy to treat patients with recurrent ovarian and breast cancer. *Cytotherapy*, 13, 1, 98-107.

Ghiringhelli, F., Menard, C., Terme, M., Flament, C., Taieb, J., Chaput, N., Puig, P.E., Novault, S., Escudier, B., Vivier, E., Lecesne, A., Robert, C., Blay, J.Y., Bernard, J., Caillat-Zucman, S., Freitas, A., Tursz, T., Wagner-Ballon, O., Capron, C., Vainchencker, W., Martin, F., and Zitvogel, L. (2005). CD4+CD25+ regulatory T cells inhibit natural killer cell functions in a transforming growth factor-beta-dependent manner. *J Exp Med*, 202, 8, 1075-1085.

Giebel, S., Locatelli, F., Lamparelli, T., Velardi, A., Davies, S., Frumento, G., Maccario, R., Bonetti, F., Wojnar, J., Martinetti, M., Frassoni, F., Giorgiani, G., Bacigalupo, A., and Holowiecki, J. (2003). Survival advantage with KIR ligand incompatibility in hematopoietic stem cell transplantation from unrelated donors. *Blood*, 102, 3, 814-819.

Gilfillan, S., Chan, C.J., Cella, M., Haynes, N.M., Rapaport, A.S., Boles, K.S., Andrews, D.M., Smyth, M.J., and Colonna, M. (2008). DNAM-1 promotes activation of cytotoxic lymphocytes by nonprofessional antigen-presenting cells and tumors. *J Exp Med*, 205, 13, 2965-2973.

Greenlee, R.T., Hill-Harmon, M.B., Murray, T., and Thun, M. (2001). Cancer statistics, 2001. *CA Cancer J Clin*, 51, 1, 15-36.

Groh, V., Wu, J., Yee, C., and Spies, T. (2002). Tumour-derived soluble MIC ligands impair expression of NKG2D and T-cell activation. *Nature*, 419, 6908, 734-738.

Guerra, N., Tan, Y.X., Joncker, N.T., Choy, A., Gallardo, F., Xiong, N., Knoblaugh, S., Cado, D., Greenberg, N.M., and Raulet, D.H. (2008). NKG2D-deficient mice are defective in tumor surveillance in models of spontaneous malignancy. *Immunity*, 28, 4, 571-580.

Haass, N.K., Smalley, K.S., Li, L., and Herlyn, M. (2005). Adhesion, migration and communication in melanocytes and melanoma. *Pigment Cell Res*, 18, 3, 150-159.

Hanna, N. (1982). Inhibition of experimental tumor metastasis by selective activation of natural killer cells. *Cancer Res*, 42, 4, 1337-1342.

Hayakawa, Y., and Smyth, M.J. (2006). NKG2D and cytotoxic effector function in tumor immune surveillance. *Semin Immunol*, 18, 3, 176-185.

Heinzerling, L., Dummer, R., Pavlovic, J., Schultz, J., Burg, G., and Moelling, K. (2002). Tumor regression of human and murine melanoma after intratumoral injection of IL-12-encoding plasmid DNA in mice. *Exp Dermatol*, 11, 3, 232-240.

Herberman, R.B., Nunn, M.E., Holden, H.T., and Lavrin, D.H. (1975). Natural cytotoxic reactivity of mouse lymphoid cells against syngeneic and allogeneic tumors. II. Characterization of effector cells. *Int J Cancer*, 16, 2, 230-239.

Hersey, P., Edwards, A., and McCarthy, W.H. (1980). Tumour-related changes in natural killer cell activity in melanoma patients. Influence of stage of disease, tumour thickness and age of patients. *Int J Cancer*, 25, 2, 187-194.

Hersey, P., Hobbs, A., Edwards, A., McCarthy, W.H., and McGovern, V.J. (1982). Relationship between natural killer cell activity and histological features of lymphocyte infiltration and partial regression of the primary tumor in melanoma patients. *Cancer Res*, 42, 1, 363-368.

Hersey, P., and Zhang, X.D. (2001). How melanoma cells evade trail-induced apoptosis. *Nat Rev Cancer*, 1, 2, 142-150.

Hill, L.L., Perussia, B., McCue, P.A., and Korngold, R. (1994). Effect of human natural killer cells on the metastatic growth of human melanoma xenografts in mice with severe combined immunodeficiency. *Cancer Res*, 54, 3, 763-770.

Hirschowitz, E.A., and Crystal, R.G. (1999). Adenovirus-mediated expression of interleukin-12 induces natural killer cell activity and complements adenovirus-directed gp75 treatment of melanoma lung metastases. *Am J Respir Cell Mol Biol*, 20, 5, 935-941.

Huang, Y., Wang, Y., Li, Y., Guo, K., and He, Y. (2011). Role of sorafenib and sunitinib in the induction of expressions of NKG2D ligands in nasopharyngeal carcinoma with high expression of ABCG(2). *J Cancer Res Clin Oncol*, 137, 5, 829-837.

Igarashi, T., Wynberg, J., Srinivasan, R., Becknell, B., McCoy, J.P., Jr., Takahashi, Y., Suffredini, D.A., Linehan, W.M., Caligiuri, M.A., and Childs, R.W. (2004). Enhanced cytotoxicity of allogeneic NK cells with killer immunoglobulin-like receptor ligand incompatibility against melanoma and renal cell carcinoma cells. *Blood*, 104, 1, 170-177.

Iguchi-Manaka, A., Kai, H., Yamashita, Y., Shibata, K., Tahara-Hanaoka, S., Honda, S., Yasui, T., Kikutani, H., Shibuya, K., and Shibuya, A. (2008). Accelerated tumor growth in mice deficient in DNAM-1 receptor. *J Exp Med*, 205, 13, 2959-2964.

Iyengar, R., Handgretinger, R., Babarin-Dorner, A., Leimig, T., Otto, M., Geiger, T.L., Holladay, M.S., Houston, J., and Leung, W. (2003). Purification of human natural killer cells using a clinical-scale immunomagnetic method. *Cytotherapy*, 5, 6, 479-484.

Jager, M.J., Hurks, H.M., Levitskaya, J., and Kiessling, R. (2002). HLA expression in uveal melanoma: there is no rule without some exception. *Hum Immunol*, 63, 6, 444-451.

Jaime-Ramirez, A.C., Mundy-Bosse, B.L., Kondadasula, S., Jones, N.B., Roda, J.M., Mani, A., Parihar, R., Karpa, V., Papenfuss, T.L., LaPerle, K.M., Biller, E., Lehman, A., Chaudhury, A.R., Jarjoura, D., Burry, R.W., and Carson, W.E., 3rd. (2011). IL-12 enhances the antitumor actions of trastuzumab via NK cell IFN-gamma production. *J Immunol*, 186, 6, 3401-3409.

Jin, G.H., Hirano, T., and Murakami, M. (2008). Combination treatment with IL-2 and anti-IL-2 mAbs reduces tumor metastasis via NK cell activation. *Int Immunol*, 20, 6, 783-789.

Jovic, V., Konjevic, G., Radulovic, S., Jelic, S., and Spuzic, I. (2001). Impaired perforin-dependent NK cell cytotoxicity and proliferative activity of peripheral blood T cells is associated with metastatic melanoma. *Tumori*, 87, 5, 324-329.

Karre, K. (1991). MHC gene control of the natural killer system at the level of the target and the host. *Semin Cancer Biol*, 2, 5, 295-309.

Kiessling, R., Klein, E., Pross, H., and Wigzell, H. (1975a). "Natural" killer cells in the mouse. II. Cytotoxic cells with specificity for mouse Moloney leukemia cells. Characteristics of the killer cell. *Eur J Immunol*, 5, 2, 117-121.

Kiessling, R., Klein, E., and Wigzell, H. (1975b). "Natural" killer cells in the mouse. I. Cytotoxic cells with specificity for mouse Moloney leukemia cells. Specificity and distribution according to genotype. *Eur J Immunol*, 5, 2, 112-117.

Kim, H., Kim, S.H., Kim, M.J., Kim, S.J., Park, S.J., Chung, J.S., Bae, J.H., and Kang, C.D. (2011). EGFR Inhibitors Enhanced the Susceptibility to NK Cell-mediated Lysis of Lung Cancer Cells. *J Immunother*, 34, 4, 372-381.

Kohga, K., Takehara, T., Tatsumi, T., Ishida, H., Miyagi, T., Hosui, A., and Hayashi, N. (2010). Sorafenib inhibits the shedding of major histocompatibility complex class I-related chain A on hepatocellular carcinoma cells by down-regulating a disintegrin and metalloproteinase 9. *Hepatology*, 51, 4, 1264-1273.

Kohno, K., Kataoka, J., Ohtsuki, T., Suemoto, Y., Okamoto, I., Usui, M., Ikeda, M., and Kurimoto, M. (1997). IFN-gamma-inducing factor (IGIF) is a costimulatory factor on the activation of Th1 but not Th2 cells and exerts its effect independently of IL-12. *J Immunol*, 158, 4, 1541-1550.

Konjevic, G., Mirjacic Martinovic, K., Vuletic, A., and Babovic, N. (2010). In-vitro IL-2 or IFN-alpha-induced NKG2D and CD161 NK cell receptor expression indicates novel aspects of NK cell activation in metastatic melanoma patients. *Melanoma Res*, 20, 6, 459-467.

Konjevic, G., Mirjacic Martinovic, K., Vuletic, A., Jovic, V., Jurisic, V., Babovic, N., and Spuzic, I. (2007). Low expression of CD161 and NKG2D activating NK receptor is associated with impaired NK cell cytotoxicity in metastatic melanoma patients. *Clin Exp Metastasis*, 24, 1, 1-11.

Kornstein, M.J., Stewart, R., and Elder, D.E. (1987). Natural killer cells in the host response to melanoma. *Cancer Res*, 47, 5, 1411-1412.

Kroger, A., Koster, M., Schroeder, K., Hauser, H., and Mueller, P.P. (2002). Activities of IRF-1. *J Interferon Cytokine Res*, 22, 1, 5-14.

Lakshmikanth, T., Burke, S., Ali, T.H., Kimpfler, S., Ursini, F., Ruggeri, L., Capanni, M., Umansky, V., Paschen, A., Sucker, A., Pende, D., Groh, V., Biassoni, R., Hoglund, P., Kato, M., Shibuya, K., Schadendorf, D., Anichini, A., Ferrone, S., Velardi, A., Karre, K., Shibuya, A., Carbone, E., and Colucci, F. (2009). NCRs and DNAM-1 mediate NK cell recognition and lysis of human and mouse melanoma cell lines in vitro and in vivo. *J Clin Invest*, 119, 5, 1251-1263.

Lamont, A.G., and Adorini, L. (1996). IL-12: a key cytokine in immune regulation. *Immunol Today*, 17, 5, 214-217.

Lanier, L.L. (2005). NK cell recognition. *Annu Rev Immunol*, 23, 225-274.

Law, T.M., Motzer, R.J., Mazumdar, M., Sell, K.W., Walther, P.J., O'Connell, M., Khan, A., Vlamis, V., Vogelzang, N.J., and Bajorin, D.F. (1995). Phase III randomized trial of interleukin-2 with or without lymphokine-activated killer cells in the treatment of patients with advanced renal cell carcinoma. *Cancer*, 76, 5, 824-832.

Le Garff-Tavernier, M., Beziat, V., Decocq, J., Siguret, V., Gandjbakhch, F., Pautas, E., Debre, P., Merle-Beral, H., and Vieillard, V. (2010). Human NK cells display major phenotypic and functional changes over the life span. *Aging Cell*, 9, 4, 527-535.

Lieberman, J. (2003). The ABCs of granule-mediated cytotoxicity: new weapons in the arsenal. *Nat Rev Immunol*, 3, 5, 361-370.

Liu, H., Lightfoot, R., and Stevens, J.L. (1996). Activation of heat shock factor by alkylating agents is triggered by glutathione depletion and oxidation of protein thiols. *J Biol Chem*, 271, 9, 4805-4812.

Ljunggren, H.G., and Karre, K. (1990). In search of the 'missing self': MHC molecules and NK cell recognition. *Immunol Today*, 11, 7, 237-244.

Ljunggren, H.G., and Malmberg, K.J. (2007). Prospects for the use of NK cells in immunotherapy of human cancer. *Nat Rev Immunol*, 7, 5, 329-339.

Long, E.O. (1999). Regulation of immune responses through inhibitory receptors. *Annu Rev Immunol*, 17, 875-904.

Long, E.O., Barber, D.F., Burshtyn, D.N., Faure, M., Peterson, M., Rajagopalan, S., Renard, V., Sandusky, M., Stebbins, C.C., Wagtmann, N., and Watzl, C. (2001). Inhibition of natural killer cell activation signals by killer cell immunoglobulin-like receptors (CD158). *Immunol Rev*, 181, 223-233.

Lotze, M.T., Rubin, J.T., and Zeh, H.J. (1992). New biologic agents come to bat for cancer therapy. *Curr Opin Oncol*, 4, 6, 1116-1123.

Loza, M.J., Zamai, L., Azzoni, L., Rosati, E., and Perussia, B. (2002). Expression of type 1 (interferon gamma) and type 2 (interleukin-13, interleukin-5) cytokines at distinct stages of natural killer cell differentiation from progenitor cells. *Blood*, 99, 4, 1273-1281.

Luci, C., Reynders, A., Ivanov, II, Cognet, C., Chiche, L., Chasson, L., Hardwigsen, J., Anguiano, E., Banchereau, J., Chaussabel, D., Dalod, M., Littman, D.R., Vivier, E., and Tomasello, E. (2009). Influence of the transcription factor RORgammat on the development of NKp46+ cell populations in gut and skin. *Nat Immunol*, 10, 1, 75-82.

Lundqvist, A., Abrams, S.I., Schrump, D.S., Alvarez, G., Suffredini, D., Berg, M., and Childs, R. (2006). Bortezomib and depsipeptide sensitize tumors to tumor necrosis factor-related apoptosis-inducing ligand: a novel method to potentiate natural killer cell tumor cytotoxicity. *Cancer Res*, 66, 14, 7317-7325.

Lundqvist, A., McCoy, J.P., Samsel, L., and Childs, R. (2007). Reduction of GVHD and enhanced antitumor effects after adoptive infusion of alloreactive Ly49-mismatched NK cells from MHC-matched donors. *Blood*, 109, 8, 3603-3606.

Lundqvist, A., Yokoyama, H., Smith, A., Berg, M., and Childs, R. (2009). Bortezomib treatment and regulatory T-cell depletion enhance the antitumor effects of adoptively infused NK cells. *Blood*, 113, 24, 6120-6127.

Ma, D., and Niederkorn, J.Y. (1995). Transforming growth factor-beta down-regulates major histocompatibility complex class I antigen expression and increases the susceptibility of uveal melanoma cells to natural killer cell-mediated cytolysis. *Immunology*, 86, 2, 263-269.

Mackensen, A., Carcelain, G., Viel, S., Raynal, M.C., Michalaki, H., Triebel, F., Bosq, J., and Hercend, T. (1994). Direct evidence to support the immunosurveillance concept in a human regressive melanoma. *J Clin Invest*, 93, 4, 1397-1402.

Marincola, F.M., Jaffee, E.M., Hicklin, D.J., and Ferrone, S. (2000). Escape of human solid tumors from T-cell recognition: molecular mechanisms and functional significance. *Adv Immunol*, 74, 181-273.

Markel, G., Lieberman, N., Katz, G., Arnon, T.I., Lotem, M., Drize, O., Blumberg, R.S., Bar-Haim, E., Mader, R., Eisenbach, L., and Mandelboim, O. (2002). CD66a interactions between human melanoma and NK cells: a novel class I MHC-independent inhibitory mechanism of cytotoxicity. *J Immunol*, 168, 6, 2803-2810.

Markel, G., Seidman, R., Besser, M.J., Zabari, N., Ortenberg, R., Shapira, R., Treves, A.J., Loewenthal, R., Orenstein, A., Nagler, A., and Schachter, J. (2009). Natural killer lysis receptor (NKLR)/NKLR-ligand matching as a novel approach for enhancing anti-tumor activity of allogeneic NK cells. *PLoS One*, 4, 5, e5597.

Markovic, S.N., and Murasko, D.M. (1991). Role of natural killer and T-cells in interferon induced inhibition of spontaneous metastases of the B16F10L murine melanoma. *Cancer Res*, 51, 4, 1124-1128.

Markovic, S.N., and Murasko, D.M. (1990). Neoadjuvant immunotherapy with interferon of the spontaneously metastasizing murine B16F10L melanoma. *Int J Cancer*, 45, 4, 788-794.

Martin-Fontecha, A., Thomsen, L.L., Brett, S., Gerard, C., Lipp, M., Lanzavecchia, A., and Sallusto, F. (2004). Induced recruitment of NK cells to lymph nodes provides IFN-gamma for T(H)1 priming. *Nat Immunol*, 5, 12, 1260-1265.

Meier, F., Satyamoorthy, K., Nesbit, M., Hsu, M.Y., Schittek, B., Garbe, C., and Herlyn, M. (1998). Molecular events in melanoma development and progression. *Front Biosci*, 3, D1005-1010.

Meyer-Monard, S., Passweg, J., Siegler, U., Kalberer, C., Koehl, U., Rovo, A., Halter, J., Stern, M., Heim, D., Alois Gratwohl, J.R., and Tichelli, A. (2009). Clinical-grade purification of natural killer cells in haploidentical hematopoietic stem cell transplantation. *Transfusion*, 49, 2, 362-371.

Miller, J.S., Soignier, Y., Panoskaltsis-Mortari, A., McNearney, S.A., Yun, G.H., Fautsch, S.K., McKenna, D., Le, C., Defor, T.E., Burns, L.J., Orchard, P.J., Blazar, B.R., Wagner, J.E., Slungaard, A., Weisdorf, D.J., Okazaki, I.J., and McGlave, P.B. (2005). Successful adoptive transfer and in vivo expansion of human haploidentical NK cells in patients with cancer. *Blood*, 105, 8, 3051-3057.

Miller, J.S., Tessmer-Tuck, J., Pierson, B.A., Weisdorf, D., McGlave, P., Blazar, B.R., Katsanis, E., Verfaillie, C., Lebkowski, J., Radford, J., Jr., and Burns, L.J. (1997). Low dose subcutaneous interleukin-2 after autologous transplantation generates sustained in vivo natural killer cell activity. *Biol Blood Marrow Transplant*, 3, 1, 34-44.

Moretta, A., Bottino, C., Vitale, M., Pende, D., Cantoni, C., Mingari, M.C., Biassoni, R., and Moretta, L. (2001). Activating receptors and coreceptors involved in human natural killer cell-mediated cytolysis. *Annu Rev Immunol*, 19, 197-223.

Morris, M.A., and Ley, K. (2004). Trafficking of natural killer cells. *Curr Mol Med*, 4, 4, 431-438.

Muller, C., Pehamberger, H., Binder, M., and Zielinski, C.C. (1989). Defective interferon-augmented natural killer cell activity in patients with metastatic malignant melanoma. *J Cancer Res Clin Oncol*, 115, 4, 393-396.

Munger, W., DeJoy, S.Q., Jeyaseelan, R., Sr., Torley, L.W., Grabstein, K.H., Eisenmann, J., Paxton, R., Cox, T., Wick, M.M., and Kerwar, S.S. (1995). Studies evaluating the antitumor activity and toxicity of interleukin-15, a new T cell growth factor: comparison with interleukin-2. *Cell Immunol*, 165, 2, 289-293.

Naume, B., Gately, M., and Espevik, T. (1992). A comparative study of IL-12 (cytotoxic lymphocyte maturation factor)-, IL-2-, and IL-7-induced effects on immunomagnetically purified CD56+ NK cells. *J Immunol*, 148, 8, 2429-2436.

Nguyen, T., Thomas, W., Zhang, X.D., Gray, C., and Hersey, P. (2000). Immunologically-mediated tumour cell apoptosis: the role of TRAIL in T cell and cytokine-mediated responses to melanoma. *Forum (Genova)*, 10, 3, 243-252.

Okamura, H., Tsutsi, H., Komatsu, T., Yutsudo, M., Hakura, A., Tanimoto, T., Torigoe, K., Okura, T., Nukada, Y., Hattori, K., and et al. (1995). Cloning of a new cytokine that induces IFN-gamma production by T cells. *Nature*, 378, 6552, 88-91.

Oppenheim, D.E., Roberts, S.J., Clarke, S.L., Filler, R., Lewis, J.M., Tigelaar, R.E., Girardi, M., and Hayday, A.C. (2005). Sustained localized expression of ligand for the activating NKG2D receptor impairs natural cytotoxicity in vivo and reduces tumor immunosurveillance. *Nat Immunol*, 6, 9, 928-937.

Osaki, T., Peron, J.M., Cai, Q., Okamura, H., Robbins, P.D., Kurimoto, M., Lotze, M.T., and Tahara, H. (1998). IFN-gamma-inducing factor/IL-18 administration mediates IFN-gamma- and IL-12-independent antitumor effects. *J Immunol*, 160, 4, 1742-1749.

Pandolfi, F., Boyle, L.A., Trentin, L., Kurnick, J.T., Isselbacher, K.J., and Gattoni-Celli, S. (1991). Expression of HLA-A2 antigen in human melanoma cell lines and its role in T-cell recognition. *Cancer Res*, 51, 12, 3164-3170.

Parrish-Novak, J., Dillon, S.R., Nelson, A., Hammond, A., Sprecher, C., Gross, J.A., Johnston, J., Madden, K., Xu, W., West, J., Schrader, S., Burkhead, S., Heipel, M., Brandt, C., Kuijper, J.L., Kramer, J., Conklin, D., Presnell, S.R., Berry, J., Shiota, F., Bort, S., Hambly, K., Mudri, S., Clegg, C., Moore, M., Grant, F.J., Lofton-Day, C., Gilbert, T., Rayond, F., Ching, A., Yao, L., Smith, D., Webster, P., Whitmore, T., Maurer, M., Kaushansky, K., Holly, R.D., and Foster, D. (2000). Interleukin 21 and its receptor are involved in NK cell expansion and regulation of lymphocyte function. *Nature*, 408, 6808, 57-63.

Paul, P., Rouas-Freiss, N., Khalil-Daher, I., Moreau, P., Riteau, B., Le Gal, F.A., Avril, M.F., Dausset, J., Guillet, J.G., and Carosella, E.D. (1998). HLA-G expression in melanoma: a way for tumor cells to escape from immunosurveillance. *Proc Natl Acad Sci U S A*, 95, 8, 4510-4515.

Pende, D., Accame, L., Pareti, L., Mazzocchi, A., Moretta, A., Parmiani, G., and Moretta, L. (1998). The susceptibility to natural killer cell-mediated lysis of HLA class I-positive melanomas reflects the expression of insufficient amounts of different HLA class I alleles. *Eur J Immunol*, 28, 8, 2384-2394.

Pende, D., Cantoni, C., Rivera, P., Vitale, M., Castriconi, R., Marcenaro, S., Nanni, M., Biassoni, R., Bottino, C., Moretta, A., and Moretta, L. (2001). Role of NKG2D in tumor cell lysis mediated by human NK cells: cooperation with natural cytotoxicity receptors and capability of recognizing tumors of nonepithelial origin. *Eur J Immunol*, 31, 4, 1076-1086.

Pende, D., Parolini, S., Pessino, A., Sivori, S., Augugliaro, R., Morelli, L., Marcenaro, E., Accame, L., Malaspina, A., Biassoni, R., Bottino, C., Moretta, L., and Moretta, A. (1999). Identification and molecular characterization of NKp30, a novel triggering receptor involved in natural cytotoxicity mediated by human natural killer cells. *J Exp Med*, 190, 10, 1505-1516.

Pende, D., Rivera, P., Marcenaro, S., Chang, C.C., Biassoni, R., Conte, R., Kubin, M., Cosman, D., Ferrone, S., Moretta, L., and Moretta, A. (2002). Major histocompatibility complex class I-related chain A and UL16-binding protein expression on tumor cell lines of different histotypes: analysis of tumor susceptibility to NKG2D-dependent natural killer cell cytotoxicity. *Cancer Res*, 62, 21, 6178-6186.

Perussia, B., Chan, S.H., D'Andrea, A., Tsuji, K., Santoli, D., Pospisil, M., Young, D., Wolf, S.F., and Trinchieri, G. (1992). Natural killer (NK) cell stimulatory factor or IL-12 has differential effects on the proliferation of TCR-alpha beta+, TCR-gamma delta+ T lymphocytes, and NK cells. *J Immunol*, 149, 11, 3495-3502.

Pogge von Strandmann, E., Simhadri, V.R., von Tresckow, B., Sasse, S., Reiners, K.S., Hansen, H.P., Rothe, A., Boll, B., Simhadri, V.L., Borchmann, P., McKinnon, P.J., Hallek, M., and Engert, A. (2007). Human leukocyte antigen-B-associated transcript 3 is released from tumor cells and engages the NKp30 receptor on natural killer cells. *Immunity*, 27, 6, 965-974.

Porgador, A., Mandelboim, O., Restifo, N.P., and Strominger, J.L. (1997). Natural killer cell lines kill autologous beta2-microglobulin-deficient melanoma cells: implications for cancer immunotherapy. *Proc Natl Acad Sci U S A*, 94, 24, 13140-13145.

Porgador, A., Tzehoval, E., Vadai, E., Feldman, M., and Eisenbach, L. (1995). Combined vaccination with major histocompatibility class I and interleukin 2 gene-transduced melanoma cells synergizes the cure of postsurgical established lung metastases. *Cancer Res*, 55, 21, 4941-4949.

Quan, W., Jr., Ramirez, M., Taylor, C., Quan, F., Vinogradov, M., and Walker, P. (2005). Administration of high-dose continuous infusion interleukin-2 to patients age 70 or over. *Cancer Biother Radiopharm*, 20, 1, 11-15.

Quereux, G., Pandolfino, M.C., Knol, A.C., Khammari, A., Volteau, C., Nguyen, J.M., and Dreno, B. (2007). Tissue prognostic markers for adoptive immunotherapy in melanoma. *Eur J Dermatol*, 17, 4, 295-301.

Romagne, F., Andre, P., Spee, P., Zahn, S., Anfossi, N., Gauthier, L., Capanni, M., Ruggeri, L., Benson, D.M., Jr., Blaser, B.W., Della Chiesa, M., Moretta, A., Vivier, E., Caligiuri, M.A., Velardi, A., and Wagtmann, N. (2009). Preclinical characterization of 1-7F9, a novel human anti-KIR receptor therapeutic antibody that augments natural killer-mediated killing of tumor cells. *Blood*, 114, 13, 2667-2677.

Rosenberg, S.A. (1997). Cancer vaccines based on the identification of genes encoding cancer regression antigens. *Immunol Today*, 18, 4, 175-182.

Rosenberg, S.A., Lotze, M.T., Muul, L.M., Chang, A.E., Avis, F.P., Leitman, S., Linehan, W.M., Robertson, C.N., Lee, R.E., Rubin, J.T., and et al. (1987). A progress report on the treatment of 157 patients with advanced cancer using lymphokine-activated killer cells and interleukin-2 or high-dose interleukin-2 alone. *N Engl J Med*, 316, 15, 889-897.

Rosenberg, S.A., Lotze, M.T., Muul, L.M., Leitman, S., Chang, A.E., Ettinghausen, S.E., Matory, Y.L., Skibber, J.M., Shiloni, E., Vetto, J.T., and et al. (1985). Observations on the systemic administration of autologous lymphokine-activated killer cells and recombinant interleukin-2 to patients with metastatic cancer. *N Engl J Med*, 313, 23, 1485-1492.

Ross, J.S., and Fletcher, J.A. (1998). The HER-2/neu Oncogene in Breast Cancer: Prognostic Factor, Predictive Factor, and Target for Therapy. *Oncologist*, 3, 4, 237-252.

Routes, J.M. (1992). IFN increases class I MHC antigen expression on adenovirus-infected human cells without inducing resistance to natural killer cell killing. *J Immunol*, 149, 7, 2372-2377.

Ruggeri, L., Capanni, M., Urbani, E., Perruccio, K., Shlomchik, W.D., Tosti, A., Posati, S., Rogaia, D., Frassoni, F., Aversa, F., Martelli, M.F., and Velardi, A. (2002). Effectiveness of donor natural killer cell alloreactivity in mismatched hematopoietic transplants. *Science*, 295, 5562, 2097-2100.

Ruggeri, L., Mancusi, A., Capanni, M., Urbani, E., Carotti, A., Aloisi, T., Stern, M., Pende, D., Perruccio, K., Burchielli, E., Topini, F., Bianchi, E., Aversa, F., Martelli, M.F., and

Velardi, A. (2007). Donor natural killer cell allorecognition of missing self in haploidentical hematopoietic transplantation for acute myeloid leukemia: challenging its predictive value. *Blood*, 110, 1, 433-440.

Santoni, A., Piccoli, M., Ortaldo, J.R., Mason, L., Wiltrout, R.H., and Herberman, R.B. (1985). Changes in number and density of large granular lymphocytes upon in vivo augmentation of mouse natural killer activity. *J Immunol*, 134, 4, 2799-2810.

Schwartz, R.H. (1990). A cell culture model for T lymphocyte clonal anergy. *Science*, 248, 4961, 1349-1356.

Seidel, M.G., Freissmuth, M., Pehamberger, H., and Micksche, M. (1998). Stimulation of natural killer activity in peripheral blood lymphocytes of healthy donors and melanoma patients in vitro: synergism between interleukin (IL)-12 and IL-15 or IL-12 and IL-2. *Naunyn Schmiedebergs Arch Pharmacol*, 358, 3, 382-389.

Shankaran, V., Ikeda, H., Bruce, A.T., White, J.M., Swanson, P.E., Old, L.J., and Schreiber, R.D. (2001). IFNgamma and lymphocytes prevent primary tumour development and shape tumour immunogenicity. *Nature*, 410, 6832, 1107-1111.

Shibuya, A., Campbell, D., Hannum, C., Yssel, H., Franz-Bacon, K., McClanahan, T., Kitamura, T., Nicholl, J., Sutherland, G.R., Lanier, L.L., and Phillips, J.H. (1996). DNAM-1, a novel adhesion molecule involved in the cytolytic function of T lymphocytes. *Immunity*, 4, 6, 573-581.

Sibbitt, W.L., Jr., Bankhurst, A.D., Jumonville, A.J., Saiki, J.H., Saiers, J.H., and Doberneck, R.C. (1984). Defects in natural killer cell activity and interferon response in human lung carcinoma and malignant melanoma. *Cancer Res*, 44, 2, 852-856.

Smyth, M.J., Hayakawa, Y., Takeda, K., and Yagita, H. (2002). New aspects of natural-killer-cell surveillance and therapy of cancer. *Nat Rev Cancer*, 2, 11, 850-861.

Smyth, M.J., Swann, J., Cretney, E., Zerafa, N., Yokoyama, W.M., and Hayakawa, Y. (2005). NKG2D function protects the host from tumor initiation. *J Exp Med*, 202, 5, 583-588.

Solana, R., Casado, J.G., Delgado, E., DelaRosa, O., Marin, J., Duran, E., Pawelec, G., and Tarazona, R. (2007). Lymphocyte activation in response to melanoma: interaction of NK-associated receptors and their ligands. *Cancer Immunol Immunother*, 56, 1, 101-109.

Soriani, A., Zingoni, A., Cerboni, C., Iannitto, M.L., Ricciardi, M.R., Di Gialleonardo, V., Cippitelli, M., Fionda, C., Petrucci, M.T., Guarini, A., Foa, R., and Santoni, A. (2009). ATM-ATR-dependent up-regulation of DNAM-1 and NKG2D ligands on multiple myeloma cells by therapeutic agents results in enhanced NK-cell susceptibility and is associated with a senescent phenotype. *Blood*, 113, 15, 3503-3511.

Spanholtz, J., Tordoir, M., Eissens, D., Preijers, F., van der Meer, A., Joosten, I., Schaap, N., de Witte, T.M., and Dolstra, H. (2010). High log-scale expansion of functional human natural killer cells from umbilical cord blood CD34-positive cells for adoptive cancer immunotherapy. *PLoS One*, 5, 2, e9221.

Srivastava, S., Salim, N., and Robertson, M.J. (2010). Interleukin-18: biology and role in the immunotherapy of cancer. *Curr Med Chem*, 17, 29, 3353-3357.

Street, S.E., Cretney, E., and Smyth, M.J. (2001). Perforin and interferon-gamma activities independently control tumor initiation, growth, and metastasis. *Blood*, 97, 1, 192-197.

Strid, J., Roberts, S.J., Filler, R.B., Lewis, J.M., Kwong, B.Y., Schpero, W., Kaplan, D.H., Hayday, A.C., and Girardi, M. (2008). Acute upregulation of an NKG2D ligand promotes rapid reorganization of a local immune compartment with pleiotropic effects on carcinogenesis. *Nat Immunol*, 9, 2, 146-154.

Talmadge, J.E., Phillips, H., Schindler, J., Tribble, H., and Pennington, R. (1987). Systematic preclinical study on the therapeutic properties of recombinant human interleukin 2 for the treatment of metastatic disease. *Cancer Res*, 47, 21, 5725-5732.

Taniguchi, K., Karre, K., and Klein, G. (1985). Lung colonization and metastasis by disseminated B16 melanoma cells: H-2 associated control at the level of the host and the tumor cell. *Int J Cancer*, 36, 4, 503-510.

Terme, M., Ullrich, E., Delahaye, N.F., Chaput, N., and Zitvogel, L. (2008). Natural killer cell-directed therapies: moving from unexpected results to successful strategies. *Nat Immunol*, 9, 5, 486-494.

Thies, A., Moll, I., Berger, J., Wagener, C., Brummer, J., Schulze, H.J., Brunner, G., and Schumacher, U. (2002). CEACAM1 expression in cutaneous malignant melanoma predicts the development of metastatic disease. *J Clin Oncol*, 20, 10, 2530-2536.

Trapani, J.A., Davis, J., Sutton, V.R., and Smyth, M.J. (2000). Proapoptotic functions of cytotoxic lymphocyte granule constituents in vitro and in vivo. *Curr Opin Immunol*, 12, 3, 323-329.

Trinchieri, G. (1998). Interleukin-12: a cytokine at the interface of inflammation and immunity. *Adv Immunol*, 70, 83-243.

Trinchieri, G., and Perussia, B. (1984). Human natural killer cells: biologic and pathologic aspects. *Lab Invest*, 50, 5, 489-513.

Tsao, H., Atkins, M.B., and Sober, A.J. (2004). Management of cutaneous melanoma. *N Engl J Med*, 351, 10, 998-1012.

Vahlne, G., Lindholm, K., Meier, A., Wickstrom, S., Lakshmikanth, T., Brennan, F., Wilken, M., Nielsen, R., Romagne, F., Wagtmann, N.R., Karre, K., and Johansson, M.H. (2010). In vivo tumor cell rejection induced by NK cell inhibitory receptor blockade: maintained tolerance to normal cells even in the presence of IL-2. *Eur J Immunol*, 40, 3, 813-823.

Velardi, A., Ruggeri, L., Mancusi, A., Aversa, F., and Christiansen, F.T. (2009). Natural killer cell allorecognition of missing self in allogeneic hematopoietic transplantation: a tool for immunotherapy of leukemia. *Curr Opin Immunol*, 21, 5, 525-530.

Vetter, C.S., Groh, V., thor Straten, P., Spies, T., Brocker, E.B., and Becker, J.C. (2002). Expression of stress-induced MHC class I related chain molecules on human melanoma. *J Invest Dermatol*, 118, 4, 600-605.

Vetter, C.S., Lieb, W., Brocker, E.B., and Becker, J.C. (2004). Loss of nonclassical MHC molecules MIC-A/B expression during progression of uveal melanoma. *Br J Cancer*, 91, 8, 1495-1499.

Wang, G., Tschoi, M., Spolski, R., Lou, Y., Ozaki, K., Feng, C., Kim, G., Leonard, W.J., and Hwu, P. (2003). In vivo antitumor activity of interleukin 21 mediated by natural killer cells. *Cancer Res*, 63, 24, 9016-9022.

Wang, R.F., and Rosenberg, S.A. (1996). Human tumor antigens recognized by T lymphocytes: implications for cancer therapy. *J Leukoc Biol*, 60, 3, 296-309.

Wen, D.R., Hoon, D.S., Chang, C., and Cochran, A.J. (1989). Variations in lymphokine generation by individual lymph nodes draining human malignant tumors. *Cancer Immunol Immunother*, 30, 5, 277-282.

Whiteman, D.C., Whiteman, C.A., and Green, A.C. (2001). Childhood sun exposure as a risk factor for melanoma: a systematic review of epidemiologic studies. *Cancer Causes Control*, 12, 1, 69-82.

Wiemann, K., Mittrucker, H.W., Feger, U., Welte, S.A., Yokoyama, W.M., Spies, T., Rammensee, H.G., and Steinle, A. (2005). Systemic NKG2D down-regulation impairs NK and CD8 T cell responses in vivo. *J Immunol*, 175, 2, 720-729.

Xu, D., Gu, P., Pan, P.Y., Li, Q., Sato, A.I., and Chen, S.H. (2004). NK and CD8+ T cell-mediated eradication of poorly immunogenic B16-F10 melanoma by the combined action of IL-12 gene therapy and 4-1BB costimulation. *Int J Cancer*, 109, 4, 499-506.

Yajima, T., Nishimura, H., Wajjwalku, W., Harada, M., Kuwano, H., and Yoshikai, Y. (2002). Overexpression of interleukin-15 in vivo enhances antitumor activity against MHC class I-negative and -positive malignant melanoma through augmented NK activity and cytotoxic T-cell response. *Int J Cancer*, 99, 4, 573-578.

Yang, Q., Hokland, M.E., Bryant, J.L., Zhang, Y., Nannmark, U., Watkins, S.C., Goldfarb, R.H., Herberman, R.B., and Basse, P.H. (2003). Tumor-localization by adoptively transferred, interleukin-2-activated NK cells leads to destruction of well-established lung metastases. *Int J Cancer*, 105, 4, 512-519.

Yee, C., Thompson, J.A., Byrd, D., Riddell, S.R., Roche, P., Celis, E., and Greenberg, P.D. (2002). Adoptive T cell therapy using antigen-specific CD8+ T cell clones for the treatment of patients with metastatic melanoma: in vivo persistence, migration, and antitumor effect of transferred T cells. *Proc Natl Acad Sci U S A*, 99, 25, 16168-16173.

Yu, X., Harden, K., Gonzalez, L.C., Francesco, M., Chiang, E., Irving, B., Tom, I., Ivelja, S., Refino, C.J., Clark, H., Eaton, D., and Grogan, J.L. (2009). The surface protein TIGIT suppresses T cell activation by promoting the generation of mature immunoregulatory dendritic cells. *Nat Immunol*, 10, 1, 48-57.

Zaidi, M.R., Davis, S., Noonan, F.P., Graff-Cherry, C., Hawley, T.S., Walker, R.L., Feigenbaum, L., Fuchs, E., Lyakh, L., Young, H.A., Hornyak, T.J., Arnheiter, H., Trinchieri, G., Meltzer, P.S., De Fabo, E.C., and Merlino, G. (2011). Interferon-gamma links ultraviolet radiation to melanomagenesis in mice. *Nature*, 469, 7331, 548-553.

Zitvogel, L., Tesniere, A., and Kroemer, G. (2006). Cancer despite immunosurveillance: immunoselection and immunosubversion. *Nat Rev Immunol*, 6, 10, 715-727.

10

Tumour-Associated Macrophages (TAMs) and Cox-2 Expression in Canine Melanocytic Lesions

Isabel Pires, Justina Prada, LuisCoelho,
Anabela Garcia and Felisbina Luisa Queiroga
CECAV, Department of VeterinarySciences,
Universidade de Trás-os-Montes e Alto Douro
Portugal

1. Introduction

Melanoma is a devastating disease frequently encountered within both veterinary and human medicine. Melanocytic tumours are relatively common in dogs and represent 4 to 7% of all canine neoplasms. It is the most common malignant neoplasm of the oral cavity and the second most frequent subungual neoplasm. Classically, body location is one criteria used to establish a prognosis of these tumours (Martínez et al., 2011; Smith et al., 2002). Cutaneous canine melanocytic lesions are usually benign. However, the canine oropharyngeal, uveal, and mucocutaneous neoplasms are aggressive and have high metastatic potential (Marino et al., 1995; Smith et al., 2002; Spangler & Kass, 2006).

In other animals species melanocytic tumours were also seen, but in cats it is not as common and carries a poor prognosis (Dorn&Priester, 1976; Goldschmidt, 1985). In white or gray horses melanoma is very common, considered almost inevitable (Johnson, 1998; Valentine, 1995). In pigs, melanoma is very frequent in some breeds, as Sinclair (Berkelhammer&Hook, 1980; Hook et al., 1982; Misfeldt & Grimm, 1994).

Generally, cutaneous melanoma in domestic animals does not share the same degree of diversity described in the medical literature. Canine cutaneous melanoma can be either benign (melanocytoma) or malignant (melanoma) and are most common in older animals with darker coats. The benign form is often referred to as melanocytic nevus or melanocytoma, and is well-defined, firm, dome-shaped, with less than 2 cm in diameter and mobile. Malignant melanomas are less frequent in the skin and appear ulcerated with a rapid grow. Most oral and mucocutaneous (except eyelid) and 50% of nail bed (subungual) melanomas are malignant (Smith et al., 2002)

Unlike humans, dogs do not seem to develop malignant melanomas due to exposure to ionizing solar radiation. With the exception of gray horses, malignant transformation of benign lesions is very uncommon in animals, and most melanomas are believed to arised "*de novo*" from melanocytes in the epidermis, dermis, ocular epithelium, and oral epithelium (Conroy, 1967; Smith et al., 2002). However, little is known about initiation of most animal melanomas. Breed and familial clustering in domestic animals suggest that genetic susceptibility, possibly resulting in a greater frequency of spontaneously mutated cells, may be critical to initiation of many of these tumours (Goldschmidt, 1985; Smith et al., 2002). Conroy described two canine cases of melanoma that arose from junctional or dermal pigmented nevi (hamartomas), although in neither case was metastatic behavior observed (Conroy, 1967). There is a single report of a primary melanoma in the skin of a dog that originated from a subcutaneous melanocytoma (Mulligan, 1961).

Cutaneous melanoma is the group of melanocytic lesions that constitute the big challenge to pathologist. The majority of the cases are benign but can be find malignant melanomas with elevated aggressiveness. Mitotic rate is highly predictive of the degree of malignancy and a mitotic rate of less than 3 per 10 high-power fields is strongly associated with benign behavior (Smith et al., 2002). Additional analysis by flow cytometry has shown a correlation between DNA ploidy and malignancy (Bolon et al., 1990). In the last years, several prognostic factors related to proliferation (Laprie et al., 2001; Roels et al., 1999), angiogenesis (Mukaratirwa et al., 2006; Taylor et al., 2007), apoptosis (Roels et al., 2001), and others have been investigated.

The incidence of melanocytic lesions is increasing among canine population. Canine malignant melanoma could have an aggressive behavior, metastasize early in the course of the disease and is resistant to most current therapeutic regimens. The role of a vaccine and the search of novel therapeutic tools are essential in the fight against this devastating disease. Furthermore, the similarities between human and canine melanoma make spontaneous canine melanoma an excellent disease model for studying the correspondent human disease (Bergman et al., 2006; Smith et al., 2002; von Euler et al., 2008).

Inflammation in tumour stroma greatly influences its development. In human cancer it has been described that tumour associated macrophages (TAMs) may promote tumour cell invasiveness and potentiate metastatic diffusion. Among the various inflammatory mediators generated by TAM, assume particular relevance the arachidonic acid metabolites, which are known to influence several biological responses involved in tumour progression, such as inflammatory and immune reactions, haemostasis and angiogenesis. Although the scientific evidence of an association between TAM and histological aggressiveness in human melanoma (Bianchini et al., 2007; Brocker et al., 1987), in the dog there are no studies concerning this subject.

Cyclooxigenase (-1 and -2) are isoenzymes that promote the transition of arachidonic acid in to different prostanoids. These isoenzymes are also the main targets of the NSAIDs (non steroid anti-inflammatory drugs). Several studies have been suggested the potential role of NSAID blocking particularly cyclo-oxygenases-2 (Cox-2) in the prevention and treatment of malignant tumours in humans (Cerella et al., 2010; Dubois et al., 1998). In dogs, there are evidences of a strong relationship between Cox-2 expression and malignancy in several types of cancers (bladder, skin, intestinal, mammary, bone, nasal) (Mohammed et al., 2004; Queiroga et al., 2007). Cox-1 and Cox-2 expression in canine melanocytic lesions has been recently published by the authors, describing that Cox-2 expression was restricted to the malignant melanoma group, being found in 11 of the 20 cutaneous malignant melanomas, in all oral malignant melanomas and in one of two ocular malignant melanomas analyzed. Authors also found that Cox-2 labeling was particularly intense in the more aggressive oral tumours (Pires et al., 2010). In human melanoma, Cox-2 has been implied in tumour progression (Chwirot&Kuzbicki, 2007; Kuzbicki et al., 2006).

The aims of the present work were: a) to describe, the number and the distribution of TAMs in canine melanocytic lesions; b) to investigate associations between TAMs and several clinicopathological characteristics; c) investigate the possible association between Cox-2 expression and the presence of TAMs in these tumours.

2. Material and methods

2.1 Tissue processing and tumour classification

Thirty seven melanocytic tumours, obtained from the UTAD Histopathology Laboratory archives were included. For the histopathologic study, 4-μm-thick tissue sections were stained with the hematoxylin and eosin with and without blanching by incubation in 0,25% potassium permanganate for 30-60 minutes, depending on the amount of pigment and then by incubation in 0,1% oxalic acid for 5-8 minutes. Each sample was re-examined by two independent pathologists (IP and JP) in order to confirm the diagnosis, according to the World Health Organization International Histological Classification of Tumours of Domestic Animals criteria (Goldschmidt et al., 1998).

2.2 Clinicopathological evaluation

The following clinicopathological features were evaluated: histological type-melanocytoma (benign), melanoma (malign); presence of ulceration; presence of necrosis; mitotic index; nuclear grade; degree of pigmentation, presence of aberrant tumoural cells; stroma; and tumoural vascular invasion. Mitotic index was calculated by counting all the mitosis present in 10 high power fields (HPF) (400x): mitotic index I (<3 mitosis in 10 HPF); mitotic index II (3-5 mitosis in 10 HPF) or mitotic index III (>5 mitosis in 10 HPF). For nuclear grade, the following grades were defined: (i) nuclear grade I when the nuclei had minimal variations in their shape and size compared to normal nuclei; (ii) nuclear grade II consisted of moderate alterations of nuclear shape; and (iii) nuclear grade III consisted of the nuclei that were irregular and larger than normal (Queiroga et al., 2010).The degree of pigmentation was estimated using a subjective scale from scant (pigment in fewer than 30% of cells), moderate (pigmentation in 31-80% of cells), and abundant (pigment in more than 80% of cells). The amount of stroma was categorized in: scant, moderate, and abundant (Ramos-Vara et al., 2000).

2.3 Immunohistochemistry

For immunohistochemical studies, 3-μm sections were cut from each specimen and mounted on silane-coated slides. MAC 387 (for macrophage immunolabelling) and Cox-2 immunoexpression were carried out by the streptavidin-biotin-peroxidase complex method, with a commercial detection system (Ultra Vision Detection System; Lab Vision Corporation, Fremont, USA) following the manufacturer's instructions, with and without blanching. Antigen retrieval was by microwave treatment in citrate buffer (pH 6.0) three times for 5 min each in a 750 W microwave oven, followed by cooling for 20 min at room temperature.

Primary antibodies were: MAC 387 (AbDSerotec, MorphoSys UK Ltd., Kidlington, Oxford,U.K.; Clone MCA 874G) diluted 1 in 100 in PBS and applied for 1 h at room temperature and COX-2 (Transduction Laboratories, Lexington, Kentucky; clone 33) diluted 1 in 40 in phosphate buffered saline (PBS; pH 7.4, 0.01 M) and applied overnight at 4°C.

Immunoreaction was visualized by incubation with 3,3'-diaminobenzidine tetrahydrochloride (DAB) at 0.05% with 0.01% H_2O_2 as the final substrate for 5 minutes. After a final washing in distilled water, the sections were counterstained with haematoxylin, dehydrated, cleared and mounted.

The primary antibody was replaced by PBS and by an irrelevant antibody for negative controls. Positive controls consisted of canine epidermis and liver for MAC 387 and sections from *macula densa* of young normal canine kidney for Cox-2.

2.4 Immunohistochemistry evaluation

Positivity was indicated by the presence of distinct brown cytoplasmic labeling. Immunoreactivity was evaluated "blindly" by two observers (IP e FLQ).

TAMs were counted in the three regions with more intense and homogeneous positivity of each of counting areas (Hussein et al., 2009). In these regions, we counted all labeled cells, evaluating a total of ten high-power fields (HPF), (400x magnification power). TAM were then categorized in three classes: 1: <20 positive macrophages (sparse); 2: 20-100 (moderate), 3: >100 positive macrophages (intense) (Piras et al., 2005).

Positive Cox-2 expression was defined when more than 10% of the tumour cells showed positive staining. The staining intensity was not scored in this method.

2.5 Statistical analysis

The statistical software SPSS version 12.0 was used for statistical analysis. The Chi-square test and the Fisher's exact test were used for studying categorical variables. In all statistical comparisons, $p < 0.05$ was accepted as denoting significant differences.

3. Results

3.1 Tumours

From the 37 tumours included in the study, 8 cases were classified as melanocytomas (benign tumours) and 29 cases as malignant melanomas (malignant tumours, Fig.1).

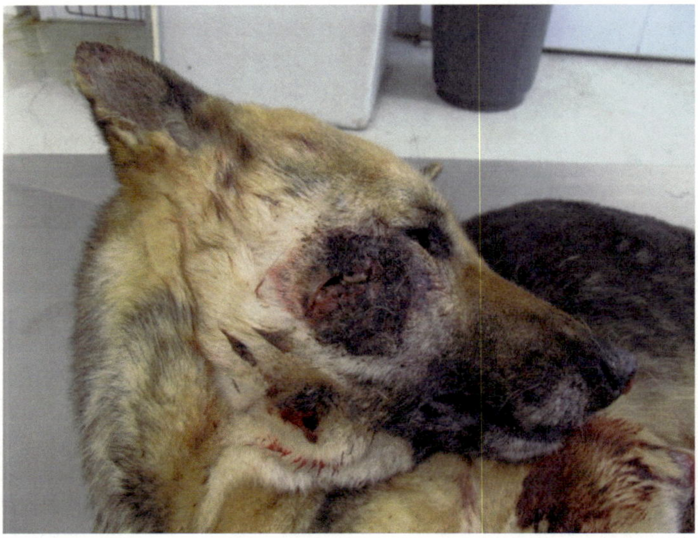

Fig. 1. Cutaneous malignant melanoma in a German Shepard dog.

3.2 Tumour- associated macrophages (TAMs) in canine melanocytic tumours

MAC 387 immunostaining was always observed in the cytoplasm of macrophages in a diffuse and homogeneous pattern. The upper layers of epidermis also stained with MAC 387.

TAMs were observed in all the samples analyzed (n=37). As shown in Table 1, all the benign lesions had sparse macrophage infiltration, while malignant melanomas presented a moderate or intense infiltration (Fig.2 and Fig.3). The number of tumoural-associated macrophages in malignant melanoma was significantly higher than the mean values in the benign counterparts (p=0,002).

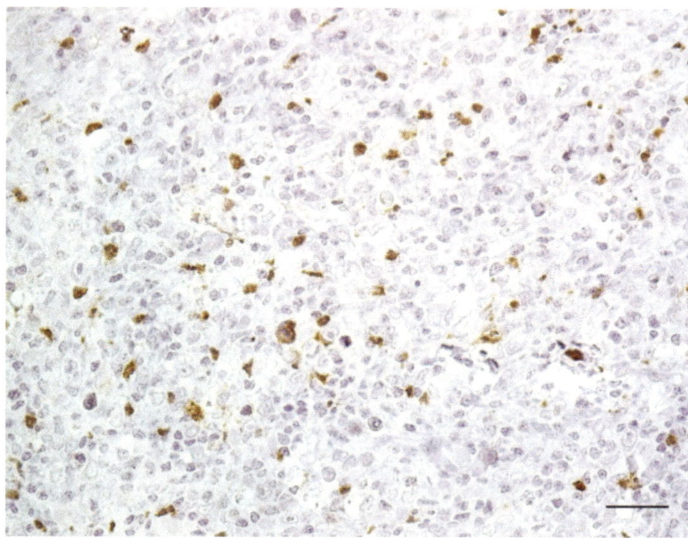

Fig. 2. Canine malignant melanoma showing a moderate number of TAMs. IHC. Bar, 30 mm.

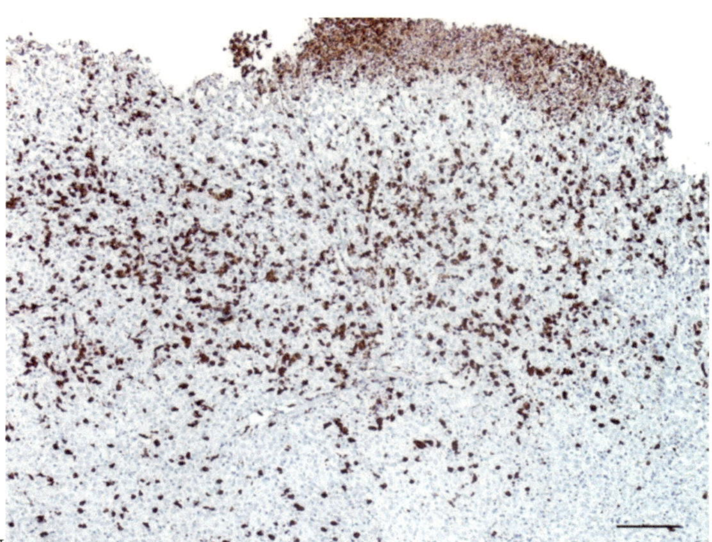

Fig. 3. Intense infiltration of macrophages in a cutaneous melanoma. IHC. Bar, 120 μm.

3.3 Cox-2 expression in canine melanocytic tumours

The expression of COX-2 was absent in 18/37 (48,6%) of the canine melanocytic tumours (Fig. 4). None of the 8 benign tumours expressed Cox-2 in tumoural cells. Among the malignant tumours, COX-2 was expressed by 19 of the 29 melanomas (65,5%), (Fig. 5 e Fig. 6). There was a significant difference in COX-2 expression between melanocytomas and malignant melanomas (p < 0,001).

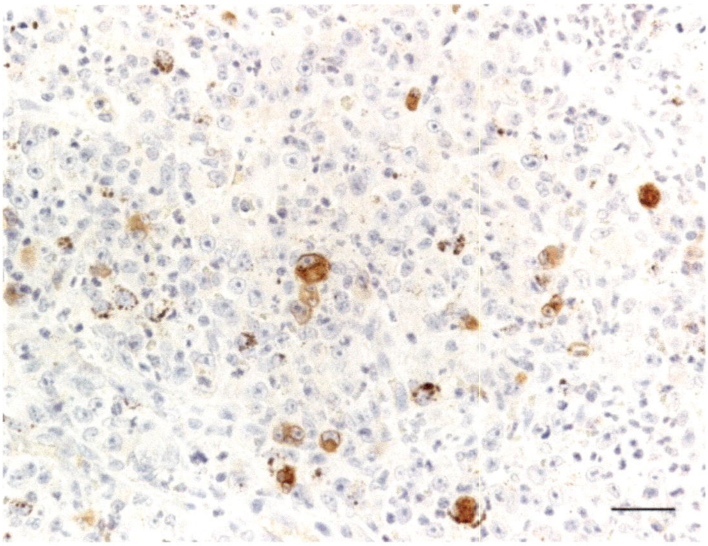

Fig. 4. Cutaneous malignant melanoma considered negative to Cox-2 (less than 10% of positive cells). IHC. Bar, 30 μm.

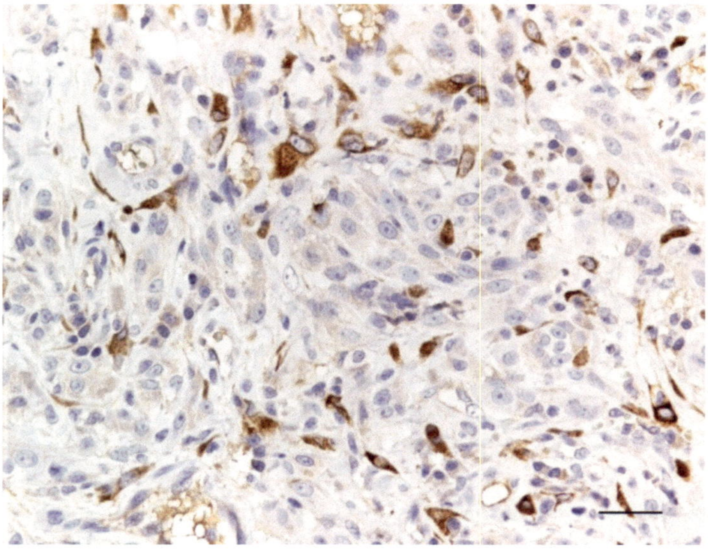

Fig. 5. Cox-2 expression in canine malignant melanoma. IHC. Bar, 30 μm.

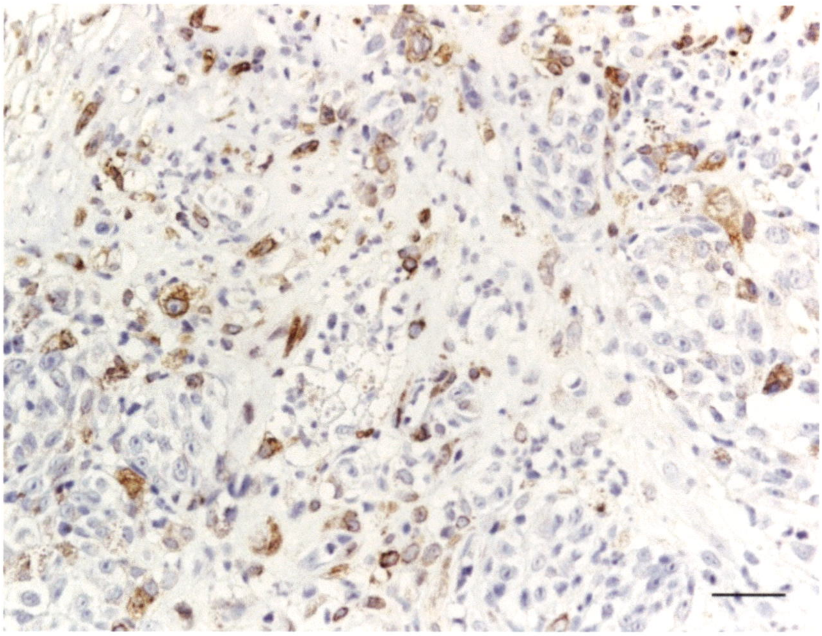

Fig. 6. Cox-2 expression in canine melanoma; positive cells invading epidermis. IHC. Bar, 30 μm.

3.4 Association between TAMs and COX-2 and clinicopathological features in canine melanocytic tumours

Table 1 presents the clinicopathological variables analyzed and its association with TAM and Cox-2 expression in canine melanocytic tumours.

The number of TAMs presented a statistical significant association with the presence of ulceration (p<0,001), presence of necrosis (0,001), nuclear grade (p=0,046), degree of pigmentation (p<0,001), tumoural aberrant cells (p=0,014), stroma (p=0,018) and tumoural embolus (p=0,011). Canine melanocytictumours with ulceration, necrosis, with a high nuclear grade, less pigmented, with the presence of tumoural aberrant cells, with a scarce or moderate stroma and with vascular invasion have a high number of macrophages associated to the tumour.

COX-2 expression was associated with ulceration (p=0,005), necrosis (p=0,003), mitotic index (p=0,029), nuclear grade (p=0,035) and degree of pigmentation (p=0,001). Cox-2 expression was observed in tumours with epithelium ulceration, necrosis, high mitotic index and nuclear grade and in less pigmented neoplasms.

3.5 Association of TAMs and COX-2 in canine melanocytic tumours

There was a significant association between the number of TAMs and COX-2 expression in canine melanocytic tumours (p=0,006). Cox2 positive tumours had a high number of TAMs. Among Cox- negative tumours, only 3 out of 18 tumours had a moderate or abundant number of TAMs. Considering only malignant melanomas, in spite of Cox-2 positive tumours had more TAMs than Cox-2 negative tumours, the association was not statistical significant.

Clinicopathological features	TAMs 1	TAMs 2	TAMs 3	p	Cox-2 -	Cox-2 +	p
Histological classification							
Melanocytoma	8	0	0	**0,020**	8	0	**0,001**
Melanoma	13	10	6		10	19	
Ulceration							
Absent	15	1	0	**<0,001**	12	4	**0,005**
Present	6	9	6		6	15	
Necrosis							
Absent	18	6	0	**0,001**	16	8	**0,003**
Present	3	4	6		2	11	
Mitotic index							
I	9	2	10	0,308	9	2	**0,029**
II	2	1	7		1	3	
III	10	7	5		8	14	
Nuclear grade							
I	10	3	0	**0,046**	10	3	**0,035**
II	2	3	2		5	8	
III	3	4	4		3	8	
Degree of pigmentation							
Scant	0	10	11	**<0,001**	1	11	**0,001**
Moderate	10	1	2		6	6	
Abundant	11	1	0		11	2	
Aberrant cells							
Absent	19	7	2	**0,014**	16	12	0,068
Present	2	3	9		2	7	
Stroma							
Scarse	3	7	2	**0,018**	4	10	0,154
Moderate	16	3	0		13	8	
Abundant	2	0	0		1	1	
Vascular invasion							
Absent	19	8	2	**0,011**	16	13	0,232
Present	2	2	4		2	6	

Table 1. Association of clinicopathological variables with TAMs and Cox-2 in canine melanocytic tumours.

Clinicopathological features	TAMs 1	2	3	p	Cox-2 -	+	p
Ulceration							
Absent	7	1	0	**0,016**	4	4	0,390
Present	6	9	6		6	15	
Necrosis							
Absent	10	6	0	**0,007**	8	8	0,114
Present	3	4	6		2	11	
Mitotic index							
I	1	2	0	0,760	1	2	**0,029**
II	2	1	1		1	3	
III	10	7	5		8	14	
Nuclear grade							
I	1	8	3	0,235	2	3	0,814
II	2	3	4		5	8	
III	10	2	4		3	8	
Degree of pigmentation							
Scant	0	7	5	**<0,001**	1	11	**0,031**
Moderate	9	1	1		5	6	
Abundant	4	2	0		4	2	
Aberrant cells							
Absent	11	7	2	0,08	8	12	0,431
Present	2	3	4		2	7	
Stroma							
Scarse	3	7	4	0,165	4	10	0,555
Moderate	9	3	2		6	8	
Abundant	1	0	0		0	1	
Vascular invasion							
Absent	11	8	2	**0,049**	8	2	0,675
Present	2	2	4		13	6	

Table 2. Association of clinicopathological variables with TAMs and Cox-2 in canine malignant melanomas.

4. Discussion

Melanoma is relatively common in dogs, accounting for 3% of all neoplasms and up to 7% of all malignant tumours. Melanocytic neoplasms that arise in the oral cavity, one of the most frequent localization of melanocytic tumours in dog, are virtually always considered malignant and constitute the most common oral malignant neoplasm (Smith et al., 2002). Much work is currently underway in to try and identify specific tumour markers, associated with malignancy. However, more studies are needed to differentiating canine benign from malignant melanocytic neoplasms or predicting survival times.

4.1 TAMs in canine melanocytic tumours

It has long been thought that inflammation and carcinogenesis are related (Le Bitoux&Stamenkovic, 2008). Macrophages belong to the innate immune system and as such constitute one of the first barriers against infection. Depending on the activation state of the macrophage, this antigen presentation may trigger a full-blown active immune response, or may suppress a potential immune reaction (Jager et al., 2011). The role of macrophages in tumour growth and development is complex and multifaceted. Whilst there is limited evidence that TAMs can be directly tumouricidal and stimulate the anti-tumour activity of T cells, there is now contrasting evidence that tumour cells are able to block or evade the activity of TAMs at the tumour site. In some cases, tumour-derived molecules even redirect TAMs activities to promote tumour survival and growth (Bingle et al., 2002).

In our study, TAMs were observed in all tumours analyzed. Melanocytomas presented few macrophages, while malignant melanoma showed generally moderate or intense macrophage infiltration. Higher number of TAMs has been associated with malignancy in different types of human tumours (Siveen&Kuttan, 2009), as breast carcinomas (Leek et al., 1996) and gliomas (Nishie et al., 1999). In human cutaneous melanoma (Torisu et al., 2000), uveal melanoma (Toivonen et al., 2004) and sinonasal melanoma (Shi et al., 2010) a high number of TAMs was closely associated with bad tumour phenotypes. These observations were in accordance with our results in canine melanocytic lesions.

In canine melanocytic tumours, a higher number of TAMs appears associated, in a statistical significant way, with ulceration ($p<0,001$), necrosis (0,001), nuclear grade ($p=0,046$), degree of pigmentation ($p<0,001$), tumoural aberrant cells ($p=0,014$), stroma ($p=0,018$) and tumoural embolus ($p=0,011$). Even considering only malignant melanomas, an association was noted between TMAs and ulceration ($p=0,016$), histological necrosis ($p=0,007$), degree of pigmentation ($p=<0,001$) and presence of vascular invasion by tumoural cells ($p=0,049$). Interestingly most of these characteristics are classically linked to higher tumoural aggressiveness and poor clinical prognosis in these neoplasias. TAMs could constitute an important marker of canine melanocytic aggressiveness; however, studies with prognostic are needed to clarify this subject.

The statistical significant association observed between tumoural necrosis and a high number of TAMs in malignant melanomas is not surprising. Indeed, in human cancer, evidence has emerged for a symbiotic relationship between tumour cells and TAMs. The pathways involved in this crosstalk could imply a response to micro-environmental factors such as hypoxia, as well as various growth factors and enzymes that stimulate tumour angiogenesis (Bingle et al., 2002). Many macrophage products released in the tumour stroma can directly stimulate the growth of tumour cells and/or promote tumour cell migration and metastasis. These include, for instance, the epidermal growth factor (EGF), cytokines like IL-6 and TNF, as well as chemokines such as CXCL12. TAMs contribute to tumour progression also by producing several factors which enhance neo-angiogenesis and the dissolution and remodeling of the interstitial matrix. Moreover TAMs are a source of potent immunosuppressive molecules, such as IL-10 and PGE2, contributing to the tumour immune-evasion (Allavena et al., 2008; Mantovani et al., 2002; Van Ginderachter et al., 2006). It is probably that similar mechanisms occur also in canine malignant melanomas.

4.2 Cox-2 labeling in canine melanocytic tumours

Cox-2 is a key enzyme controlling the conversion of arachidonic acid to prostaglandin H2, the precursor of various molecules, including prostaglandins, prostacyclins and tromboxanes. Cox-2 is commonly undetectable in normal tissues, but can be induced through several stimuli, including mitogens, growth factors, hormones, and cytokines (Dubois et al., 1998). In recent years, many molecular pathways have been suggested to explain how increased Cox-2 and the resultant prostaglandin overproduction might contribute to carcinogenesis (Hu et al., 2009; Singh-Ranger et al., 2008; Wu&Liou, 2009). These pathways included stimulation of tumoural angiogenesis, decreased tumoural apoptosis, increased invasion and metastasis, immune suppression and tumour associated inflammation (Ghosh et al., 2010). Various studies indicate a link between high Cox-2 expression and malignancy in both human (Balan et al., 2011; Costa et al., 2002; Lee et al., 2011) and canine tumours (Queiroga et al., 2007; Queiroga et al., 2010). In the dog, Cox-2 "up-regulation" has been investigated in different tumours, including prostate (L'Eplattenier et al., 2007), ovarian (Borzacchiello et al., 2007), bladder (Khan et al., 2000), intestinal (McEntee et al., 2002), mammary (Queiroga et al., 2005; Queiroga et al., 2007; Dias Pereira et al., 2009), nasal carcinomas (Impellizeri & Esplin, 2008) and sarcomas, including osteosarcoma and oral fibrosarcoma (Heller et al., 2005; Mullins et al., 2004). In human cancer, Cox-2 expression has been detected in a considerable number of epithelial tumours as breast, lung, colon, prostate, head and neck, gastric, ovary, among many others (Ghosh et al., 2010; Menczer, 2009; Wu et al., 2010).

Concerning malignant melanoma, in humans it was recently reported that changes in Cox-2 expression levels were correlated with development and progression of human melanoma (Goulet et al., 2003; Kuzbicki et al., 2006). COX-2 expression arises as a potential immunohistochemical marker for distinguishing human cutaneous melanomas from benign melanocytic lesions (Minami et al., 2011; Pires et al., 2010). Additionally, Cox-2 expression appears as a useful prognostic marker being related with histological and clinical malignant melanoma aggressiveness (Becker et al., 2009).

In canine melanocytic tumours, Cox-2 expression was recently described (Paglia et al., 2009; Pires et al., 2010). Cox-2 over-expression was related with a tumoural malignant behavior (Pires et al., 2010) and with a poor overall survival (Martínez et al., 2011). In the present work, Cox-2 expression was associated with ulceration (p=0,005), necrosis (p=0,003), mitotic index (p=0,029), nuclear grade (p=0,035) and degree of pigmentation (p=0,001). These associations could represent the higher aggressiveness of Cox-2 positive melanocytic tumours. Curiously, these associations lost their statistical significance when we consider for statistical analysis only the group of malignant melanomas. However, an association with mitotic index is observed, that suggests that Cox-2 is associated with a higher cellular proliferation. The real significance of these results needs to be clarified. Clinical studies, with follow-up information and proliferation markers will be necessary to clarify if Cox-2 could be more important in early phases of carcinogenesis or also in tumour progression.

4.3 Relationship between TAMs and Cox-2 expression in canine melanocytic tumours

Tumour associated macrophages and high COX-2 expression have been both associated with malignancy in canine melanocytic tumours, but their potential interdependence has not yet been evaluated. The present study showed that there is a close relationship between TAMs and Cox-2 expression in canine melanocytic lesions. This is the first time, to our best knowledge, that a similar relationship was investigated in tumours of domestic animals. This crosstalk is referred in human tumours, as colorectal carcinoma (Naghshvar et al., 2009), urotelial carcinoma (Chen et al., 2009), basal cell carcinoma (Tjiu et al., 2009) and in breast cancer cells (Hou et al., 2011). The pathways involved in this relationship are diverse, and remain to be completed elucidated. In human basal cell carcinoma, macrophages induced COX-2-dependent release of matrix metalloproteinase-9 and subsequent increased invasion and induced COX-2-dependent secretion of basic fibroblast growth factor and vascular endothelial growth factor-A, and increased angiogenesis (Tjiu et al., 2009). Macrophage-mediated induction of COX-2 in breast cancer cells is a consequence of IL-1β-mediated stimulation of ROS→Src→MAP kinase→AP-1 signaling. IL-1β-dependent induction of COX-2 in breast cancer cells provides a mechanism whereby macrophages contribute to tumour progression (Hou et al., 2011). Another mechanism proposed could involve Cox-2 induced angiogenesis through increasing TAM infiltration or hypoxia-inducible factor-1alpha by hypoxia (Chen et al., 2009).

Considering only malignant melanomas, the association was not significant that could suggested that this cross-talk (between TAMs and Cox-2 positive tumoural cells) could be decisive in carcinogenesis but not in tumour progression. Only more studies could help to investigate the meaning of these findings. In turn, in human oral squamous cell carcinoma, Cox-2 and TAMs are not related (Boas et al., 2010).

The development of therapeutic targeting of cancer promoting inflammatory reactions is crucially dependent on defining the underlying cellular and molecular mechanisms in relevant systems (Allavena et al., 2008). By inhibiting the release of prostaglandins from the tumour and by blocking COX activity in immune effector cells, NSAIDs may also bias the function of immune cells towards a more tumouricidal phenotype (Lang et al., 2006).

5. Conclusion

In conclusion, this study presents a close relationship of TAM and Cox-2 expression in canine melanocytic lesions. It is possible that proinflammatory cytokines released by intratumoural macrophages, up-regulate Cox-2 tumour cells expression stimulating tumour progression. Additionally, the differences observed between benign and malignant melanocytic lesions may suggest that TAM and Cox-2 are implicated in the progression of melanocytic precursor lesions to malignant melanoma.

6. Acknowledgment

The authors thank Mrs. Lígia Bento for expert technical assistance.

7. References

Allavena, P., Sica, A., Solinas, G., Porta, C.&Mantovani, A. (2008). The inflammatory micro-environment in tumor progression: the role of tumor-associated macrophages. *Critical Reviews Oncology Hematology*, Vol. 66, No. 1, (April 2008), pp. 1-9, ISSN 1040-8428

Balan, R., Amalinei, C., Giusca, S. E., Ditescu, D., Gheorghita, V., Crauciuc, E.&Caruntu, I. D. (2011). Immunohistochemical evaluation of COX-2 expression in HPV-positive cervical squamous intraepithelial lesions. *Romanian Journal of Morphology Embryology*, Vol. 52, No. 1, 2011), pp. 39-43, ISSN 1220-0522

Becker, M. R., Siegelin, M. D., Rompel, R., Enk, A. H.&Gaiser, T. (2009). COX-2 expression in malignant melanoma: a novel prognostic marker? *Melanoma Research*, Vol. 19, No. 1, (February 2009), pp. 8-16, ISSN 1473-5636

Bergman, P. J., Camps-Palau, M. A., McKnight, J. A., Leibman, N. F., Craft, D. M., Leung, C., Liao, J., Riviere, I., Sadelain, M., Hohenhaus, A. E., Gregor, P., Houghton, A. N., Perales, M. A.&Wolchok, J. D. (2006). Development of a xenogeneic DNA vaccine program for canine malignant melanoma at the Animal Medical Center. *Vaccine*, Vol. 24, No. 21, (May 22 2006), pp. 4582-5, ISSN 0264-410X

Berkelhammer, J.&Hook, R. R., Jr. (1980). Growth of Sinclair swine melanoma in the hamster cheek pouch. *Transplantation*, Vol. 29, No. 3, (March 1980), pp. 193-5, ISSN 0041-1337

Bianchini, F., Massi, D., Marconi, C., Franchi, A., Baroni, G., Santucci, M., Mannini, A., Mugnai, G.&Calorini, L. (2007). Expression of cyclo-oxygenase-2 in macrophages associated with cutaneous melanoma at different stages of progression. *Prostaglandins & Other Lipid Mediators*, Vol. 83, No. 4, (June 2007), pp. 320-8,

Bingle, L., Brown, N. J.&Lewis, C. E. (2002). The role of tumour-associated macrophages in tumour progression: implications for new anticancer therapies. *Journal of Pathology*, Vol. 196, No. 3, (March 2002), pp. 254-65, ISSN 0022-3417

Boas, D. S., Takiya, C. M., Coelho-Sampaio, T. L., Moncao-Ribeiro, L. C., Ramos, E. A., Cabral, M. G.&dos Santos, J. N. (2010). Immunohistochemical detection of Ki-67 is not associated with tumor-infiltrating macrophages and cyclooxygenase-2 in oral squamous cell carcinoma. *Journal of Oral Pathology & Medicine*, Vol. 39, No. 7, (August 2010), pp. 565-70, ISSN 1600-0714

Bolon, B., Calderwood Mays, M. B.&Hall, B. J. (1990). Characteristics of canine melanomas and comparison of histology and DNA ploidy to their biologic behavior. *Veterinary Pathology*, Vol. 27, No. 2, (March 1990), pp. 96-102, ISSN 0300-9858

Borzacchiello, G., Russo, V.&Russo, M. (2007). Immunohistochemical expression of cyclooxygenase-2 in canine ovarian carcinomas. *Journal of Veterinary Medicine Series A*, Vol. 54, No. 5, (Jun 2007), pp. 247-9, ISSN 1439-0442

Brocker, E. B., Zwadlo, G., Suter, L., Brune, M.&Sorg, C. (1987). Infiltration of primary and metastatic melanomas with macrophages of the 25F9-positive phenotype. *Cancer Immunology & Immunotherapy*, Vol. 25, No. 2, 1987), pp. 81-6,

Cerella, C., Sobolewski, C., Dicato, M.&Diederich, M. (2010). Targeting COX-2 expression by natural compounds: a promising alternative strategy to synthetic COX-2 inhibitors for cancer chemoprevention and therapy. *Biochemical Pharmacology*, Vol. 80, No. 12, (December 15 2010), pp. 1801-15,

Chen, W. T., Hung, W. C., Kang, W. Y., Huang, Y. C., Su, Y. C., Yang, C. H.&Chai, C. Y. (2009). Overexpression of cyclooxygenase-2 in urothelial carcinoma in conjunction with tumor-associated-macrophage infiltration, hypoxia-inducible factor-1alpha expression, and tumor angiogenesis. *APMIS*, Vol. 117, No. 3, (March 2009), pp. 176-84, ISSN 1600-0463

Chwirot, B. W.&Kuzbicki, L. (2007). Cyclooxygenase-2 (COX-2): first immunohistochemical marker distinguishing early cutaneous melanomas from benign melanocytic skin tumours. *Melanoma Research*, Vol. 17, No. 3, (June 2007), pp. 139-45,

Conroy, J. D. (1967). Melanocytic tumors of domestic animals with special reference to dogs. *Archives of Dermatology*, Vol. 96, No. 4, (October 1967), pp. 372-80, ISSN 0003-987X

Conroy, J. D. (1967). Melanocytic tumors of domestic animals with special reference to dogs. *Archives of Dermatology*, Vol. 96, No. 4, (October 1967), pp. 372-80, ISSN 0003-987X

Costa, C., Soares, R., Reis-Filho, J. S., Leitao, D., Amendoeira, I.&Schmitt, F. C. (2002). Cyclo-oxygenase 2 expression is associated with angiogenesis and lymph node metastasis in human breast cancer. *Journal of Clinical Pathology*, Vol. 55, No. 6, (June 2002), pp. 429-34, ISSN 0021-9746

Dias Pereira, P., Lopes, C. C., Matos, A. J., Santos, M., Gartner, F., Medeiros, R.&Lopes, C. (2009). COX-2 Expression in Canine Normal and Neoplastic Mammary Gland. *Journal of Comparative Pathology*, Vol.140, No.4. (May 2009),

Dorn, C. R.&Priester, W. A. (1976). Epidemiologic analysis of oral and pharyngeal cancer in dogs, cats, horses, and cattle. *Journal of the American Veterinary Medical Association*, Vol. 169, No. 11, (December 1 1976), pp. 1202-6, ISSN 0003-1488

Dubois, R. N., Abramson, S. B., Crofford, L., Gupta, R. A., Simon, L. S., Van De Putte, L. B.&Lipsky, P. E. (1998). Cyclooxygenase in biology and disease. *Faseb Journal*, Vol. 12, No. 12, (September 1998), pp. 1063-73,

Ghosh, N., Chaki, R., Mandal, V.&Mandal, S. C. (2010). COX-2 as a target for cancer chemotherapy. *Pharmacological Reports*, Vol. 62, No. 2, (March-April 2010), pp. 233-44, ISSN 1734-1140

Goldschmidt, M., Dunstan, R.&Stannard, A. (1998). *Histological Classifcation of Epithelial and Melanocytic Tumors of the Skin of Domestic Animals (WHO International Classification of Tumors of Domestic Animals,* Armed Forces Institute of Pathology, American Registry of Pathology, Washington D.C.

Goldschmidt, M. H. (1985). Benign and malignant melanocytic neoplasms of domestic animals. *American Journal of Dermatopathology*, Vol. 7 Suppl, No. 1985), pp. 203-12, ISSN 0193-1091

Goulet, A. C., Einsphar, J. G., Alberts, D. S., Beas, A., Burk, C., Bhattacharyya, A., Bangert, J., Harmon, J. M., Fujiwara, H., Koki, A.&Nelson, M. A. (2003). Analysis of cyclooxygenase 2 (COX-2) expression during malignant melanoma progression. *Cancer Biology & Therapy*, Vol. 2, No. 6, (November-December 2003), pp. 713-8,

Heller, D. A., Clifford, C. A., Goldschmidt, M. H., Holt, D. E., Manfredi, M. J.&Sorenmo, K. U. (2005). Assessment of cyclooxygenase-2 expression in canine hemangiosarcoma, histiocytic sarcoma, and mast cell tumor. *Veterinary Pathology*, Vol. 42, No. 3, (May 2005), pp. 350-3,

Hook, R. R., Jr., Berkelhammer, J.&Oxenhandler, R. W. (1982). Melanoma: Sinclair swine melanoma. *American Journal of Pathology*, Vol. 108, No. 1, (July 1982), pp. 130-3, ISSN 0002-9440

Hou, Z., Falcone, D. J., Subbaramaiah, K.&Dannenberg, A. J. (2011). Macrophages induce COX-2 expression in breast cancer cells: Role of IL-1{beta} auto-amplification. *Carcinogenesis*, [Epub ahead of print] (February 10 2011), ISSN 1460-2180

Hu, M., Peluffo, G., Chen, H., Gelman, R., Schnitt, S.&Polyak, K. (2009). Role of COX-2 in epithelial-stromal cell interactions and progression of ductal carcinoma in situ of the breast. *Proceedings of the National Academy of Sciences U S A*, Vol. 106, No. 9, (March 3 2009), pp. 3372-7, ISSN 1091-6490

Hussein, M. R., Al-Assiri, M.&Musalam, A. O. (2009). Phenotypic characterization of the infiltrating immune cells in normal prostate, benign nodular prostatic hyperplasia and prostatic adenocarcinoma. *Experimental Molecular Pathology*, Vol. 86, No. 2, (April 2009), pp. 108-13,

Impellizeri, J. A.&Esplin, D. G. (2008). Expression of cyclooxygenase-2 in canine nasal carcinomas. *Veterinary Journal*, Vol. 176, No. 3, (June 2008), pp. 408-10,

Jager, M. J., Ly, L. V., El Filali, M.&Madigan, M. C. (2011). Macrophages in uveal melanoma and in experimental ocular tumor models: Friends or foes? *Progress in Retin and Eye Research*, Vol. 30, No. 2, (March 2011), pp. 129-46, ISSN 1873-1635

Johnson, P. J. (1998). Dermatologic tumors (excluding sarcoids). *Veterinary Clinics of North America Equine Practice*, Vol. 14, No. 3, (December 1998), pp. 625-58, ISSN 0749-0739

Khan, K. N., Knapp, D. W., Denicola, D. B.&Harris, R. K. (2000). Expression of cyclooxygenase-2 in transitional cell carcinoma of the urinary bladder in dogs. *American Journal of Veterinary Research*, Vol. 61, No. 5, (May 2000), pp. 478-81,

Kuzbicki, L., Sarnecka, A.&Chwirot, B. W. (2006). Expression of cyclooxygenase-2 in benign naevi and during human cutaneous melanoma progression. *Melanoma Research*, Vol. 16, No. 1, (February 2006), pp. 29-36,

L'Eplattenier, H. F., Lai, C. L., van den Ham, R., Mol, J., van Sluijs, F.&Teske, E. (2007). Regulation of COX-2 expression in canine prostate carcinoma: increased COX-2 expression is not related to inflammation. *Journal of Veterinary Internal Medicine*, Vol. 21, No. 4, (July-August 2007), pp. 776-82,

Lang, S., Picu, A., Hofmann, T., Andratschke, M., Mack, B., Moosmann, A., Gires, O., Tiwari, S.&Zeidler, R. (2006). COX-inhibitors relieve the immunosuppressive effect of tumor cells and improve functions of immune effectors. *International Journal Immunopathology Pharmacology*, Vol. 19, No. 2, (April-June 2006), pp. 409-19, ISSN 0394-6320

Laprie, C., Abadie, J., Amardeilh, M. F., Net, J. L., Lagadic, M.&Delverdier, M. (2001). MIB-1 immunoreactivity correlates with biologic behaviour in canine cutaneous melanoma. *Veterinary Dermatology*, Vol. 12, No. 3, (June 2001), pp. 139-47, ISSN 0959-4493

Le Bitoux, M. A.&Stamenkovic, I. (2008). Tumor-host interactions: the role of inflammation. *Histochemical Cell Biology*, Vol. 130, No. 6, (December 2008), pp. 1079-90, ISSN 0948-6143

Lee, C. H., Roh, J. W., Choi, J. S., Kang, S., Park, I. A., Chung, H. H., Jeon, Y. T., Kim, J. W., Park, N. H., Kang, S. B.&Song, Y. S. (2011). Cyclooxygenase-2 Is an Independent Predictor of Poor Prognosis in Uterine Leiomyosarcomas. *International Journal of Gynecological Cancer*, Vol. No. (March 15 2011), ISSN 1525-1438

Leek, R. D., Lewis, C. E., Whitehouse, R., Greenall, M., Clarke, J.&Harris, A. L. (1996). Association of macrophage infiltration with angiogenesis and prognosis in invasive breast carcinoma. *Cancer Research*, Vol. 56, No. 20, (October 15 1996), pp. 4625-9, ISSN 0008-5472

Mantovani, A., Sozzani, S., Locati, M., Allavena, P.&Sica, A. (2002). Macrophage polarization: tumor-associated macrophages as a paradigm for polarized M2 mononuclear phagocytes. *Trends in Immunology*, Vol. 23, No. 11, (November 2002), pp. 549-55, ISSN 1471-4906

Marino, D. J., Matthiesen, D. T., Stefanacci, J. D.&Moroff, S. D. (1995). Evaluation of dogs with digit masses: 117 cases (1981-1991). *Journal of the American Veterinary Medical Association*, Vol. 207, No. 6, (September 15 1995), pp. 726-8, ISSN 0003-1488

Martínez CM Dr, Peñafiel-Verdú C, Vilafranca M, Ramírez G, Méndez-Gallego M, Buendí A AJ&J., S. (2011). Cyclooxygenase-2 Expression Is Related With Localization, Proliferation, and Overall Survival in Canine Melanocytic Neoplasms. *Veterinary Pathology*, Vol. February 3. [Epub ahead of print], No. 2011),

McEntee, M. F., Cates, J. M.&Neilsen, N. (2002). Cyclooxygenase-2 expression in spontaneous intestinal neoplasia of domestic dogs. *Veterinary Pathology*, Vol. 39, No. 4, (July 2002), pp. 428-36,

Menczer, J. (2009). Cox-2 expression in ovarian malignancies: a review of the clinical aspects. *European Journal of Obstetrics & Gynecology and Reproductive Biology*, Vol. 146, No. 2, (October 2009), pp. 129-32, ISSN 1872-7654

Minami, S., Lum, C. A., Kitagawa, K. M.&Namiki, T. S. (2011). Immunohistochemical expression of cyclooxygenage-2 in melanocytic skin lesions. *International Journal of Dermatology*, Vol. 50, No. 1, (January 2011), pp. 24-29, ISSN 0011-9059

Misfeldt, M. L.&Grimm, D. R. (1994). Sinclair miniature swine: an animal model of human melanoma. *Veterinary Immunology & Immunopathology*, Vol. 43, No. 1-3, (October 1994), pp. 167-75, ISSN 0165-2427

Mohammed, S. I., Khan, K. N., Sellers, R. S., Hayek, M. G., DeNicola, D. B., Wu, L., Bonney, P. L.&Knapp, D. W. (2004). Expression of cyclooxygenase-1 and 2 in naturally-occurring canine cancer. *Prostaglandins Leukot Essent Fatty Acids*, Vol. 70, No. 5, (May 2004), pp. 479-83,

Mukaratirwa, S., Chikafa, L., Dliwayo, R.&Moyo, N. (2006). Mast cells and angiogenesis in canine melanomas: malignancy and clinicopathological factors. *Veterinary Dermatology*, Vol. 17, No. 2, (April 2006), pp. 141-6, ISSN 0959-4493

Mulligan, R. M. (1961). Melanoblastic tumors in the dog. *American Journal of Veterinary Research*, Vol. 22, No. (May 1961), pp. 345-51, ISSN 0002-9645

Mullins, M. N., Lana, S. E., Dernell, W. S., Ogilvie, G. K., Withrow, S. J.&Ehrhart, E. J. (2004). Cyclooxygenase-2 expression in canine appendicular osteosarcomas. *Journal of Veterinary Internal Medicine*, Vol. 18, No. 6, (November-December 2004), pp. 859-65,

Naghshvar, F., Torabizadeh, Z., Emadian, O., Enami, K.&Ghahremani, M. (2009). Correlation of cyclooxygenase 2 expression and inflammatory cells infiltration in colorectal cancer. *Pakistan Journal of Biological Sciences*, Vol. 12, No. 1, (January 1 2009), pp. 98-100, ISSN 1028-8880

Nishie, A., Ono, M., Shono, T., Fukushi, J., Otsubo, M., Onoue, H., Ito, Y., Inamura, T., Ikezaki, K., Fukui, M., Iwaki, T.&Kuwano, M. (1999). Macrophage infiltration and heme oxygenase-1 expression correlate with angiogenesis in human gliomas. *Clinical Cancer Research*, Vol. 5, No. 5, (May 1999), pp. 1107-13, ISSN 1078-0432

Paglia, D., Dubielzig, R. R., Kado-Fong, H. K.&Maggs, D. J. (2009). Expression of cyclooxygenase-2 in canine uveal melanocytic neoplasms. *American Journal of Veterinary Research*, Vol. 70, No. 10, (October 2009), pp. 1284-90, ISSN 0002-9645

Piras, F., Colombari, R., Minerba, L., Murtas, D., Floris, C., Maxia, C., Corbu, A., Perra, M. T.&Sirigu, P. (2005). The predictive value of CD8, CD4, CD68, and human leukocyte antigen-D-related cells in the prognosis of cutaneous malignant melanoma with vertical growth phase. *Cancer*, Vol. 104, No. 6, (September 15 2005), pp. 1246-54,

Pires, I., Garcia, A., Prada, J.&Queiroga, F. L. (2010). COX-1 and COX-2 expression in canine cutaneous, oral and ocular melanocytic tumours. *Journal of Comparative Pathology*, Vol. 143, No. 2-3, (August-October 2010), pp. 142-9, ISSN 1532-3129

Queiroga, F. L., Alves, A., Pires, I.&Lopes, C. (2007). Expression of Cox-1 and Cox-2 in canine mammary tumours. *Journal of Comparative Pathology*, Vol. 136, No. 2-3, (February-April 2007), pp. 177-85,

Queiroga, F. L., Perez-Alenza, M. D., Silvan, G., Pena, L., Lopes, C.&Illera, J. C. (2005). Cox-2 levels in canine mammary tumors, including inflammatory mammary carcinoma:

clinicopathological features and prognostic significance. *Anticancer Research*, Vol. 25, No. 6B, (November-December 2005), pp. 4269-75, ISSN 0250-7005

Queiroga, F. L., Pires, I., Parente, M., Gregorio, H.&Lopes, C. S. (2010). COX-2 over-expression correlates with VEGF and tumour angiogenesis in canine mammary cancer. *The Veterinary Journal*, Vol. No. (July 30 2010), ISSN 1532-2971

Ramos-Vara, J. A., Beissenherz, M. E., Miller, M. A., Johnson, G. C., Pace, L. W., Fard, A.&Kottler, S. J. (2000). Retrospective study of 338 canine oral melanomas with clinical, histologic, and immunohistochemical review of 129 cases. *Veterinary Pathology*, Vol. 37, No. 6, (November 2000), pp. 597-608, ISSN 0300-9858

Roels, S., Tilmant, K.&Ducatelle, R. (1999). PCNA and Ki67 proliferation markers as criteria for prediction of clinical behaviour of melanocytic tumours in cats and dogs. *Journal of Comparative Pathology*, Vol. 121, No. 1, (July 1999), pp. 13-24, ISSN 0021-9975

Roels, S., Tilmant, K.&Ducatelle, R. (2001). p53 expression and apoptosis in melanomas of dogs and cats. *Research in Veterinary Science*, Vol. 70, No. 1, (February 2001), pp. 19-25, ISSN 0034-5288

Shi, L., Lei, D., Ma, C., Xu, F., Li, Y., Wang, Y., Cong, N., Liu, D.&Pan, X. L. (2010). Clinicopathological Implications of Tumour-associated Macrophages and Vascularization in Sinonasal Melanoma. *Journal of International Medical Research*, Vol. 38, No. 4, (July-August 2010), pp. 1276-1286, ISSN 0300-0605

Singh-Ranger, G., Salhab, M.&Mokbel, K. (2008). The role of cyclooxygenase-2 in breast cancer: review. *Breast Cancer Research and Treatment*, Vol. 109, No. 2, (May 2008), pp. 189-98, ISSN 0167-6806

Siveen, K. S.&Kuttan, G. (2009). Role of macrophages in tumour progression. *Immunology Letters*, Vol. 123, No. 2, (April 27 2009), pp. 97-102, ISSN 1879-0542

Smith, S. H., Goldschmidt, M. H.&McManus, P. M. (2002). A comparative review of melanocytic neoplasms. *Veterinary Pathology*, Vol. 39, No. 6, (November 2002), pp. 651-78, ISSN 0300-9858

Spangler, W. L.&Kass, P. H. (2006). The histologic and epidemiologic bases for prognostic considerations in canine melanocytic neoplasia. *Veterinary Pathology*, Vol. 43, No. 2, (March 2006), pp. 136-49, ISSN 0300-9858

Taylor, K. H., Smith, A. N., Higginbotham, M., Schwartz, D. D., Carpenter, D. M.&Whitley, E. M. (2007). Expression of vascular endothelial growth factor in canine oral malignant melanoma. *Veterinary and Comparative Oncology*, Vol. 5, No. 4, (December 2007), pp. 208-18, ISSN 1476-5829

Tjiu, J. W., Chen, J. S., Shun, C. T., Lin, S. J., Liao, Y. H., Chu, C. Y., Tsai, T. F., Chiu, H. C., Dai, Y. S., Inoue, H., Yang, P. C., Kuo, M. L.&Jee, S. H. (2009). Tumor-associated macrophage-induced invasion and angiogenesis of human basal cell carcinoma cells by cyclooxygenase-2 induction. *Journal of Investigative Dermatology*, Vol. 129, No. 4, (April 2009), pp. 1016-25, ISSN 1523-1747

Toivonen, P., Makitie, T., Kujala, E.&Kivela, T. (2004). Microcirculation and tumor-infiltrating macrophages choroidal and ciliary body melanoma and corresponding metastases. *Investigative Ophthalmology & Visual Science*, Vol. 45, No. 1, (January 2004), pp. 1-6, ISSN 0146-0404

Torisu, H., Ono, M., Kiryu, H., Furue, M., Ohmoto, Y., Nakayama, J., Nishioka, Y., Sone, S.&Kuwano, M. (2000). Macrophage infiltration correlates with tumor stage and angiogenesis in human malignant melanoma: Possible involvement of TNF alpha and IL-1 alpha. *International Journal of Cancer*, Vol. 85, No. 2, (January 15 2000), pp. 182-188, ISSN 0020-7136

Valentine, B. A. (1995). Equine melanocytic tumors: a retrospective study of 53 horses (1988 to 1991). *Journal of Veterinary Internal Medicine*, Vol. 9, No. 5, (September-October 1995), pp. 291-7, ISSN 0891-6640

Van Ginderachter, J. A., Movahedi, K., Hassanzadeh Ghassabeh, G., Meerschaut, S., Beschin, A., Raes, G.&De Baetselier, P. (2006). Classical and alternative activation of mononuclear phagocytes: picking the best of both worlds for tumor promotion. *Immunobiology*, Vol. 211, No. 6-8, 2006), pp. 487-501, ISSN 0171-2985

von Euler, H., Sadeghi, A., Carlsson, B., Rivera, P., Loskog, A., Segall, T., Korsgren, O.&Totterman, T. H. (2008). Efficient adenovector CD40 ligand immunotherapy of canine malignant melanoma. *Journal of Immunotherapy*, Vol. 31, No. 4, (May 2008), pp. 377-84, ISSN 1524-9557

Wu, K. K.&Liou, J. Y. (2009). Cyclooxygenase inhibitors induce colon cancer cell apoptosis Via PPARdelta --> 14-3-3epsilon pathway. *Methods in Molecular Biology*, Vol. 512, No. 2009), pp. 295-307, ISSN 1064-3745

Wu, R., Abramson, A. L., Symons, M. H.&Steinberg, B. M. (2010). Pak1 and Pak2 are activated in recurrent respiratory papillomas, contributing to one pathway of Rac1-mediated COX-2 expression. *International Journal of Cancer*, Vol. 127, No. 9, (November 1 2010), pp. 2230-7, ISSN 1097-0215

Part 3

Disease Management and Clinical Cases

11

Surgical Management of Malignant Melanoma of Gastrointestinal Tract

Thawatchai Akaraviputh and Atthaphorn Trakarnsanga
Division of General Surgery, Department of Surgery, Faculty of Medicine Siriraj Hospital, Mahidol University, Bangkok, Thailand

1. Introduction

Malignant melanoma of gastrointestinal (GI) tract is a less common condition especially in eastern countries and can be either primary or metastasis. Most of the cases are secondary melanoma. GI metastases are frequently found during autopsy, only small proportion of the patients can be detected while living (2-5% of the patients). Clinically, a primary GI malignant melanoma is suggested if the patient has no obvious primary cutaneous lesion or other extra-intestinal disease especially the ocular system. Malignant melanoma of anorectum is the most common site of the primary tumor of GI tract. For metastasis, small bowel is the most frequently site followed by stomach, large bowel and esophagus. Mucosal melanoma pursued more aggressive nature and poorer prognosis than other subsets of melanomas. Prognosis of malignant melanoma of GI tract is very poor because of difficult to diagnosis.

Malignant melanoma of GI tract can present as abdominal pain, upper or lower GI tract bleeding, obstructive jaundice, obstruction or perforation. Several case reports demonstrated small bowel obstruction from intussusceptions of malignant melanoma. The diagnosis can be made by GI endoscopy or imaging radiographic studies. The definite diagnosis is the pathological examination. Management of GI malignant melanoma depends on the location and number of the lesion. Surgical resection for primary melanoma of GI tract is the mainstay treatment and provides a chance for cure. For metastatic disease, multidisciplinary approach is the best option. Surgery is the alternative way to use in selected patient.

2. Diagnosis and staging

Melanoma originates from melanocyte, a pigmented, dendritic-like cell located in epidermis of skin, eye, epithelium of the nasal cavity, oropharynx, anus and genitourinary system. The diagnosis of melanoma includes assessment of the architectural and cytological features combine with the clinical examination. The only staging system of malignant melanoma is used for cutaneous melanoma because of the high incidence rate compare to non-cutaneous group, accounts about 90% of all melanoma. Of the remaining forms of melanoma, ocular melanoma accounts for 5%, mucosal melanoma for 1% and melanoma of unknown origin for 2%. Within the mucosal subgroup, half of them are head and neck origin followed by anorectal, female genital, and urinary tract tumors respectively. The pathological staging of primary tumor uses the tumor thickness and ulceration. Ulceration is defined as the absence of the intact epithelium overlying a major portion of the tumor. Ulceration is the result of the thickness of tumor and has a strong correlation to survival.

Recently, American Joint Committee on Cancer (AJCC) presented the 7th edition of the melanoma staging system in 2009. Differences from the 6th edition (2002) included the used of mitotic rate to classify stage 1a and 1b, used of immunochemical detection of nodal metastasis and no lower threshold to define positive nodal status. For stage IV disease, the staging system is not change. The site(s) of metastases and elevated serum levels of lactate dehydrogenase (LDH) are used to divided M stage to three categories; M1a, M1b and M1c. The definition and survival were shown in table 1.

M stage	Site	Serum LDH	One-year survival rates	
			%	*p*
M0	No distant metastases	NA	NA	
M1a	Distant skin, subcutaneous, or nodal metastases	Normal	62	<0.0001
M1b	Lung metastases	Normal	53	
M1c	All other visceral metastases Any distant metastases	Normal Elevated	33	

Table 1. Modification of the 7th AJCC classification of metastatic melanoma.

Most of melanoma in GI tract is metastases. Only 2-15% of all GI melanomas are primary. Whenever a seemingly primary melanoma is detected in GI tract, it is prudent to conduct a through clinical investigation to consider the possibility of metastatic disease including history, physical examination and investigations. Carefully history taking and comprehensive physical examination are the initial crucial step of the approach. Skin and eye examination should be mandatory examination in all patients. Gynecological and abdominal examination include rectal examination should be performed for the next step.

Ozdemir et al. proposed criteria for diagnosis primary bronchial melanoma to be defined as a primary lesion that can apply to GI melanoma as well. The criteria including (1) there is only single lesion in the surgical specimen (2) there must be no previously excised skin tumor (3) no previous ocular tumor (4) morphology must be compatible with primary tumor (5) there must be no other demonstrable melanomas at the time of surgery (6) findings should be confirmed by careful autopsy. The lesions that not fulfill these criteria should be termed secondary. The problem of the criteria is we could know the exact diagnosis after the autopsy when patient passed away. Then, these criteria did not have an impact to the treatment, only for the epidemiology. Blecker et al. suggested the following criteria for a diagnosis of primary intestinal melanoma: 1) no evidence of concurrent melanoma or atypical melanocytic lesion of the skin, 2) absence of extraintestinal metastatic spread of melanoma, and 3) presence of intramucosal lesions in the overlying or adjacent intestinal epithelium.

3. Investigation

3.1 Endoscopy

Small bowel is the most common site of GI melanoma and bleeding is one of the most frequent presentations of the patients. Therefore, a GI endoscopy with magnification should be the procedure of choice to diagnose malignant melanoma of GI tract. Multiple black, depressed lesions (1+ 5 mm in diameter) with a "bull's eye" appearance are usually viewed in the GI mucosa (Figure 1). At present endoscopic ultrasonography (EUS) guided fine needle aspiration (FNA) may play an important role for cytological diagnosis in the patients with advanced disease (Figure 2).

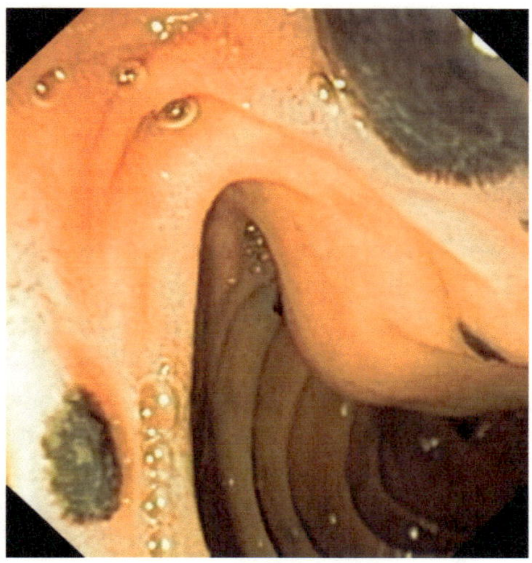

Fig. 1. Endoscopic view showed multiple typical black color lesions in the second part of duodenum.

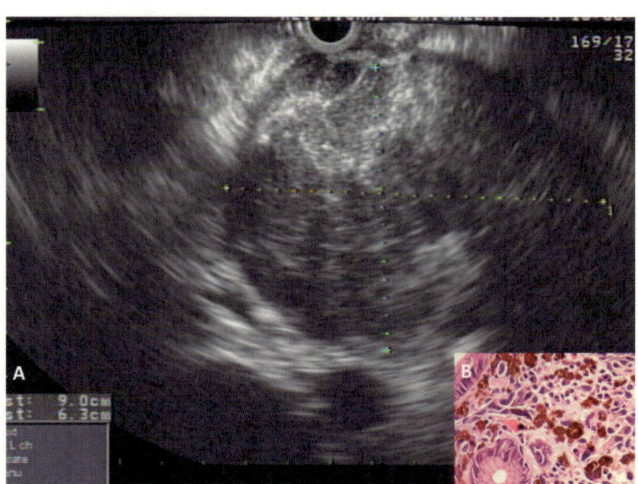

Fig. 2. EUS-guided (A) FNA for cytological confirmation (B) in the patient with advanced malignant melanoma.

3.2 Barium study and capsule endoscopy

Small bowel metastatic may present as varying sized single or multiple nodules that can have polypoid or infiltrating appearance. Central ulceration can occur when lesions outgrow their blood supply, giving a "target" appearance on barium study. The target sign can be found with other hematogenous metastases such as lymphoma or sarcoma. For small bowel metastatic, the lesion can be intraluminal involvement and act as leading point for intussusceptions.

Capsule endoscopy (CE) is the current standard and one of the most sensitive investigations for detection of small bowel lesion. The finding could be a polypoid lesion with central umbilication or an ulcerative lesion with bleeding. Prakosa et al. reported a series of 21 patients diagnosed malignant melanoma and underwent positron emission tomography (PET) scanning and CE. They suggested that CE could identify and provide confirmation of small-bowel involvement in patients with metastatic melanoma after PET scanning. These two investigations are recommended as part of the work-up of all patients with or without GI symptoms.

3.3 Computed tomography (CT) and magnetic resonance imaging (MRI)

Computed tomography (CT) is the most commonly used imaging technique for staging and follow up in the malignant melanoma patients. Two studies have compared staging with Positron emission tomography (PET) and CT scan in all stages. Both studies found PET to be superior in terms of sensitivity and specificity to CT in all stages of Melanoma. In the contrary, Krug et al. demonstrated inferiority of PET to CT for the detection of lung and liver metastases.

Magnetic resonance imaging (MRI) is a good investigation for detection of brain and bone metastases. For anorectal region, MRI and endorectal ultrasonography are the good investigational methods for preoperative evaluation both of primary tumor and local nodal status. In one prospective study of 64 patients, whole-body MRI has been reported to have an overall accuracy for the detection of lesion slightly lower than PET-CT (78.8% vs. 86.7%), but the sensitivity for the detection of bone and liver metastases was better than PET-CT.

3.4 Positron emission tomography (PET)

Positron emission tomography (PET) is an advanced diagnostic imaging technique. This technique exploits the increased metabolism of glucose in malignant viable cells. ^{18}F-fluorodeoxyglucose (FDG) is one of the most commonly used radioisotopes. FDG is transported into tumor cells like glucose molecule. There is a many-fold increase in glucose metabolism in malignant tumors as compared with normal cells, therefore, the different in metabolism of tumor call and normal tissue can be detected by this technique. The potential benefits of FDG-PET for melanoma included the detection of locoregional and distant metastasis for staging.

The presence or absence of regional lymph node metastases is an important prognostic factor for patients with melanoma. FDG-PET has shown a limitation of sensitivity and wide variation of the data from previous studies. The sensitivity of FDG-PET is varied from 8% to 100%. Moreover, in the subgroup of subclinical nodal disease in stage I and II melanoma, the sensitivity of FDG-PET is only 14-17% whereas, sentinel node biopsy reached 86-94%. Crippa *et al.* identified the correlation between size of lymph node and sensitivity; sensitivity is 23%, 83% and 100% for lymph node less than 5mm, 6-10mm and greater than

10 mm in diameter, respectively. Therefore, FDG-PET might not be the investigation of choice for locoregional evaluation especially for clinically nonpalpable group.

For the distant metastatic evaluation especially in curative intent resected patients, the precise identification of the location and number of metastatic lesions could be important for surgical planning. From several studies, FDG-PET has been shown to be more accurate than conventional modalities such as ultrasonography, CT, and MRI. Then, FDG-PET is most commonly used for suspected or known distant metastases. The sensitivity is varied from 79% to 92% and specificity is varied from 86% to 90%. Several reports identified the influence of therapy by FDG-PET, 17- 48% of patients were changed their treatment plan. In the same way, FDG-PET is highly sensitive and specific for detection or restaging of melanoma. Prichard *et al.* reported the sensitivity and specificity of FDG-PET for detection of recurrent melanoma, 74-100% and 67-100%, respectively. Figure 2 is the one example of PET scan of intraabdominal metastatic of melanoma.

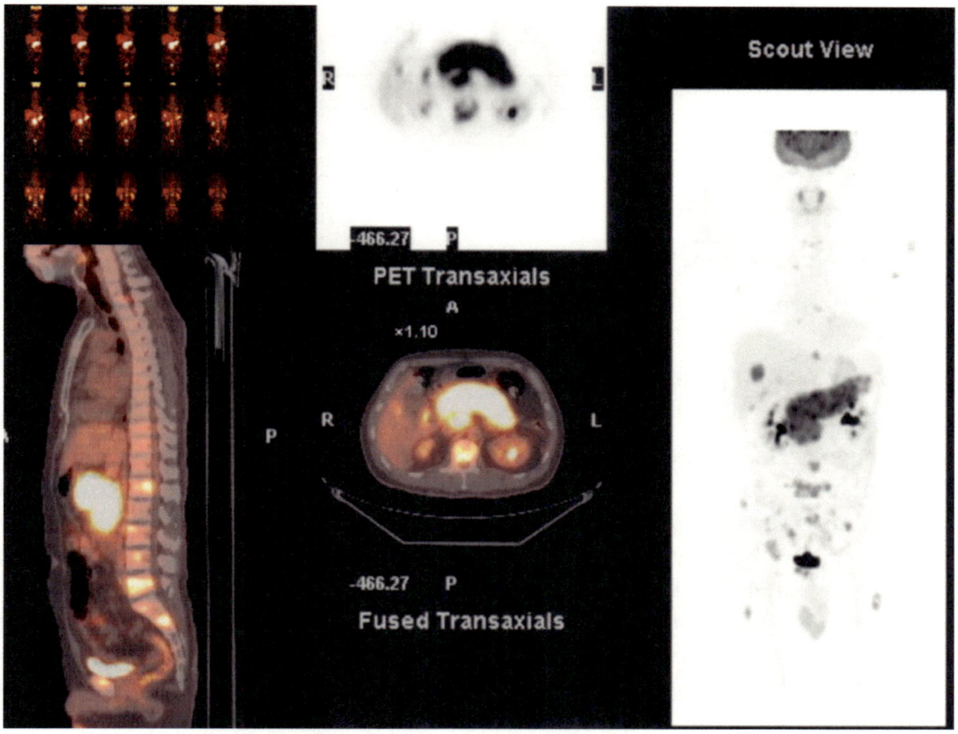

Fig. 3. PET scan revealed multiple metastasis lesions of malignant melanoma of gastrointestinal tract such as pancreas, liver and small bowel.

4. Introduction to primary malignant melanoma of GI tract

GI tract is not the normal organ that contain of melanocytes. Then, how be possible primary melanoma can develop in GI tract? One explanation is neural crest cells that demonstrated in the intestines, these cells have a potential to develop to mature melanocyte. Another reason, the aberrant migration of melanocytes that usually migrate from neural crest to the epidermis, hair follicles, oral cavity, nasopharynx, uvea, leptomeninges, and inner ear during early embryogenesis. These are the reasons that why melanoma can be found in the gastrointestinal tract.

Primary GI melanoma can arise in various GI mucosal sites, including oral cavity, esophagus, stomach, small bowel, colon and anorectum. Distinguish between primary and metastatic from an unknown or regressed cutaneous melanoma may be difficult. Clinically, a primary GI melanoma is suggested if the patient has no obvious primary cutaneous melanoma from history and physical examination. Moreover, the patient has an isolated GI lesion without extraintestinal metastases. For histologically, the presence of atypical melanocytic cells in the basal layer of the epithelium and extending in a pagetoid fashion in to more superficial epithelium, may be reported in 40-100% of primary GI melanoma. The surgical treatment and the outcomes were depended on the organ of tumor involvement. Then, we divided primary melanoma in this section to organ specific. Summarized of the survivals was showed in the table 2.

Organ	Median survival (months)	5-year survival
Oral cavity	27-38.9	30-40%
Esophagus	12-13.4	4.2-14 %
Stomach	5-12	0
Small intestine	16	10%
Colon	27.5	21-56%
Anorectum	15-28.6	17-30.6%
Gallbladder and biliary tract	20.1-41	29 %

Table 2. Summarized of survivals divided by primary organ involvement.

5. Surgery of primary malignant melanoma of GI tract

5.1 Esophagus

Primary malignant melanoma of esophagus is the rare condition, accounts only 0.1-0.2% of primary esophageal tumors. Whereas, cadaveric study from De la Pava *et al.* demonstrated the presence of melanocytes in 4% of all esophageal specimen examined. Then, there are other entities of melanotic condition that can be found in esophagus. One benign condition called esophageal melanocytosis need to differentiate from the esophageal melanoma. This condition described the distribution of melanocytes in the basal layer of the esophageal squamous epithelium. The incidence is about 0.07-2.1% from previous reports. For primary esophageal melanoma is commonest in older males and more found in the middle and lower esophagus.

Patients may present with symptoms of dysphagia, retrosternal discomfort, weight loss, regurgitation or melena. After careful history and physical examination, barium swallow and/or endoscopy is the next investigation same as all esophageal lesions. The characteristic endoscopic appearance of primary malignant melanoma is a polypoid, irregularly pigmented, obstructive esophageal tumor. The tumor most often is polypoid; the nonpolypoid form is extremely rare. The color of the tumor may vary from black to white. An ulcerative lesion of the mucosa can be found in some case, then some tumors may be difficult to differentiate from esophageal carcinoma. Most of the cases are grossly pigmentation, but not almost always. The endoscopic biopsy can diagnose only half of the patients due to submucosal nature of the tumor. Up to 25% of all esophageal melanomas are amelanotic. Presence of associated benign melanocytes or in situ melanoma from pathological examination favors the diagnosis of primary, rather than metastatic. If primary malignant melanoma is suspected at endoscopy, immunohistochemical staining of biopsy specimens is essential for diagnosis.

Regard to difficulty of the diagnosis, half of the patients are stage IV when diagnosed. The median survival is about one year and 5-year survival varied from 4.2% to 14%. The mainstay of the treatment is still surgical resection with dissection of the regional lymph nodes. Compared with other esophageal tumors, wider margins of resection are required. For early-localized lesion, radical resection had a significantly longer survival compare to local excision. Radiation can increased the mean survival rate from 14.2 months to 16.7 months, while adjuvant chemotherapy have a limited benefit. Only some case reports that demonstrated the long-term survival from surgical resection combine with chemotherapy. There are some alternative techniques such as endoscopic mucosal resection and localized ablative approaches were proposed in case report but the data still limited.

5.2 Stomach

Primary melanoma of stomach is the very rare disease entity and related to poor outcomes. Most of the reports are the case report then, the data is quite limited. The presenting symptoms of gastric melanoma are non-specific including nausea, vomiting, abdominal pain, weight loss and anemia. Perforation and/or upper GI bleeding can be presented as an initial diagnosis in some patients. Barium study, endoscopy and CT scan are the most common investigational methods. In the same way of esophageal melanoma, pigmentation of the lesion is the most clues for diagnosis and found in the majority. The median survival is usually less than 1 year. Cheung *et al.* reported 18 cases of primary gastric melanomas with the median survival is only 5 months without 5-year survival. Regard to limitation of the data, it is difficult to conclude that which operations are the appropriate surgical procedures of primary gastric melanoma.

5.3 Gallbladder and biliary tract

Primary melanoma of gallbladder is extremely rare condition as well as isolated metastasis to gallbladder. Regard to clinical presentation, involvement of the gallbladder rarely produces symptoms. Some case reports presented acalculous cholecystitis as a clinical presentation of these patients. Therefore, it is difficultly to diagnose melanoma of gallbladder preoperatively. Abdominal ultrasonography is a useful, easy, and inexpensive modality for assessing a gallbladder lesion. CT scan and Magnetic resonance cholangiography may add more information. Surgical resection of gallbladder is the treatment of both primary and metastatic lesions. The mean survival times for primary gallbladder melanoma is 20.1 months and for metastatic is 8.4 months, with few patients surviving longer than 2 years.

In 1963, Zaide first described primary malignant melanoma of common bile duct. This is also rarely disease entity same as the others primary GI melanoma. The existence of melanocytes in bile duct tissue is truly possible. Melanocytes derive from cells of the neural crest and can migrate throughout the body. They have been definitely identified in areas of endodermal origin, including gallbladder. The symptoms of this tumor mostly presented with obstructive jaundice. In most of the cases, the diagnosis can be made after the time of surgery. Wagner *et al.* reported the review of 6 cases of primary malignant melanoma of common bile duct from 1963 to 2000.

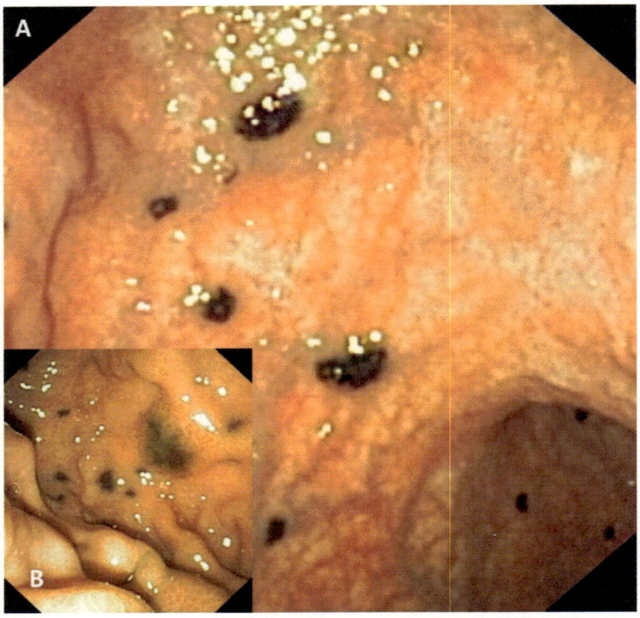

Fig. 4. Gastroscopy revealed multiple lesions of metastasis malignant melanoma in the stomach (A&B).

All of the patients underwent surgery including 4 Whipple operations, 2 partial hepatectomies and one resection of common bile duct. Three of them (2 Whipple and 1 hepatectomy) dead within 6-18 months from distant metastasis whereas three of patients didn't mention about follow up period. Therefore, it is not possible to conclude the optimal surgical option for this disease due to very limited of the data. There are also had a few literatures that reported the extremely rare primary malignant melanoma of intrahepatic duct and liver in a case report format. Because of the limitation of the data, then we not presented the detail of these disease entities in this chapter.

5.4 Small bowel

Cutaneous melanoma is the most common types of the tumor metastasis to GI tract which small intestine is the most common site of metastatic melanoma in the GI tract. However primary melanoma of small intestine is not common. Small bowel lesion can present with bleeding, abdominal pain, obstruction, weight loss and malabsorption. Intussusception can be a presenting symptom of small bowel melanoma. Diagnosis of small intestine lesion is typically made by contrast imaging study (small bowel follow-through), CT scan, endoscopy (push, single or double balloon and capsule endoscopy) and PET. Primary intestinal melanoma tends to be more aggressive and worse prognosis than cutaneous origin. The possible reasons are due to late diagnosis and rapidly growth of the tumor in the rich vascular and lymphatic supply of the intestinal mucosa.

Surgery is the treatment of choice in patients with primary or metastatic intestinal melanoma. Segmental resection with adequate free margins is a recommended procedure. Morbidity and mortality of this type of surgery is very low. Systemic adjuvant therapy has a limited role for this disease. The median survival rate is 16 months and 5-year survival rate is 10%.

5.5 Colon

Primary melanoma of the colon is also a rare clinical entity. Khalid *et al.* (2011) reported their review study of 12 patients with primary melanoma of colon. Right-sided colon is the most common location of the disease; about 65% of the patients. Lower GI bleeding is the most common presentation (50%) followed by abdominal pain (20%), obstruction (20%), and weight loss (16%). Amelanocytic colon melanoma is found in 14% of the cases.

For localized disease, surgical resection is the mainstay of the treatment. We cannot conclude that what is the standard of the operation because of the limitation of the data. Most of the patients in the previous studies underwent the oncologic colon resection same as adenocarcinoma. The prognosis of primary malignant melanoma of the colon seems to be better than other types of primary mucosal melanomas. However, colon melanoma is still aggressive than cutaneous origin. One-year and five-year survival rates are 37-60% and 21-33%, respectively and the median survival is 27.5 months.

5.6 Anus and rectum

In 1857, Moore first described anorectal melanoma, a rare and very aggressive tumor with the extremely poor prognosis. The incidence is less than 1% of all melanomas and about 2 - 4% of all anal malignancies. Majority about two-third of all lesions are pigmented. Two-third of anorectal melanoma is located within the anal canal or at the anal verge and the others demonstrated in the rectum. Presentation is often nonspecific symptoms and indistinguishable from other conditions in this area such as rectal bleeding, palpable of anal mass, anal pain or discomfort. Some of the patients underwent an excision due to misinterpreted as a thrombosed hemorrhoid or anal polyp. Anorectal melanoma is diagnosed histologically by melanin pigment. However, immunohistochemical staining of melanoma antigen such as HMB-45 and S-100 protein are adjunctive for diagnosis.

Unlike cutaneous melanoma, noncutaneous origin are more likely to be found metastasized to locoregional lymph node or distal organ when the time of diagnosis. For anorectal melanoma, incidence rate for locoregional lymph node is 61% and distant metastases are 29%. Surgery still is the mainstay of the treatment for primary anorectal melanoma. The extent of resection (wide local excision versus radical resection) and extent of lymphadenectomy remain debated. Early some studies proposed radical resection like abdominoperineal resection was associated with the better outcomes. Unfortunately, other studies have reported similar patterns of recurrence and survival in patients undergoing local excision. Unlike anorectal adenocarcinoma, in the study from Memorial Sloan-Kettering, demonstrated lymph node metastases did not predict outcome of patients undergoing radical resection. Moreover, prophylactic bilateral inguinal lymphadenectomy in the patients with clinically non-palpable lymph node has not shown to improve survival. The details of results from previous studies were summarized in the table 3.

Change of practice patterns over the time depend on the new data that suggested local recurrence and survival are not associated with extent of resection. Moreover, recurrences of primary anorectal melanoma after surgery are more commonly distant and lethal. Then, local excision is the appropriate surgical management for localized primary anorectal melanoma. More radical resection and nodal resection may be needed in selected patients with clinically bulky tumor, involved sphincter complex or nodal positive including locoregional and inguinal area.

Author	Year	N	Abdominoperineal resection vs. Local excision			Entire Series	
			Overall recurrence	DFS	OS	DFS	OS
Slingluff et al. (1990)	1974-1990	24	-	-	-	*6.7*	-
Weinstock (1993)	1973-1987	55	-	-	-	*16*	*22*
Brady et al. (1995)	1929-1993	85	-	*NS p=0.11 (27 vs. 5)*	-	*9.4*	*12*
Pessaux et al. (2004)	1977-2002	40	-	-	*NS (30 vs. 19)*	14	*17*
Yeh et al. (2006)	1984-2003	46	*NS (26 vs. 26)*	-	*NS (32 vs.35)*	-	*35*
Ishizone et al. (2008)	1997-2006	79	-	-	*NS*	-	*28.8*
Nilsson et al. (2009)	1960-1999	251	*NS*	-	*NS (7 vs. 15)*	-	*13.6*

Table 3. Summarized of previous studies of primary anorectal melanoma (DFS: Disease free survival, OS: Overall survival, NS: not significant).

6. Surgery of secondary malignant melanoma of GI tract

Survival rate of stage IV melanoma patient is really worse, typically measured in months rather than years. Recurrence is identified about one-third of the patients, most of them recur at the regional nodes. For distant metastasis, almost major organ and tissue can be a site of metastases. Commonly of metastatic image is a wide spreading disease then role of surgical management is often palliative. In a retrospective review of 4,426 patients with stage IV melanoma treated at the John Wayne Cancer Institute, only 35% of all cases underwent surgical resection. These patients had a 5-year overall survival of 23% compared with 6% in those who were not surgical candidates ($p < 0.001$). Surgery with the intent of providing long-term survival should be considered only when all sites of disease can be completely removed. Therefore, a careful evaluation is an importance step of management and for looking to exclude others organ involvement. Regard to palliative intent, patient's status, comorbidities, symptoms and life expectancy are the clues to decide the operative procedure.

Preoperative evaluations include history taking, physical examination and assessment investigation such as ultrasonography, CT scan and MRI are a useful tool to evaluate status of the patients. CT scan is the most commonly used staging modality and has sensitivity about 60%. PET scan seems to have more sensitivity than CT scan, previously the sensitivity was reported in range from 70-100%. There are some reports proposed that the precise preoperative imaging can change surgical decision making 17-48%.

The GI tract is an uncommon site for malignant metastases, only 2-5% of these patients can be detected clinically. However, melanoma is one of the most common tumors that metastasis to GI tract. Small intestine is the most common size. GI metastases are usually associated with disseminated disease. From previously studies, the median survival time is only 5-11 months in secondary GI melanoma and estimated 5-year survival is usually less than 10%. Depend on the nature of the disease, the intent of surgical treatment usually for palliation. Surgery can relive the symptoms about 70-90% of the group especially obstruction, bleeding and perforation. The morbidities and mortalities of GI surgery are acceptable usually mortality less than 5% from previous studies.

One paper from Memorial Sloan-Kettering Cancer Center reported 68 patients, who underwent surgical exploration for metastatic GI melanoma from total 7965 melanoma patients. The most common presentations are anemia (60%), abdominal pain (59%) and bleeding (44%). Sixty-two from 68 of patients had small bowel involvement. The median survival was estimated to be 8.2 months (6.9-11.4 months). The 1-, 2- and 5-year survivals were 35%, 23% and 18%, respectively. The significant factors from multivariate analysis were included preoperative serum LDH ($p < 0.01$) and residual disease ($p = 0.03$). Ninety percent of the patients had palliation of symptom after surgery.

Another large series of secondary abdominal melanoma from M.D. Anderson, 251 patients was enrolled from the year 1970-1991. The common metastatic organs are small bowel (62%), mesenteric lymph nodes (45%), liver (37%) and stomach and duodenum (31%). The median of interval time after diagnosis was 38.5 months (1-258 months) and 13% of the cases developed intraabdominal recurrence during the first year of follow-up period. The median survival is 8 months in only intestinal metastatic group, 5 months in only visceral metastatic group and 4 months in both metastatic organs group. For palliative surgical resection, the median survival was increase significantly from 5 months in non-surgical group to 11 months in surgical group ($p < 0.0001$). This benefit of the palliative surgical resection is concordant to our study that previously reported. In the 86 patients' subgroup that had severely symptoms, surgergical approach was associated with longer symptom-free periods compared with non-surgical approach significantly ($p < 0.0001$). The multivariate analysis revealed that complete tumor removal, only intestinal metastasis and interval time of recurrence after diagnosis greater than 48 months were significance associated to better overall survival ($p = 0.0001$, $=0.002$, $=0.005$, respectively). Concomitant to most of the reports that supported complete resection, GI tract as a first site of metastasis, longer of disease free interval or interval from diagnosis, and lower level of LDH were associated to better outcomes. Summarized of favorable factors from multivariate analysis was in table 4.

Favorable factors
- Complete removal of the tumor
- Intestinal metastasis without others abdominal visceral involvement
- Interval time of recurrence after diagnosis greater than 48 months
- GI tract as a first site of metastasis
- Presence of extra-abdominal disease
- Preoperative serum LDH level < 200 u/L

Table 4. Summarized of favorable factors from multivariate analysis.

From these data, we can summarized that for secondary GI melanoma, particularly if the GI tract is the first site of metastasis, the curative surgical resection should be strongly considered not only for palliation of symptoms but also for improvement in survival. Although, improvement of survivals is only in the number of months, but surgery can provide significant improvement in quality of life of the patients with acceptable operative morbidity and mortality.

7. Non-surgical management

Over the past 50 years, more than 100 randomized clinical trials have investigated cytotoxic chemotherapeutic agents and immunostimulants such as Bacille Calmette-Guerin (BCG), *Corynebacterium parvum*, and levamisole. Interestingly, nonspecific immunotherapy declined as more active immunostimulatory cytokines, in particular interferon (IFN), came to clinical practice. In this chapter, we briefly presented the alternative management of surgery including chemotherapy, immunotherapy, vaccination and radiation in the setting of adjuvant and metastatic treatment.

7.1 Chemotherapy

Most of the data are in the setting of treatment of metastatic disease. Apart form IL-2, Dacarbazine (DTIC) is one of the two agents that were approved from U.S. Food and Drug Administration (US-FDA) for the treatment of advanced melanoma. The response rate was 19-28% from previous studies. Unfortunately, no any studies demonstrated the benefit of overall survival of DTIC compare to supportive care in the advanced melanoma patients. Temozolomide (TMZ), an analog of DTIC with similar activity, the potential benefit over DTIC is available in oral form. Several studies suggested TMZ is active against CNS metastases. Therefore, TMZ should be considered in the patient with brain metastases although, no difference of overall survival compare to DTIC.

The combination of chemotherapeutic agents have been developed including BOLD (Bleomycin, Vincristine, Lomustine, and DTIC), CVD (Cisplatin, Vinblastine, and DTIC), The Dartmouth regimen (DTIC, Cisplatin, Carmustine, and Tamoxifen). The response rate was improved, but no difference in survivals compare to DTIC alone. Moreover, the toxicity was increased when used of the combine regimens.

7.2 Immunotherapy

High dose of the Interferon α-2b (IFN α-2b) is the only adjuvant therapy for stages II and III cutaneous melanoma that got the approval form US-FDA. Relapse-free survival was significantly prolonged ($p= 0.006$, HR= 1.30) compared to observational group. Unfortunately, the data did not show a survival benefit. The toxicities considerably affect quality of life over the course of the treatment. The most common toxicity is neutropenia. Interleukin-2 (IL-2) was approved by US-FDA for the treatment of adults with advanced metastatic melanoma. IL-2 toxicity can involve multiple organ system, most significantly cardiovascular, respiratory, and excretory system. Most of the toxicity is related to the capillary leak syndrome. To improve the activity of immunotherapy, combining different chemotherapy agents (Biochemotherapy, BCT) and vaccines has been reported. All of studies concluded that BCT is associated with increased toxicity and the highest response rate is about 50%. A metaanalysis of BCT by the Cochrane Collaboration included 2,625 patients. The response rate is increased in the group of BCT, but no difference in overall survival. ($p= 0.31$, HR 0.89)

7.3 Vaccines

Melanoma has a unique relationship to the immune system with the development of spontaneous tumor-specific immune responses in patients. For this reason, melanoma has been a frequently targeted disease in the development of cancer vaccines. The various vaccines were used in the treatment of melanoma including DNA vaccine, dendritic cell vaccines, peptide-based vaccines, and viral vaccines. Although vaccines have been demonstrated to produce immunologic responses, unfortunately, no clinical benefit has been demonstrated in the previous large randomized vaccine trials performed in melanoma in the adjuvant setting.

7.4 Emerging therapeutic agents

Despite of increasing understanding the biology of melanoma, the novel therapeutic agents that developed based on the new knowledge with some demonstrated promising antitumor effect in several clinical trials. Ipilimumab (MDX-010) is an IgG1 antibody. The several of phrase II trials of ipilimumab demonstrated a promising 1-year OS of over 47% and a 2-year OS of over 30% (compare to 25% of 1-year survival from meta-analysis). A double-blinded phrase III randomized study is ongoing. The in depth other agents such as Bevacizumab, Thalidomide is beyond the scope of this review.

The discovery of *BRAF, NRAS, PTEN* and *KIT* alterations in melanoma has supported the development of various rational therapeutic approaches. Sorafenib, PLX4032, and GSK2118436 are the effective *BRAF* inhibitors. Most of the studies still ongoing, hopefully these new agents may be a novel effective treatment options for the patients with advanced melanoma in the near future.

7.5 Radiotherapy

Although, melanoma is a relatively radio-resistance tumor, undoubtedly, radiation is an effective palliative treatment for the 40 -50% of patients who develop unresectable, locally recurrent, and/or metastatic disease resulting in bone pain, spinal core compression, tumor hemorrhage, and central nervous system dysfunction secondary to cerebral metastases.

8. Conclusion

Malignant melanoma of GI tract is uncommon especially primary GI melanoma. History taking and careful physical examination is the first step of approach to rule out the primary other sources. Skin, eye and rectal examination should be mandatory performed. Investigation including endoscopy, ultrasonography, contrast GI studies, CT scan, MRI, and PET scan can be used for different purposed. Prognosis is quite poor, particularly in secondary GI melanoma. Anorectal melanoma and small bowel is the most common site in the primary and metastatic GI melanoma respectively. Surgery is still the mainstay of the treatment for localized primary disease. Extensive surgical resection is reserved for selected patients. Melanoma is one of the most common tumors that metastasis to GI tract. The median survival is usually less than year and estimated 5-year survival is less than 10%. Palliative surgical resections are recommended for symptoms relieved. Moreover, it can be prolonged survival in the subgroup that completely tumor removal was achieved. Unfortunately, most of the cases after resection will experience recurrence of the diseases. Then, the current adjuvant treatment such as immunotherapy, chemotherapy, targeted therapy, and vaccination may play the important role in this setting.

9. References

Agrawal S, Yao TJ, Coit DG. (1999) Surgery for melanoma metastatic to the gastrointestinal tract. *Annals of Surgical Oncology*, Vol. 6, No. 4, (June 1999), pp. 336-344.

Agrawal D, Tannous GC, Chak A. (2010) Primary malignant melanoma of the hepatic duct: a case report. *Gastrointestinal Endoscopy*, Vol. 72, No. 4, (October 2010), pp. 845-846.

Akaraviputh T, Arunakul S, Lohsiriwat V, Iramaneerat C, Trakarnsanga A. (2010) Surgery for gastrointestinal malignant melanoma: experience from surgical training center. *World Journal of Gastroenterology*, Vol. 16, No. 6, (February 2010), pp. 745-748.

Albert JG, Gimm O, Stock K, Bilkenroth U, Marsch WC, Helmbold P. (2007) Small bowel endoscopy is crucial for diagnosis of melanoma metastases to the small bowel: a case of metachronous small bowel metastases and review of the literature. *Melanoma Research*, Vol. 17, (2007), pp. 335-338.

Avital S, Romaguera RL, Sands L, Marchetti F, Hellinger MD. (2004) Primary malignant melanoma of right colon. *The American Surgeon*, Vol. 70, No. 7, (July 2004), pp. 649-651.

Balch CM, Gershenwald JE, Soong SJ, et al. (2009) Final Version of 2009 AJC Melanoma Staging and Classification. *Journal of Clinical Oncology*, Vol. 27, No. 36, (December 2009), pp. 6199-6206.

Bastiaannet E, Hoekstra HJ, Hoekstra OS. (2011) Melanoma, Positron Emission Tomography. *Methods in Molecular Biology*, Vol. 727, (May 2011), pp. 123-139.

Bender GN, Maglinte DD, McLarney JH, Rex D, Kelvin FM. (2001) Malignant melanoma: patterns of metastasis to the small bowel, reliability of imaging studies, and clinical relevance. *The American Journal of Gastroenterology*, Vol. 96, No. 8, (August 2001), pp. 2392-2400.

Blecker D, Abraham S, Furth EE, Kochman ML. (1999) Melanoma in the gastrointestinal tract. *The American Journal of Gastroenterology*, Vol. 94, No. 12, (December 1999), pp. 3427-3433.

Brady MS, Kavolius JP, Quan SH. (1995) Anorectal melanoma. A 64-year experience at Memorial Sloan-Kettering Cancer Center. *Diseases of the Colon and Rectum*, Vol. 38, No. 2, (February 1995), pp. 146-151.

Cadili A. (2009) Primary melanoma of the esophagus: A rare and challenging problem. *Southern Medical Journal*, Vol. 102, No. 9, (September 2009), pp. 883-884.

Cagir B, Whiteford MH, Topham A, Rakinic J, Fry RD. (1999) Changing epidemiology of anorectal melanoma. *Diseases of the Colon and Rectum*, Vol. 42, No. 9, (September 1999), pp. 1203-1208.

Caudie AS, Ross MI. (2011) Metastectomy for stage IV melanoma: for whom and how much? *Surgical Oncology Clinics of North America*, Vol. 20, No. 1, (January 2011), pp. 133-144.

Chalkiadakis G, Wihlm JM, Morand G, Weill-Bousson M, Witz JP. (1985) Primary malignant melanoma of the esophagus. *The Annals of Thoracic Surgery*, Vol. 39, No. 5, (May 1985), pp. 472-475.

Chang F, Deere H. (2006) Esophageal melanocytosis morphologic features and review of the literature. *Archives of Pathology & Laboratory Medicine*, Vol. 130, No. 4, (April 2006), pp. 552-557.

Cheung MC, Perez EA, Molina MA, Jin X, Gutierrez JC, Franceschi D, Livingstone AS, Koniaris LG. (2008) Defining the role of surgery for primary gastrointestinal tract melanoma. *Journal of Gastrointestinal Surgery*, Vol. 12, No. 4, (April 2008), pp. 731-738.

Chong AE, Karnell LH, Menck HR. (1998) The National Cancer Data Base report on cutaneous and noncutaneous melanoma: a summary of 84,836 cases from the past decade. The American College of Surgeons Commission on Cancer and the American Cancer Society. *Cancer*, Vol. 83, No. 8, (October 1998), pp. 1664-1678.

Crippa F, Leutner M, Belli F, Gallino F, Greco M, Pilotti S, Cascinelli N, Bombardieri E. (2000) Which kinds of lymph node metastases can FDG PET detect? A clinical study in melanoma. *Journal of Nuclear Medicine*, Vol. 41, No. 9, (September 2000), pp. 1491-1494.

Crippa S, Bovo G, Romano F, Mussi C, Uggeri F. (2004) Melanoma metastatic to the gallbladder and small bowel: report of a case and review of the literature. *Melanoma Research*, Vol. 14, No. 5, (October 2004), pp. 427-430.

Dasgupta T, Brasfield R. (1964) Metastatic Melanoma. A clinicopathological study. *Cancer*, Vol. 17, (October 1964), pp. 1323-1339.

Davies MA, Gershenwald JE. Targeted therapy for melanoma: a primer. *Surgical Oncology Clinics of North America*, Vol. 20, No. 1, (January 2010), pp. 165-180.

De la Pava S, Nigogosyan G, Pickren JW, et al. (1963) Melanosis of the esophagus. *Cancer*, Vol. 16, (1963), pp. 48-50.

Essner R. (2003) Surgical Treatment of malignant melanoma. *The Surgical Clinics of North America*, Vol. 83, No. 1, (February 2003), pp. 109-156.

Essner R, Lee J, Wanek LA, Itakura H, Morton DL. (2004) Contemporary surgical treatment of advanced-stage melanoma. *Archives of Surgery*, Vol. 139, No. 9, (September 2004), pp.961-966.

Galloro G, Inzirillo A, Magno L, Diamantis G, Inzirillo M, Pastore A, Ruggiero S, Mosella G. (2011) Multiple nodular lesions by colonic metastatic malignant melanoma. *Digestive and Liver Disease*, Vol. 41, No. 2, (February 2009), pp. 169.

Gabali AM, Priebe P, Ganesan S. (2008) Primary melanoma of small intestine masquerading as gastrointestinal stromal tumor: a case report and literature review. *The American Surgeon*, Vol.74, No. 4, (April 2008), pp. 318-321.

Garrett K, Kalady MF. (2010) Anal neoplasms. *Surgical Oncology Clinics of North America*, Vol. 90, No. 1, (February 2010), pp. 147-161.

Gong L, Li YH, Zhao JY, Wang XX, Zhu SJ, Zhang W. (2008) Primary malignant melanoma of the liver: A case report. *World Journal of Gastroenterology*, Vol. 14, No. 31, (August 2008), pp. 4968-4971.

Gutman H, Hess KR, Kokotsakis JA, Ross MI, Guinee VF, Balch CM. (2001) Surgery of abdominal metastases of cutaneous melanoma. *World Journal of Surgery*, Vol. 25, No. 6, (June 2001), pp. 750-758.

Homsi J, Grimm JC, Hwu P. (2010) Immunotherapy of melanoma: an update. *Surgical Oncology Clinics of North America*, Vol. 20, No. 1, (January 2010), pp. 145-163.

Hulshof MC, Van Haaren PM, Zum Vörde Sive Vörding PJ, Krishnadath S, Marsman WA, Van Berge Henegouwen MI, Geijsen ED, Crezee J. (2010) Radiotherapy combined with hyperthermia for primary malignant melanomas of the esophagus. *Disease of the Esophagus*, Vol. 23, No. 8, (November 2010), pp. E42-47.

Ishizone S, Koide N, Karasawa F, Akita N, Muranaka F, Uhara H, Miyagawa S. (2008) Surgical treatment for anorectal malignant melanoma: report of five cases and review of 79 Japanese cases. *International Journal of Colorectal Disease*, Vol. 23, no. 12, (December 2008), pp.1257-62.

Joob AW, Haines GK, Kies MS, Shields TW. (1995) Primary malignant melanoma of the esophagus. *The Annals of Thoracic Surgery*, Vol. 60, No. 1, (July 1995), pp. 217-222.

Katz SC, Bowne WB, Wolchok JD, Busam KJ, Jaques DP, Coit DG. (2007) Surgical management of melanoma of the gallbladder: a report of 13 cases and review of the literature. *American Journal of Surgery*, Vol. 193, No. 4, (April 2007), pp. 493-497.

Kenny B, Dotto J, Homer R, Shafi N, Davydova L. Primary malignant melanoma of the transverse colon: Report of a case and review of the literaure. *International Journal of Surgical Pathology*, Vol. 15, No. 4, (October 2007), 401-407.

Khalid U, Saleem T, Imam AM, Khan MR. (2011) Pathogenesis, diagnosis and management of primary melanoma of the colon. *World Journal of Surgical Oncology*, Vol. 9, No. 14, (February 2011), pp. 1-9.

Kim HS, Kim EK, Jun HJ, Oh SY, Park KW, Lim do H, Lee SI, Kim JH, Kim KM, Lee DH, Lee J. (2010) Noncutaneous malignant melanoma: a prognostic model from a retrospective multicenter study. *BMC Cancer*, Vol. 28,No. 10, (April 2010), pp. 1-8.

Kimura H, Kato H, Sohda M, Nakajima M, Fukai Y, Miyazaki T, Masuda N, Manda R, Fukuchi M, Ojima H, Tsukada K, Kuwano H. (2005) Flat-type primary malignant melanoma of the esophagus treated by EMR: case report. *Gastrointestinal Endoscopy*, Vol. 61, No. 6, (May 2005), pp. 787-789.

Klas JV, Rothenberger DA, Wong WD, Madoff RD. (1999) Malignant tumors of the anal canal: the spectrum of disease, treatment, and outcomes. *Cancer*, Vol. 85, No. 8, (April 1999), pp. 1686-1693.

Kranzfelder M, Seidl S, Dobritz M, Brücher BL. (2008) Amelanotic esophageal malignant melanoma: case report and short review of the literature. *Case Reports in Gastroenterology*, Vol. 2, No. 2, (July 2008), pp. 224-231.

Kumar R, Alavi A. (2005) Clinical applications of fluorodeoxyglucose--positron emission tomography in the management of malignant melanoma. *Current Opinion in Oncology*, Vol. 17, No. 2, (March 2005), pp. 154-159.

Lagoudianakis EE, Genetzakis M, Tsekouras DK, Papadima A, Kafiri G, Toutouzas K, Katergiannakis V, Manouras A. (2006) Primary gastric melanoma: a case report. *World Journal of Gastroenterology*, Vol. 12, No. 27, (July 2006), pp. 4425-4427.

Lens M, Bataille V, Krivokapic Z. (2009) Melanoma of the small intestine. *The Lancet Oncology*, Vol. 10, No. 5, (May 2009), pp. 516-521.

Li B, Lei W, Shao K, Zhang C, Chen Z, Shi S, He J. (2007) Characteristics and prognosis of primary malignant melanoma of the esophagus. *Melanoma Research*, Vol. 17, No. 4, (August 2007), pp. 239-242.

Liang KV, Sanderson SO, Nowakowski GS, Arora AS. (2006) Metastatic malignant melanoma of the gastrointestinal tract. *Mayo Clinic Proceedings*, Vol. 81, No. 4, (April 2006), pp. 511-516.

Manola J, Atkins M, Ibrahim J, Kirkwood J. (2000) Prognostic factors in metastatic melanoma: a pooled analysis of Eastern Cooperative Oncology Group trials. *Journal of Clinical Oncology*, Vol. 18, No. 22, (November 2000), pp. 3782-3793.

Manouras A, Genetzakis M, Lagoudianakis E, Markogiannakis H, Papadima A, Kafiri G, Filis K, Kekis PB, Katergiannakis V. (2007) Malignant gastrointestinal melanomas of unknown origin: should it be considered primary? *World Journal of Gastroenterology*, Vol. 13, No. 29, (August 2007), pp. 4027-4029.

Martinez SR, Young SE. (2008) A rational surgical approach to the treatment of distant melanoma metastases. *Cancer Treatments Reviews*, Vol. 34, No. 7, (November 2008), pp. 614-620.

Moore WD. (1857) Recurrent melanosis of the rectum after previous removal from the verge of the anus in a man aged 65. *Lancet*, Vol. 1, (1857), pp. 290-294.

Nilsson PJ, Ragnarsson-Olding BK. (2010) Importance of clear resection margins in anorectal malignant melanoma. *The British Journal of Surgery*, Vol. 97, No. 1, (January 2010), pp. 98-103.

Ollila DW, Hsueh EC, Stern SL, Morton DL. (1999) Metastasectomy for recurrent stage IV melanoma. *Journal of Surgical Oncology,* Vol. 71, No. 4, (August 1999) pp. 209-213.

Panagiotou I, Brountzos EN, Bafaloukos D, Stoupis C, Brestas P, Kelekis DA. (2002) Malignant melanoma metastatic to the gastrointestinal tract. *Melanoma Research,* Vol. 12, No. 2, (April 2002), pp. 169-173.

Pantalone D, Taruffi F, Paolucci R, Liguori P, Rastrelli M, Andreoli F. (2000) Malignant melanoma of the rectum. *The European Journal of Surgery,* Vol. 166, No. 7, (July 2000), pp. 583-584.

Patnana M, Bronstein Y, Szklaruk J, Bedi DG, Hwu WJ, Gershenwald JE, Prieto VG, Ng CS. (2011) Multimethod imaging, staging, and spectrum of manifestations of metastatic melanoma. *Clinical Radiology,* Vol. 66, No. 3, (March 2011), pp. 224-236.

Pessaux P, Pocard M, Elias D, Duvillard P, Avril MF, Zimmerman P, Lasser P. (2004) Surgical management of primary anorectal melanoma. *The British Journal of Surgery,* Vol 91, No. 9, (September 2004), pp.1183-1187.

Poggi S, McNiff JFM, Hwu WJP, Bayar S, Salem RR. (2000) Colonic melanoma, primary or regressed primary. *Journal of Clinical Gastroenterology,* Vol. 30, No. 4, (June 2000), pp. 441-444.

Pommer B, Probst A, Messmann H. (2008) Gastric metastases from malignant melanoma. *Endoscopy,* Vol. 40, Suppl. 2, (September 2008), E30-1.

Prakoso E, Fulham M, Thompson JF, Selby WS. (2011) Capsule endoscopy versus positron emission tomography for detection of small: a pilot study. *Gastrointestinal Endoscopy,* (Febuary 1) (Epub ahead of print)

Prichard RS, Hill AD, Skehan SJ, O'Higgins NJ. (2002) Positron emission tomography for staging and management of malignant melanoma. *The British Journal of Surgery,* Vol. 89, No. 4, (April 2002), pp. 389-396.

Row D, Weiser MR. (2009) Anorectal Melanoma. Clinics in Colon and Rectal Surgery, Vol. 22, No. 2, (May 2009), pp 120-126.

Sabanathan S, Eng J, Pradhan GN. (1989) Primary malignant melanoma of the esophagus. *American journal of Gastroenterology,* Vol. 84, No. 2, (December 1989), pp. 1475-1481.

Sachs DL, Lowe L, Chang AE, Carson E, Johnson TM. (1999) Do primary small intestinal melanomas exist? Report of a case. *Journal of the American Academy of Dermatology,* Vol. 41, No. 6, (December 1999), pp. 1042-1044.

Safioleas M, Agapitos E, Kontzoglou K, Stamatakos M, Safioleas P, Mouzopoulos G, Kostakis A. (2006) Primary melanoma of the gallbladder: Does it exist? *World Journal of Gastroenterology,* Vol. 12, No. 26, (July 2006), pp. 4259-4261.

Sanchez AA, Wu TT, Prieto VG, Rashid A, Hamilton SR, Wang H. (2008) Comparison of primary and metastatic malignant melanoma of the esophagus: clinicopathologic review of 10 cases. *Archives of Pathology & Laboratory Medicine,* Vol. 132, No. 10, (October 2008), pp. 1623-1629.

Sanki A, Scolyer RA, Thompson JF. (2009) Surgery for melanoma metastases of the gastrointestinal tract: indications and results. *European Journal of Surgical Oncology,* Vol. 35, No. 3, (March 2009), pp. 313-319.

Schuchter LM, Green R, Fraker D. (2000) Primary and metastatic diseases in malignant melanoma of the gastrointestinal tract. *Current Opinion in Oncology,* Vol. 12, No. 2, (March 2000), pp. 181-185.

Shia J. (2010) An update on tumors of the anal canal. *Archives of Pathology & Laboratory Medicine,* Vol. 134, No. 11, (November 2010), pp. 1601-1611.

Slingluff CL Jr, Vollmer RT, Seigler HF. (1990) Anorectal melanoma: clinical characteristics and results of surgical management in twenty-four patients. *Surgery*, Vol. 107, No. 1, (January 1990), pp.1-9.

Sondak VK, Gonzalez RJ, Kudchadkar R. Adjuvant therapy for melanoma: a surgical perspective. *Surgical Oncology Clinics of North America*, Vol. 20, No. 1, (January 2011), pp. 105-114.

Spanknebel K, Kaufman HL. (2004) Surgical treatment of stage IV melanoma. *Clinics in Dermatology*, Vol. 22, No. 3, (May 2004), pp. 240-250.

Stringa O, Valdez R, Beguerie JR, Abbruzzese M, Lioni M, Nadales A, Iudica F, Venditti J, San Roman A. (2006) Primary amelanotic melanoma of the esophagus. *International Journal of Dermatology*, Vol. 45, No. 10, (October 2006), pp. 1207-1210.

Suzuki H, Nakanishi Y, Taniguchi H, Shimoda T, Yamaguchi H, Igaki H, Tachimori Y, Kato H. (2008) Two cases of early-stage esophageal malignant melanoma with long-term survival. *Pathology International*, Vol. 58, No. 7, (July 2008), pp. 432-435.

Tanaka K, Toyoda H, Hamada Y, Aoki M, Kosaka R, Noda T, Katsurahara M, Nakamura M, Ninomiya K, Inoue H, Imoto I. (2008) Duodenal metastasis of malignant melanoma observed by magnification endoscopy. *Endoscopy*, Vol. 40, Suppl. 2, (September 2008), E6-7.

Tessier DJ, McConnell EJ, Young-Fadok T, Wolff BG. (2003) Melanoma metastatic to the colon: case series and review of the

literature with outcome analysis. *Diseases of the Colon and Rectum*, Vol. 46, No. 4, (April 2003), pp. 441-447.

Thibault C, Sagar P, Nivatvongs S, Ilstrup DM, Wolff BG. (1997) Anorectal melanoma--an incurable disease? *Diseases of the Colon and Rectum*, Vol. 40, No. 6, (June 1997), pp. 661-618.

Wagner MS, Shoup M, Pickleman J, Yong S. (2000) Primary malignant melanoma of the common bile duct: a case report and review of the literature. *Archives of Pathology & Laboratory Medicine*, Vol. 124, No. 3, (March 2000), pp. 419-422.

Weinstock MA. (1993) Epidemiology and prognosis of anorectal melanoma. *Gastroenterology*, Vol. 104, No. 1, (January 1993), pp. 174-178.

Wong SL, Coit DG. (2004) Role of surgery in patients with stage IV melanoma. *Current Opinion in Oncology*, Vol. 16, No. 2, (March 2000), pp. 150-160.

Wood TF, DiFronzo LA, Rose DM, Haigh PI, Stern SL, Wanek L, Essner R, Morton DL. (2001) Does complete resection of melanoma metastatic to solid intra-abdominal organs improve survival? *Annals of Surgical Oncology*, Vol. 8, No. 8, (September 2001), pp. 658-662.

Yeh JJ, Shia J, Hwu WJ, Busam KJ, Paty PB, Guillem JG, Coit DG, Wong WD, Weiser MR. (2006) The role of Abdomino -perineal resection as surgical therapy for anorectal melanoma. *Annals of Surgery*, Vol. 244, No. 6, (December 2006), pp. 1012-1017.

Young SE, Martinez SR, Essner R. (2006) The role of surgery in treatment of stage IV melanoma. *Journal of Surgical Oncology*, Vol. 94, No. 4, (September 2006), pp. 344-351.

Zaide EC. (1963) Melanoma maligno do coledoco. Arq Oncol, Vol. 5, (1963), pp. 254-255.

12

Surgical Treatment of Pulmonary Metastases from Melanoma: Emerging Options

Pier Luigi Filosso, Alberto Sandri, Enrico Ruffini, Paolo Olivo Lausi, Maria Cristina Bruna and Alberto Oliaro
University of Torino; Department of Thoracic Surgery, Torino, Italy

1. Introduction

Malignant melanoma (MM) is rapidly becoming a major health problem in the USA and in Europe. It has been estimated that more than 55,000 Americans developed MM in 2004, and that about 8,000 ultimately died of it (1).

More than one third of patients operated for MM develop tumor recurrence; melanoma patients' annual risk of death in Stage IV of the American Joint Committee on Cancer (AJCC) has been estimated to be about 20% during the first 3 years (2). The site of relapse is a very important predictor of survival. Regional lymph node recurrences in fact, may be surgically resected and 5-year survival rate have been reported to be between 20% and 50% (3-4). Distant metastases (MTS), both in visceral and non-visceral sites, reported a 5-year survival of approximately 5% (5-7); for these patients surgery is not often feasible and systemic treatment (chemotherapy, immunotherapy, radiotherapy) is sometimes the curative option.

Lung is the second most common site for metastatic MM spread (8). The annual probability of developing lung MTS progressively increases from 10% at 5 years to 17% at 15 years after the resection of the primary tumor (9). Lung MTS are usually asymptomatic, sometimes multiple, occasionally detected with radiological imaging during patient follow-up.

Once lung MTS has developed, the possible surgical treatment remains controversial. Even if a clear clinical advantage in overall survival (OS) after resection of pulmonary MTS from osteogenic sarcoma, soft tissue sarcoma, non-seminomatous testicular neoplasms, colorectal and renal cell carcinoma has been demonstrated, 5-year survival rates in melanoma patients were lower, ranging between 5% and 31% (10-12). These ranges indicate how a preoperative patient selection is mandatory. In fact, only 10-35% of all metastatic melanoma patients are suitable for a complete surgical resection (13).

Systemic treatments including chemotherapy, radiotherapy, immunotherapy and more recently molecular target agents, demonstrated a partial clinical response only, with severe adverse effect and a dramatic impact on patient's quality of life (QOL), providing little, if any, attested survival benefit. Chemotherapy regimens may include: dacarbazine, cisplatin and carmusine, alone or in combination with a variety of immunotherapies, including cytokines, monoclonal antibodies and vaccination strategies with synthetic peptides, naked DNA, dendritic cells and recombinant viruses (14-17). Unfortunately, results are presently discouraging: <20% of patients treated with such therapeutic options present with a partial response rate and very few are long-term survivors.

Due to these reasons, surgery remains the treatment of choice to improve OS in Stage IV melanoma patients; anyway, surgery cannot be offered to all of metastatic patients. The need for a correct patient preoperative clinical assessment, in order to avoid incomplete surgical resections, has been demonstrated by many studies.

The aim of this paper is to underline the prognostic factors which influence survival in melanoma patients with pulmonary metastases undergoing surgical resection. The first part regards the experience of the Thoracic Surgery Department of the University of Torino; lastly we discuss our results at the light of those of the most important series published in Literature.

2. Surgical treatment of pulmonary metastases: indications and results

2.1 *Oliaro-Filosso et al.* – University of Torino (2000-2008)

In 2010 our group, a dedicated high-volume thoracic surgical team with long time experience in the management of pulmonary metastases, published its experience on the surgical treatment of pulmonary metastases from MM (18). Twenty-six patients were operated between January 2000 and December 2008. Table 1 shows patients clinical characteristics.

Gender (male/female)	14/12
Mean age (years)	62 (range 28-79)
Localization of the lung MTS	
Left lung	8
Right lung	16
Bilateral	2
Number of pulmonary MTS	
1 node	14
2 nodes	5
>2 nodes	7
Median DFI (months)	36
Type of surgical resection	
Wedge/segmental resection	23
Lobectomy	3

From Oliaro A, Filosso PL et.al: J.Thorac.Oncol. 2010;5(suppl.6):S187-S191 with permission

Table 1. University of Torino Department of Thoracic Surgery Stage IV melanoma metastatic to the lung: patients characteristics (number: 26).

Our patients' inclusion criteria were: 1) complete resection of the primary tumor; 2) no evidence of any other extrapulmonary MTSs; 3) resectable lung MTS; 4) predicted post-resection lung volumes compatible with the anticipated pulmonary resection.

In all cases lung MTSs were discovered with a routine chest X-ray during the follow-up program. The lesion/s was/were confirmed by a thoracic CT scan; since 2003, PET scan was available in our centre and routinely used.

Lung represented the first metastatic site in the majority of our patients (17; 65%); in 9 patients, lung MTS developed after metastatic spread in other viscera. A single pulmonary nodule was observed in 14 cases; 5 patients had 2 nodules and multiple nodules were observed in the remaining 7.

All patients received adjuvant or neoadjuvant systemic therapy (either chemotherapy or immunotherapy). The mean disease-free interval (DFI) was of 36 months.

Lung wedge resection was the commonest surgical procedure performed (23 cases) whereas lobectomy was necessary in 3 patients. A complete surgical resection was accomplished in all patients and it was confirmed by the histological examination. There was no postoperative mortality.

One, 3 and 5-year survival rates were 72%, 36% and 23% respectively.

The Cox regression analysis identified the female gender (p=0.05) as the only independent prognostic factor related to patients survival. This result can be attributed to the limited number of our patients and to their preoperative selection: these factors may explain why the number of pulmonary MTS and/or the DFI did not reach a statistical significance in our analysis (18).

A formal search in literature results in several small and out of date series, and many case reports regarding unusual clinical manifestations of pulmonary MTS from MM.

In order to analyze the results and to recognize possible prognostic factors we summarize the most interesting ones, comparing them to our data.

2.2 *Tafra et al.* - John Wayne cancer institute (1971 - 1993)

Tafra et al. (12) reviewed the John Wayne Cancer Institute's melanoma series: among 6129 patients treated from 1971 to 1993, 2167 had distant MTS and 984 presented with pulmonary nodules. Of these, only 106 (11%) were submitted to a surgical resection and received an overall of 117 procedures. All operations were performed through thoracotomy.

Wedge resection was performed in 71 cases (61%), lobectomy in 25 and pneumonectomy in 6. Fifteen patients received an extrapulmonary intrathoracic resection (not otherwise clarified).

More than half of patients (56/106) had a single pulmonary MTS; 23 had 2 or 3 nodules and 28 more than 3. In 41 patients (38.7%) an incomplete resection was performed.

Authors concluded that patients with complete resection survived longer than those with an incomplete one, even if this data did not reach statistical significance.

There was a trend towards a better survival in patients receiving a lobectomy when compared to those submitted to a wedge and for those with a single pulmonary lesion, but also these results were not statistically significant.

2.3 *Olilla et al.* - John Wayne cancer institute (1971 - 1994)

Olilla et al. (15) reconsidered the John Wayne Cancer Institute series of metastatic melanoma patients between 1971 and 1994 (129 cases) and pointed out the importance of the Tumor Doubling Time (TDT). TDT was calculated for each patient comparing successive chest radiographs in order to measure the changing diameters of each pulmonary nodule. When a patient presented with more than a nodule, TDT was calculated by measuring the fastest-growing one. Forty-five patients had at least two preoperative chest X-rays to compare, and only those were included in the study. Again, most of patients had a solitary nodule

(33,73%). A complete resection was accomplished in 38 cases (84.4%): wedge resection was the commonest surgical procedure (32, 71.1%), followed by lobectomy (11, 24.4%). The median TDT for these 45 patients was 66.9 days (range: 13.7-287.4 days). Sixty days was the TDT cut-off value decided by Authors.

A radical surgical resection ($p=0.04$) and a TDT≥60 days ($p=0.01$) were the two statistically positive prognostic factors. In particular, for patients with a TDT≥60 days, the median survival was 29.2 months with 20.7% 5-year survival rate.

2.4 *Leo et al.* - International registry of lung metastases (1945-1995)

Leo et al. (19) reconsidered 328 patients with pulmonary MTS from MM, previously collected by Pastorino *et al.*, including them into the International Registry of Lung Metastases which gathered data from 18 mayor Thoracic Surgical centres from Europe, USA and North America (20).

Thoracotomic surgical approach was the commonest proposed in Leo's series (247 patients); sternotomy was performed in 74 and video-assisted thoracic surgery (VATS) in 7, only. Bilateral interventions were proposed in 74 patients. Wedge resection was the most common surgical procedure (230), followed by lobectomy (4) and pneumonectomy (14). An extrapulmonary resection (chest wall, pleura, diaphragm, liver, mediastinal structures) was required in 50 cases (15.2%). A complete surgical resection (R0) was accomplished in 282 patients (85.9%).

Patients receiving a R0 resection survived longer than others in whom an incomplete one (R1-2) was performed (22% 5-year and 16% 10-year survival rates for R0 patients; 0% 5-year survival for R1-2 ones, $p<0.01$). Considering R0 patients only, a DFI>36 months (30% 5-year, 22% 5-year, $p<0.01$) and a single lesion (25% 5-year and 22% 10-year, $p=0.03$) statistically influenced patients survival.

Leo proposed four prognostic groups of patients, according to his multivariate analysis results, which were: 1) R0 metastasectomy and no adverse factor (only 1 lesion *and* DFI>36 months); 2) R0 metastasectomy and 1 unfavourable factor (more than 1 pulmonary nodule *or* DFI<36 months); 3) R0 metastasectomy and 2 unvavourable factors; 4) R1-2 metastasectomy.

It was thus demonstrated that differences in survival among these groups were statistically highly significant: 29% 5-year survival rate and 26% 10 year for Group 1; 20% 5-year and 10% 10 year for Group 2; 7% 5-year and 0% 10 year for Group 3; no 5 year survivors in Group 4.

Leo concluded that a complete surgical resection and a DFI>36 months were the most important positive prognostic factors.

2.5 *Andrews et al.* - Lee Moffitt cancer center (1988-2005)

Andrews and Coll. (21) reported Lee Moffitt Cancer Center's experience of patients with pulmonary MTS from MM between 1988 and 2005. An overall of 86 cases (64 men) were enrolled in this study. Preoperative patient assessment included thoracic CT scan and brain magnetic resonance imaging (MRI) to confirm the number and location of pulmonary nodules seen at the chest radiograph, and also to exclude possible extrathoracic malignancies. PET scan was used in 27 patients. A complete resection was achieved in all cases. Wedge resection (35, 22 of which through VATS procedures) was the most frequent surgical procedure performed. Ten were the segmental resections and 9 the lobectomies, all of these performed with a thoracotomy.

The estimated 5-year survival rate was 33%.
While a long DFI did not statistically affect survival, only the number of pulmonary lesions (1 vs 2-4) was a statistical prognostic factor (41 months vs. 21, p=0.05).

2.6 *Neumann et al.* - Memorial Sloan-Kettering cancer center

Neumann and Coll. (22) studied 122 pulmonary MTS treated at the Memorial Sloan-Kettering Cancer Center (MSKCC). Of these, only 26 patients (21%) received a surgical resection while others were treated with systemic therapy (82) or did not receive any sort of treatment (14); a complete resection was accomplished in all operated patients (a wedge resection, most frequently). Metastasectomy was associated with improved survival (median 40 months vs 11 months in non-operated patients); in operated patients, Authors pointed out an estimated 29% 5-year survival rate.
At the Cox regression analysis, a solitary metastasis (HR 1.9, 95%CI 1.1-3.2, p<0.0005) and the absence of extrathoracic disease (HR 1.9, 95% CI 1.2-3.1, p=0.01) were strong positive predictors of long-term survival. The lung resection itself was an independent factor predictive of survival (HR 0.42, 95%CI 0.21-0.87, p=0.02).

2.7 *Petersen et al.* - Duke comprehensive cancer center (1970 – 2004)

Finally, *Petersen et al.* (23) retrospectively reviewed the experience with lung MTS from MM patients treated in the Duke Comprehensive Cancer Center between years 1970 and 2004. An overall of 1720 patients were recorded: those submitted to surgery were only 318 (18.5%) while others received a systemic treatment. Two hundred forty-nine (78%) of operated patients received a radical resection; those receiving an incomplete resection were more likely to have multiple pulmonary lesions. Patients receiving curative resections had 19 months median survival and 21% 5-year survival rate, compared to 11 months and 13% of those with an incomplete one (p<0.0001).
The univariate analysis highlighted that lymph nodes metastases (p=0.001), 2 or more pulmonary MTS (p<0.001), a short DFI (p<0.001) and the presence of extrathoracic MTS (p<0.001) were significant negative prognostic factors.
The number of pulmonary MTS (p=0.012), a short DFI (p<0.001) and the presence of extrathoracic MTS (p<0.001) were found to be independent predictors of survival at the multivariate analysis. Table 2 and 3 summarize the series results and their prognostic factors, respectively.

Author (%)	*Year*	*#pts*	*Median survival (months)*	*5-year survival rate*
Tafra	1995	63	25	-
Olilla	1998	38	26	-
Leo	2000	282	19	22 %
Andrews	2006	86	35	33 %
Neuman	2007	26	40	29 %
Petersen 2007		249	19	21 %
Oliaro-Filosso	2010	26	-	23 %

Table 2. Survival after complete resection of pulmonary MTS.

Author	*year*	*# pts*	*Prognostic factors*
Tafra	1995	63	n° MTS; no extrathoracic MTS; TDT
Olilla	1998	38	TDT
Leo	2000	282	n°MTS; DFI; complete resection
Andrews	2006	86	n° MTS
Neuman	2007	26	n° MTS; no extrathoracic MTS
Petersen 2007		249	complete resection; n° MTS; DFI; no extrathoracic MTS
Oliaro-Filosso	2010	26	female gender

Legenda: *TDT: Tumor Doubling Time; DFI: Disease Free Interval; MTS: metastases*

Table 3. Prognostic factors in the cited series.

3. Discussion and conclusions

One may observe, by means of a formal search in literature of surgical series of resected pulmonary MTS from MM, that only few papers have been published in a long interval of time; the most recent series were taken into consideration in order to obtain the most comparable results as possible.

Preoperative patient assessment in the oldest series (*Tafra*, *Olilla* and *Leo*) presented some limitations, especially due to the lack of new generation radiological imaging which are mandatory to avoid the risk of incomplete/non-radical resections. Percentages of reported non curative procedures were 38.7% (41/106) in Tafra, 15.6% (7/45) in Olilla and 14% (46/328) in Leo.

A preoperative patient assessment is fundamental: thoracic and abdominal CT scan, brain MRI and whole body PET scan should be proposed in all. In those patients with lung MTS and concomitant extrathoracic lesions, surgery is contraindicated: those patients should receive systemic therapy alone.

When prognostic factors are evaluated, the importance of the number of lung MTS has been emphasized by many Authors. In almost all series, a higher survival rate of patients with 1 lesion was observed. The role and the importance of the type of surgical procedure (wedge resection vs lobectomy) was not important; generally when the MTS is peripherally located, it can be easily removed with a wedge resection or a segmentectomy (Fig. 1). Instead, lobectomy is reserved to those deeply located lesions within the lung parenchyma, in which the risk of non-free resection margins of tumoral tissue may be high if a non-anatomic resection is performed. Also, the procedure used to perform the limited resection (thoracotomy or a VATS) did not influence the survival rate. With the development of mini-invasive thoracic procedures and of the technologies to it dedicated, the role of VATS (and of robotics in the next future) is rapidly growing. Patients operated in such manner face a limited surgical impact, less pain and may have a shorter postoperative course, which can also reduce the overall recovery health costs. Furthermore, if a limited pulmonary resection is performed, patients' postoperative respiratory function is conserved: this leads to a better tolerated adjuvant systemic therapy and the chance to propose a redo-surgery in case of possible tumor relapse, which unfortunately is not infrequent.

The importance of a strict follow-up is brought to evidence by the majority of Authors. The common follow-up should include a chest X-ray; thoracic CT scan should be performed

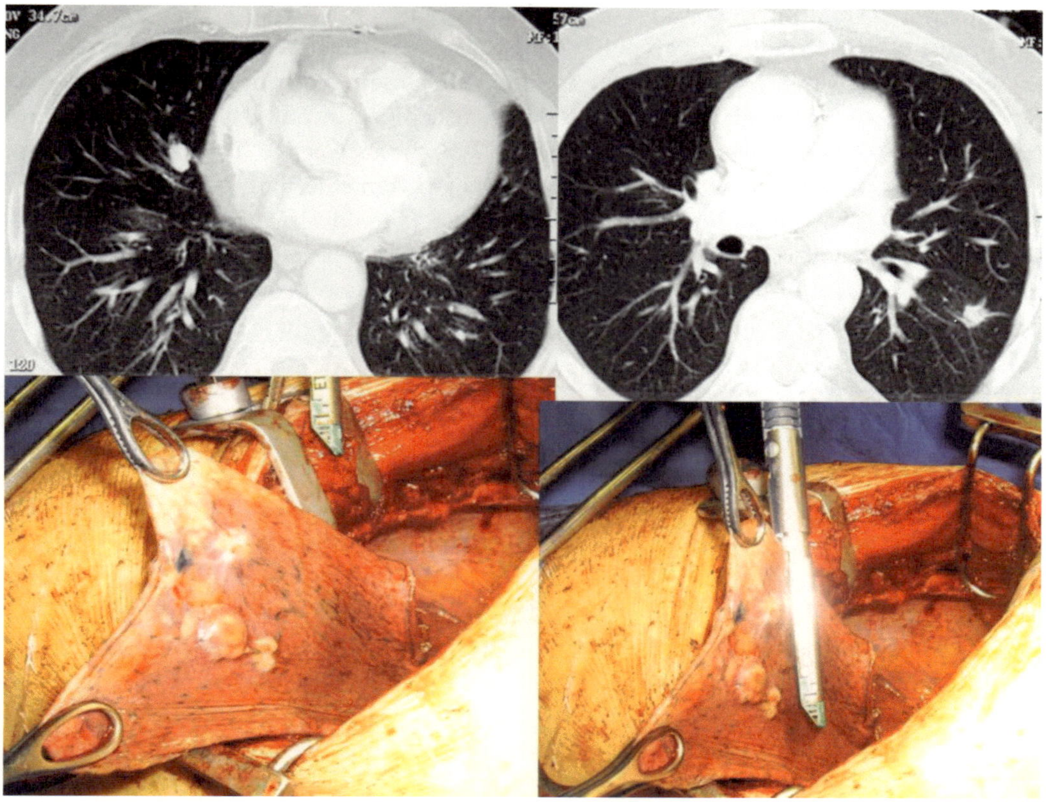

Fig. 1. Preoperative radiological and intraoperative images of resected pulmonary MTS from malignant melanoma.

whenever a nodule is detected. In case of its positivity at the PET scanning, surgery should be proposed immediately. We suggest to avoid repeated radiological controls of the nodule due to the high risk of possible tumor spreading.
Prognostic factors are almost the same: limited number of pulmonary MTS, a short DFI, absence of extrathoracic MTS, completeness of surgical resection (Table 3).
The role of the lymphadenectomy is not always put in evidence. We believe that lymph node sampling should be performed in all cases; many Author statistically demonstrated the significance of lymph node MTS as a prognostic factor: it's evident that patients with metastatic nodes have lower survival rate when compared to N0 patients. This data itself may suggest the role and importance of lymphadenectomy.
In conclusion, even if patients with pulmonary MTS from melanoma have a poor prognosis, those in whom a surgical resection can be proposed present a longer life expectancy than others treated with systemic therapy alone. In order to avoid incomplete surgical resections (in whom the survival is similar to chemotherapy) a selective preoperative patient assessment is mandatory. Surgical resection (wedge/segmentectomy) should be limited whenever possible and lymph nodal sampling should be routinely performed. Postoperative adjuvant therapy (chemotherapy, immunotherapy, radiotherapy) must always be proposed and a strict follow-up scheduled; in case of new pulmonary lesions developing, surgery should be planned, if feasible.

4. References

Jemal A, Tiwari RC, Murray T, Ghafoor A, Samuels A, Ward E, Feuer EJ, Thun MJ; American Cancer Society: cancer statistics, 2004. *CA Cancer J.Clin. 2004;54:8-29*

Slingluff CL, Dodge RK, Stanley WE,Seigler HF: The annual risk of melanoma progression. *Cancer 1992;70:1917-1927*

Morton DL, Wanek L, Nizze JA; Elashoff RM, Wong JH: Improved long-term survival after lymph-adenectomy of melanoma metastatic to regional nodes. Analysis of prognostic factors in 1134 patients from the John Wayne Cancer Clinic. *Ann.Surg. 1991;214:491-499*

Coit DG, Rogatko A, Brennan MF: Prognostic factors in patients with melanoma metastatic to axillary or inguinal lymph nodes. A multivariate analysis. *Ann.Surg. 1991;214:627-636*

Amer MH, Sarraf M, Vaitkevicius VK: Clinical presentation, natural history and prognostic factors in advanced malignant melanoma. *Surg.Gynecol.Obstet. 1991;149:687-692*

Roses DF, Karp NS, Oratz R, Dubin N, Harris MN, Speyer J, Boyd A, Golomb FM, Ransohoff J, Dugan M: Survival with regional and distant metastases from cutaneous malignant melanoma. *Surg.Gynecol.Obstet. 1991;172:262-268*

Balch CM, Soong SJ, Gershenwald JE, Thompson JF, Reintgen DS, Cascinelli N, Urist M, McMasters KM, Ross MI, Kirkwood JM, Atkins MB, Thompson JA, Coit DG, Byrd D, Desmond R, Zhang Y, Liu PY, Lyman GH, Morabito A: Prognostic factors analysis of 17,600 melanoma patients: validation of the American Joint Commettee on Cancer melanoma staging system. *J.Clin.Oncol. 2001;19:3622-3634*

Balch CM, Milton GW: Diagnosis of metastatic melanoma at distant sites. *In Cutaneous melanoma: clinical management and treatment results worldwide. 1985:222 Philadelphia: Lippincott*

Harpole DH, Johnson CM, Wolfe WG, George SL, Seigler HF: Analysis of 945 cases of pulmonary metastastatic melanoma. *J.Thorac.Cardiovasc.Surg. 1992;103:743-750*

Cahan WG: Excision of melanoma metastases to lung: problems in diagnosis and management. *Ann.Surg. 1973;178:703-709*

Gorenstein LA, Putnam JB, Natarajan G, Balch CA, Roth JA: Improved survival after resection of pulmonary metastases from malignant melanoma. *Ann.Thorac.Surg. 1991;52.201-210*

Tafra L, Dale PS, Wanek LA, Ramming KP, Morton DL: Resection and adjuvant immunotherapy for melanoma metastatic to the lung and thorax.*J.Thorac.Cardiovasc.Surg. 1995,110:119-129*

Essner R, Lee JH, Wanek LA, Itakura H, Morton DL: Contemporary surgical treatment of advanced-stage melanoma. *Arch.Surg. 2004;139:961-967*

Sasse A, Sasse E, Clark L, Ulloa L, Clark O: Chemoimmunotherapy versus chemotherapy for metastatic malignant melanoma. *Cochrane database Syst.rev. 2007;1):CD005 413*

Olilla DW, Stern SL, Morton DL: Tumor doubling time: a selection factor for pulmonary resection of metastatic melanoma. *J.Surg.Oncol. 1998;69:206-211*

Tarhini AA, Agarwala SS: Interleukin-2 for the treatment of melanoma. *Curr.Opin.Investig.Drugs 2005;6:1234-1239*

Riker AI, Jove R, Daud AI: Immunotherapy as a part of a multidisciplinary approach to melanoma treatment. *Front.Biosci. 2006;11:1-14*

Oliaro A; Filosso PL, Bruna MC, Mossetti C, Ruffini E: Pulmonary metastasectomy for melanoma. *J.Thorac.Oncol. 2010;5(S6):S187-S191.*

Leo F, Cagini L, Rocmans P, Cappello M, Van Geel AN, Maggi G, Goldstraw P, Pastorino U: Lung metastases from melanoma: when is surgical treatment warranted? *Br.J.Cancer 2000;83:569-572*

Pastorino U, Buyse M, Friedel G, Ginsberg RJ, Girard P, Goldstraw P, Johnston M, McCormack P, Pass H, Putnam JB: Long-term results of lung metastasectomy: prognostic analysis based on 5206 cases. *J.Thorac.Cardiovasc.Surg. 1997;113:37-} 49*

Andrews S, Robinson L, Cantor A, DeConti RC: Survival after surgical resection of isolated pulmonary metastases from malignant melanoma. *Cancer Control 2006;13:218-223*

Neumann HB, Patel A, Hanlon C, Wolchok JD, Houghton AN, Coit DG: Stage IV melanoma and pulmonary metastases: factors predictive of survival. *Ann.Surg.Oncol. 2007;14:2847-2853*

Petersen RP, Hanish SI, Haney JC, Miller III CC, Burfeind WR, Tyler DS, Seigler HF, Wolfe W, D'Amico TA, Harpole Jr DH: Improved survival with pulmonary metastasectomy: an analysis of 1270 patients with pulmonary metastatic melanoma. *J.Thorac.Cardiovasc.Surg. 2007;133:104-110*

13

Melanoma-Predisposing CDKN2A Mutations in Association with Breast Cancer: A Case-Study and Review of the Literature

Klára Balogh et al.*
Department of Dermatology and Allergology,
University of Szeged
Hungary

1. Introduction

The authors present the case of a 33-year-old female patient who developed melanoma, ductal adenocarcinoma of the breast and primary pancreas adenocarcinoma nearly simultaneously, but independently of each other. Past medical history of the patient was unremarkable, however, in her family history gastric, laryngeal and breast cancer was noted on the paternal side. The occurrence of multiple primary tumours in a relatively young individual, together with the family history of different malignancies, suggested that there might be genetic predisposition to the development of multiple tumours. In this chapter we present the case of the young female patient suffering from three independent primary tumours and review current data on the germ-line mutations detected to date in the CDKN2A gene, in view of the association not only with melanoma, but also with additional malignant diseases, such as pancreas carcinoma and breast cancer.

2. Case presentation and review of the literature

2.1 Clinical observations and management

The 33-year-old female patient presented with a lesion which had the clinical appearance of a verrucous pigmented nevus on the left lower back for the preceeding 2 years. Histology of the excised lesion showed a pT2b stage malignant melanoma consisting of exulcerated nodular (Fig. 1a) and superficial (Fig. 1b) areas with 1.524 mm Breslow's thickness and Clark's level II-III. Based on the above results, reexcision and sentinel lymph node biopsy were performed. Histological examination of the sentinel lymph nodes from the left axillary

*Edina Nemes[1], Gabriella Uhercsák[2], Zsuzsanna Kahán[2], György Lázár[3], Gyula Farkas[3], Hilda Polyánka[4], Erika Kiss[1], Rolland Gyulai[1], Erika Varga[1], Erika Keresztné Határvölgyi[5], László Kaizer[6], Lajos Haracska[5], László Tiszlavicz[6], Lajos Kemény[1,4], Judit Oláh[1],Márta Széll[4],
1 Department of Dermatology and Allergology,
2 Department of Oncology,
3 Department of Surgery,
4 Dermatological Research Group of the Hungarian Academy of Sciences,
5 Institute of Genetics, Biological Research Centre of the Hungarian Academy of Sciences
6 Department of Pathology, all at the University of Szeged,

and left inguinal regions did not reveal any metastases. Staging investigations - chest x-ray, ultrasound scan of the abdomen, pelvis, left axillary and left inguinal regions - did not find any regional lymph node or internal organ involvement. Results of laboratory tests, including serum lactate dehydrogenase levels, were all normal. The patient received low dose (3 MIU - 3 times a week sc.) interferon-α 2a treatment for one year.

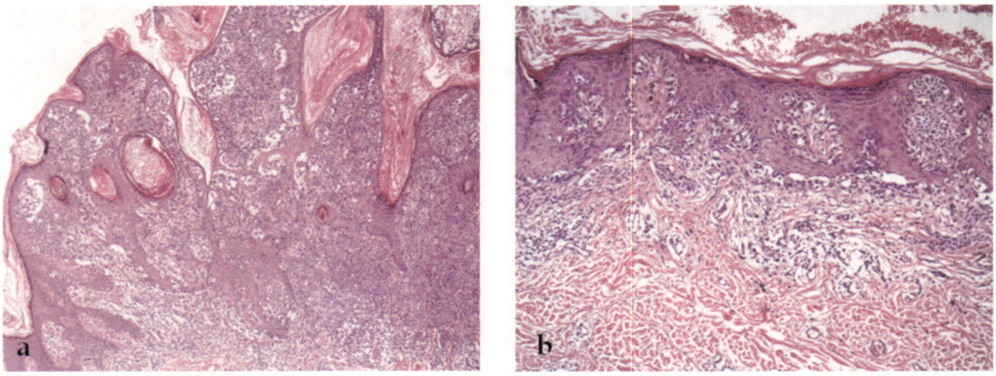

Fig. 1. Histology of primary malignant melanoma. Hematoxylin-eosin staining of the excised lesion revealed its combined nature having nodular (a) and superficial (b) parts.

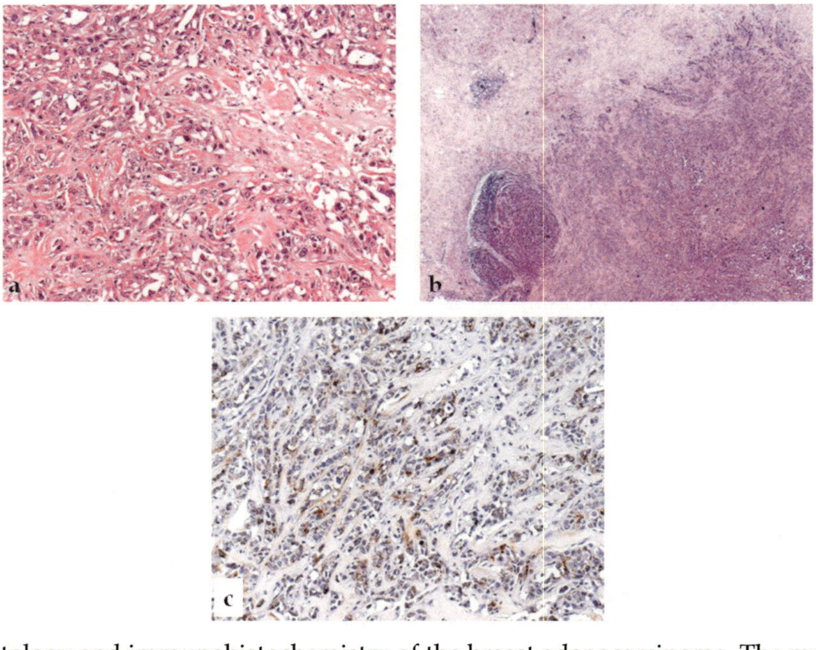

Fig. 2. Histology and immunohistochemistry of the breast adenocarcinoma. The marked nuclear polymorphism, lack of tubular forming and high number of mitoses indicated the diagnosis of ductal adenocarcinoma (a). Two of the excised 14 lymph nodes proved to have metastases with capsular invasion (b). HMF-G staining indicated a poorly differentiated breast adenocarcinoma (c).

Fifteen months after the completion of interferon treatment, the patient noted a firm nodule in the lateral area of the left breast which was biopsied. Histological examination revealed four foci of Grade III invasive ductal adenocarcinoma (Fig. 2a). Grading was based on the marked nuclear polymorphism, lack of tubular forming and high number of mitoses. In view of the multifocal malignant enhancement seen on the MRI and the histology report of the core biopsy, the patient underwent left mastectomy with radical left axillary lymph node dissection. Metastases infiltrating the capsule were found in 2 out of the 14 lymph nodes examined (Fig. 2b).

With regards to the diagnosis of breast cancer, PET CT was performed in order to exclude dissemination. The PET CT suggested the presence of a malignant lesion in the region of the pancreas. Abdominal MRI revealed a neoplasm of 2 cm in diameter in the caudal part of the pancreas (Fig. 3a). Laboratory investigations showed elevated CA 19-9 and serum amylase levels. On explorative laparotomy, an irresectable tumour mass involving the pancreas, liver and the regional lymph nodes was found. The tumour was biopsied and was initially described as metastatic adenocarcinoma (Fig. 3b). However, further immunohistochemical (CK20 and CK7) and mucin staining (MUC5AC) of the specimens from the breast (Fig. 2c) and abdominal mass (Fig. 3c), clearly differentiated two tumours: 1. poorly differentiated [CK7+/CK20-/MUC5AC-] breast adenocarcinoma, 2. moderately differentiated [CK7+/CK20+/MUC5AC+]) pancreas adenocarcinoma. This verified the gastrointestinal origin of the primary tumour i.e. the abdominal mass originated from the primary pancreas adenocarcinoma.

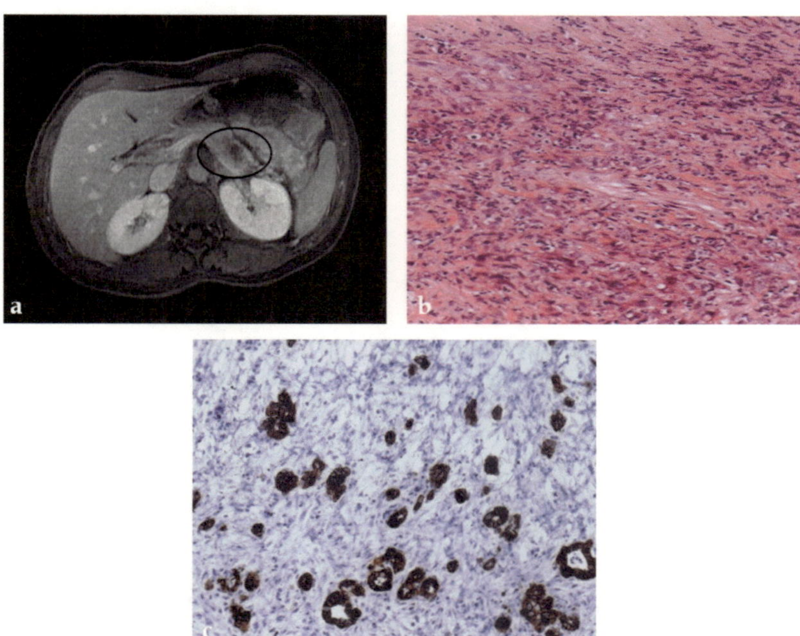

Fig. 3. Diagnosis of pancreas adenocarcinoma. Abdominal MRI showed a neoplasm in the caudal part of the pancreas (a). Hematoxylin-eosin staining indicated the malignant nature of the excised tumour (b). CK-20 immunohistochemistry indicated a moderately differentiated metastatic adenocarcinoma with globular components in the pancreas (c).

With regards to the case of multiple primary tumours, the patient received gemcitabine plus cisplatin combined chemotherapy. Repeated laparotomy performed on follow up after the treatment course noted complete regression of the previously detected primary tumours and tumour-free abdominal organs. Subsequently, the results of all re-staging investigations were negative and tumour markers returned to the normal range.

2.2 Genetic investigations

During the course of the patient's treatment, her family history for tumours was investigated. She reported that her father was suffering from gastric and laryngeal carcinoma and that her father's sister had died from breast cancer at a young age several decades ago. (Fig. 4a). We therefore set out to perform genetic investigations and check whether there are any cancer predisposing factors, causing the high prevalence of simultaneously appearing independent primary malignancies in the patient and in her family. The blood samples used in this study were taken after written informed consent of the patient and family members. The protocol was approved by the Local Ethics Committee in adherence to the Helsinki guidelines. Two ml of venous blood was taken, genomic DNA was isolated using the QIAmp DNA Blood Mini Kit (Qiagen, Hilden, Germany) and exons 1α, 1β, 2 and 3 of the CDKN2A gene were amplified with the Resequencing Amplicon probe system (http://www.ncbi.nlm.nih.gov/genome/probe/reports/probereport; probe IDs: RSA001284450, RSA000045423, RSA000942236, RSA000942233). The PCR products were purified using the Quantum Prep PCR Kleen Spin Columns (Bio-Rad, Hercules, CA, USA). The genetic analysis revealed that the patient and her father both carried the R24P CDKN2A mutation in a heterozygote form (Fig. 4b). The mutation is located in exon 1a, therefore only the $p16^{INK4a}$ transcript variant is affected (Fig. 4c).

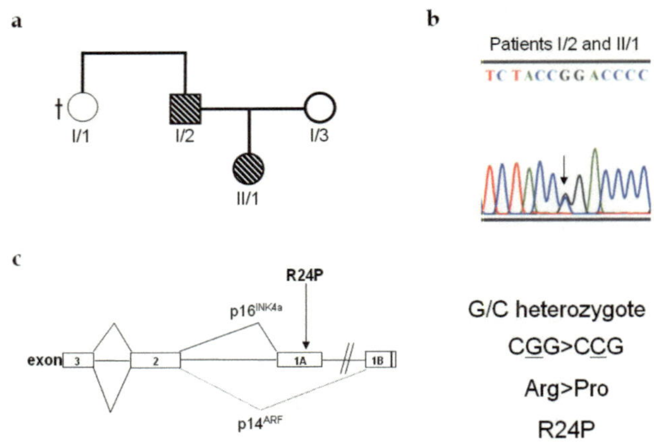

Fig. 4. Genetic analysis of the patient and her family. The 33-year-old female patient (II/1, melanoma, breast and pancreas carcinoma), her father (I/2; gastric and laryngeal carcinoma) and her mother (I/3; without any malignant diseases) were investigated. The father's sister (I/1) had died from breast cancer at a young age several decades ago, therefore her genetic investigation could not be performed (a). Sequence analysis revealed that probands I/2 and II/1 carried a missense mutation (G/C) in exon 1a of the CDKN2A gene (b), causing an arginine to proline amino acid change in codon 24 (R24P) affecting only the $p16^{INK4a}$ transcript variant (c).

Because of the occurrence of breast adenocarcinoma in our patient's medical history, it was also tested whether she carried mutations in the BRCA1 and BRCA2 genes. The 15 most commonly occurring (so-called "hot spot") BRCA mutations were studied (Table 1), but according to the sequencing data, none of them could be detected in the case of the female patient. After having received these data, we did not perform the BRCA1 and BRCA2 examinations on the genetic material of her father.
Based on these results, we hypothesize that the detected R24P mutation of the CDKN2A gene may be responsible for the melanoma and pancreas carcinoma of the 33-year-old female patient. At the same time, it may have contributed to the genetic predisposition for the breast cancer of our patient and her late aunt, as well as to the gastric and laryngeal carcinoma of her father. In the coming chapter we review current literature data about the possible breast cancer predisposing nature of CDKN2A mutations in general and the R24P mutation in particular.

2.3 The R24P mutation of CDKN2A has been worldwide implicated as a melanoma-predisposing genetic factor

The R24P germline mutation of the CDKN2A gene was first described by Australian authors. Holland et al. (Holland et al., 1995) reported on a survey performed on 17 melanoma-prone families in 1995 and they identified this mutation in one of the studied families. Since that time many independent studies proved the melanoma-predisposing nature of this mutation being one of the most widespread among the so-far identified disease-associated mutations of the CDKN2A gene. Soon after the first detection, the R24P mutation was also identified in US melanoma-prone families as early as in 1998 (Monzon et al., 1998) and its function was also assessed by yeast two-hybrid assay. According to the results, the R24P missense mutation almost completely abrogates the binding activity of the protein, thus explaining the disease-predisposing nature of the mutation. Following the "New World" publications of the R24P mutation, authors also reported it in European melanoma-prone families: it was reported in 1998 in the UK (MacKie et al., 1998) in the case of a relatively young (y31) male patient with multiple primary melanomas and in the case of two unrelated melanoma-prone kindreds in France (Soufir et al., 1998). This is why review papers from the mid-2000s refer to the R24P mutation as one of the most widespread CDKN2A mutations in the World, contributing to the genetic predisposition to familial, as well as multiple primary melanoma. To our best knowledge, ours is the first report on the identification of the R24P mutation in a Central-European family.
Taken together, the above summary well reflects that the R24P CDKN2A mutation is a relatively frequent one all over the World. Whether it is an ancient founder mutation that was spread to many geographical locale in the past, or independent mutation events happened, would be interesting to investigate (Table 2). There have been already very good examples provided where similar intriguing questions were addressed. Hashemi et al. (Hashemi et al., 2001) demonstrated that the 113insR CDKN2A mutation found only in Southern Scandinavia is a founder mutation that arose approximately 98 generations ago. Similarly, the G101W mutation that is frequent in Northern Italy, Southern Germany and France, is also a founder mutation that arose approximately 97 generations ago (Ciotti et al., 2000). Although the mutations appeared around the same time, the latter one is spread worldwide, while the Scandinavian 113insR could not be so far identified in any other geographical locale apart from Sweden. In view of these findings, it would also be very interesting to perform the haplotype mapping of R24P carrier patients to figure out whether it is also a founder mutation and if so, when it occurred in the past.

Gene and Mutation	Primers
BRCA1 3135delCATT	TCTGGGTCCTTAAAGAAACAAAGTC
	ACTTGGAATGTTCTCATTTCCC
BRCA1 3153delAG	CATCTCAGTTCAGAGGCAACG
	TGCATGACTACTTCCCATAGGC
BRCA1 3875delGTCT	TCACCCATACACATTTGGCTC
	AATCCATGCTTTGCTCTTCTTG
BRCA1 4184delTCAA	CGTTGCTACCGAGTGTCTGTC
	GACGTCCTAGCTGTGTGAAGG
BRCA1 185delAG	GGTTGGCAGCAATATGTGAAA
	TGCAGAACCAATCAAGACAGA
BRCA1 300T>G	GGCTCTTAAGGGCAGTTGTG
	AGAAAGGCAGTAAGTTTCTAATACCTG
BRCA1 1294del40	TGTAATGATAGGCGGACTCCC
	CTCAGGATGAAGGCCTGATG
BRCA1 2382GT	GACATGACAGCGATACTTTCCC
	TGTTGCACATTCCTCTTCTGC
BRCA1 5382insC	GTGTCTGCTCCACTTCCATTG
	CGAGACGGGAATCCAAATTAC
BRCA2 6079delAGTT, 6174delT, 6274delT	GTTGTTACGAGGCATTGGATG
	GGAAACTTGCTTTCCACTTGC
BRCA2 8034insAG	TATGGCAGATTTAGCAGGAGG
	TCGAGAGACAGTTAAGAGAAGAAAGA
BRCA2 8138delCCTTT	CTGGCCTCAAGCAATCCTC
	TTGACATGGAAGTCACAGACTACAC
BRCA2 9326insA	TCCACTACTAATGCCCACAAAG
	CACCTCAGAACAAGATGGCTG

Table 1. Hotspot mutations of the BRCA1 and BRCA2 genes and the primers used for the amplification of the surrounding gene regions.

Cancer-prone families identified to carry the R24P CDKN2A mutation			
Cancer types detected in the pedigrees	**Geographic locale**	**Authors**	**Date of publication**
Melanoma	Australia	Holland et al.	1995.
Melanoma	Canada	Monzon et al	1998.
Melanoma	France	Soufir et al.	1998.
Melanoma	U.K.	Mackie et al.	1998.
Sarcoma Melanoma* Cancer of the esophagus* Pancreas carcinoma* Carcinoma of the mouth and throat* Colon carcinoma* Lung carcinoma* Cancer of the gallbladder* Breast carcinoma*	North America	Lynch et al.	2002.
Melanoma Bladder cancer	Italy	Landi et al.	2004.

* The mutation was not identified in the late carcinoma patients but in a descendant with sarcoma.

Table 2. Publications on the R24P CDKN2A mutation and cancer types detected in the R24P families.

2.4 CDKN2A germline mutations in multiple primary malignancies

The idea that CDKN2A mutations may contribute to the predisposition of other primary malignancies beside melanoma came early in the middle of 90s, right after the identification of the gene's role in melanoma predisposition. Monzon et al. (Monzon et al., 1998) performed epidemiology and genetic studies on multiple primary melanoma cases and melanoma cases associated with multi-organ primary malignancies. They found that about 5 percent of patients have one or more additional primary lesions. This higher-than-expected prevalence of multiple primary melanomas may be due to excessive sun exposure, but according to the authors, genetic basis may also lay behind the phenomena. As supporting data, Monzon et al. claimed that patients with multiple primary melanomas very often have a family history of the disease. From epidemiology studies it was already known at that time that approximately 10 percent of melanoma cases have family background, which suggested genetic predisposition. Moreover, in 20 percent of the familial melanoma cases CDKN2A mutations could also be detected. The authors also claimed that in such families pancreas cancer also has a higher prevalence (Monzon et al., 1998).

The first in-depth analysis of this topic was reported in 1995 (Goldstein et al., 1995) by Goldstein and colleagues who compared the prevalence of other tumours in melanoma-prone families harboring or not harboring CDKN2A mutations. According to their analysis, CDKN2A mutation-harbouring melanoma-prone families have a 13-fold increased risk to develop pancreas cancer compared to those who do not carry such mutations. There was only one breast cancer patient mentioned in the paper who carried a mutant CDKN2A allele, while no breast cancer case could be detected in the group of melanoma-prone families with wild type CDKN2A alleles. The authors cited previous contrasting data demonstrating that the incidence of other types of cancers in melanoma-prone families in the US is not increased (Bohn et al., 2010). Moreover, another workgroup in the 80s suggested that patients with familial melanoma even had fewer other types of cancers than those suffering from sporadic melanoma (Kopf et al., 1986). These early data had been overwritten since and it is mainly due to the combined in-depth epidemiological and genetic studies performed within this special group of melanoma patients in the last 20 years.

As CDKN2A mutation studies became more and more intensive with the enrolment of centres from all over the world from Australia to the US through Europe, not only the genetic predisposition of familial melanoma but also its co-morbidities became recognized. This is a bright example of how genetic examinations can inspire epidemiological studies and shed light to connections of different diseases and their common predisposing factors. With reviewing several relevant papers we aim to demonstrate the above notion.

As early as 1999, Ghiorzo et al. (Ghiorzo et al., 1999) reported that the most prevalent malanoma-predisposing mutation of the Mediterranian, the G101W, was associated not only with a higher incidence of pancreatic malignancies, but also with breast cancer. In contrast, melanoma-prone families from the same geographical locale without CDKN2A mutations did not exhibit any non-melanoma neoplasias. The authors emphasized that the clinical-epidemiological study was conducted in a small geographical region where the sun and other types of environmental exposures of the individuals were approximately the same, therefore, differences of environmental factors could not account for the differential appearance of disease phenotypes. The authors therefore suggested that determining the underlying CDKN2A mutation in melanoma-prone families may have important implications not only for melanoma but also for further non-melanoma risk assessments.

In 2002, Lynch et al (Lynch et al., 2002) published the results of a survey where they aimed to elucidate the genetic background of the so-called FAMMM-pancreas carcinoma syndrome. They reported that their familial pancreas carcinoma database comprises of 159 families, of which 19 (12%) showed the FAMMM cutaneous phenotype. Lynch and co-workers studied the family tree, the history and the genetic background of eight families in detail. Most of the families had five-generation history of cancer where pancreas carcinoma predominated, but many other types of cancers were also prominent. A female patient of one of the families exhibited very similar multiple primary tumours as our 33-year-old patient: she had melanoma malignum, pancreas carcinoma and breast cancer with an onset at the age of 51, 56 and 61, respectively. Although the two patients exhibited a very similar pattern of tumours, there are two striking differences. The patient in the US study was already over the age 50 when her "march" of diseases started, while the Hungarian patient we are reporting now was only at the beginning of her 30s when the multiple primary tumours started. The other difference is that in the case of the Hungarian patient a melanoma-predisposing CDKN2A mutation could be detected, while in the case of the US female patient no such mutation was apparent. At the same time, Lynch et al. could also detect the previously described R24P mutation in another family of the study. In that extended family, a broad spectrum of cancers was apparent with the dominancy of pancreas carcinoma and malignant melanoma. In the case of a female family member, breast carcinoma was detected at her age of 60, but there was no report on any other malignancies. Whether she had any other predisposing genetic factors (eg BRCA1 or BRCA2 mutations) or her case was considered as a sporadic one is not discussed in the paper. Lynch et al. drew the conclusion that the cancer spectrum of the studied families in concert with CDKN2A mutations suggest a new putative hereditary carcinoma syndrome referred to as FAMMM-PC. The big variety of other types of cancers they demonstrated in the eight studied families raise the possibility that the predisposing CDKN2A mutations may contribute not only to FAMMM and PC but also to other types of malignancies, too. In this respect the case we present in this paper is also a supporting one to confirm the notion of Lynch et al.

Since Lynch and co-workers provided the first genetic study in FAMMM-PC syndrome (Lynch et al., 2002), the existence of such an entity became widely accepted and recent papers from various geographical locale were published in this topic. Bartsch and co-workers performed a survey in German pancreas cancer-prone families. Out of 110 such families, they identified 18 in which both melanoma and pancreas cancer occurred. The 18 families could be divided into two subgroups: five families with FAMMM-PC syndrome and 13 PC/melanoma families without the multiple mole phenotype (PCMS families). The authors found that the co-occurrance of pancreas carcinoma and melanoma was similar in the two subgroups; however, the prevalence of other tumour types, especially breast carcinoma was significantly higher in the latter group. Bartsch et al. checked CDKN2A germline mutations and mutations of genes contributing to breast cancer susceptibility. They identified CDKN2A mutations in 2 of the PCMS families but they could not identify any breast cancer susceptibility ones, only a co-segregating BRCA2 variant in a PCMS family without breast cancer. The conclusion they drew from the above was that families with an accumulation of pancreas cancer and melanoma show a large variety of phenotypic expression. Finally, the authors warn that more PC/melanoma families need to be analysed to clarify whether they represent a variation of the FAMMM-PC syndrome or there are two distinct hereditary cancer syndromes. The case we present in this paper may be considered as a reflection to their call since the family we studied does not show the multiple mole phenotype. It may be classified as a PCMS family with an apparent CDKN2A mutation that is responsible for the malignant melanoma and pancreas carcinoma and possibly also contributing to breast carcinoma.

In an extended study performed in Southern Scandinavia, Borg et al. (Borg et al., 2000) found that patients carrying the 113insArg melanoma-predisposing founder mutation, pancreas carcinoma and as the second most frequent malignancy, breast carcinoma can also be frequently detected. The authors studied nine 113insArg mutation-carrying families and 42 CDKN2A mutation-free melanoma-prone families. The incidence of multiple primary malignancies was significantly higher in 113insArg families compared to those free of any genetic alteration in the CDKN2A gene. Borg et al. therefore claimed that the CDKN2A 113insArg mutation carriers have an increased risk not only to malignant melanoma but also to pancreas and breast cancer.

Prowse et al. presented a very elegant work in 2003 (Prowse et al., 2003) with an approach from the opposite direction. They studied BRCA1 and BRCA2 mutation-free breast cancer-prone families presenting multiple cases of early onset breast cancer and tried to find out what type of other gene mutations could predispose them to develop the disease. According to their estimation, only one third of breast cancer-prone families carry either BRCA1 or BRCA2 mutations, therefore other candidate genes contributing to disease predisposition must also be considered. The fact that eight families out of the 31 reported multiple cases of pancreas cancer and malignant melanoma prompted the authors to study the CDKN2A gene in detail. In one of the studied families, a novel CDKN2A mutation was identified: the IVS1-1G>C intronic mutation. The nucleotide substitution occurs at a highly conserved base in the 3′ splice junction of intron 1, thus both $p16^{INK4a}$ and $p14^{ARF}$ transcript variants are affected. The authors performed a functional analysis to prove that the mutation indeed causes the emergence of an aberrant splice variant. Owing to the fact that two proteins playing pivotal role in cell cycle regulation are affected by the same mutation, it is plausible to hypothesize that it may be of key importance in predisposition to various forms of malignancies.

Up to this point rare mutations of the CDKN2A gene were discussed in relation to predisposition to melanoma and other malignant diseases. However, a Polish workgroup also provided data on a relatively common variation of the same gene, the A148T polymorphism also contributed to disease pathogenesis. Debniak and co-workers (Debniak et al., 2005b) first showed that the A148T variant having a 3% allele frequency in the general Polish population was a melanoma-predisposing factor with an odds ratio of 2.5. Next they studied whether the same variant exhibits breast-cancer-predisposing nature too and found that the odds ratio associated with the CDKN2A allele for women diagnosed with breast cancer before the age of 50 was 1.5 and after the age of 50 it was 1.3. The effect was the strongest for women diagnosed at or before the age of 30 (Debniak et al., 2005a), suggesting a role of the A148T polymorphism in breast cancer predisposition. As a next step, the workgroup performed a population-based study where they compared the genotypes and the allele frequency of the A148T polymorphism in the group of 3,583 unselected cancer cases and 3,000 random controls. They found a positive association between the A148T variant and lung cancer and colorectal cancer with odds ratios of 2.0 and 1.5, respectively. The authors concluded that the A148T variant of the CDKN2A gene may contribute to multi-organ cancer risk (Debniak et al., 2006). How this variant reveals its disease-predisposing effect is still unclear. It has been demonstrated that the A148T allele did not have a major effect on the protein function (Ranade et al., 1995; Lilischkis et al., 1996);

however, according to Debniak and co-workers (Debniak et al., 2005a) we can not exclude the possibility that it subtly affects p16^{INK4a} function or reduces its level of expression. Moreover, they could demonstrate that the A148T variant is in strong linkage disequilibrium with a promoter polymorphism of the CDKN2A gene, the P493 variant (Debniak et al., 2005b). Taken together, the Polish workgroup provided a very demonstrative set of data suggesting that beside the rare variants with high penetrance, a relatively common low-penetrance CDKN2A variant may also contribute to the pathogenesis of various cancer types. These findings may gain importance in the discovery of the pathogenesis of both familial and sporadic cancers.

The melanoma-predisposing nature of the A148T CDKN2A polymorphism have so far been most extensively studied in the Polish population, but sporadic data on the same variant exist in other populations. For example, Nagore and co-workers (Nagore et al., 2009) reported on the identification of two women in the Spanish population carrying the same A148T CDKN2A polymorphism and one of them having a hereditary breast/ovarian cancer family pedigree. At the same time, the authors claim that they could not find a significant difference in the allele frequency of the A148T variant in the general Spanish population and the studied breast cancer/melanoma patients' population. Nagore et al. could identify two more CDKN2A mutations in their study population: the V59G and the A85T, both of them frequently occurring in women suffering from both malignant melanoma and breast carcinoma. As a conclusion, the authors claim that because CDKN2A mutations are infrequent in female patients with melanoma and breast cancer, other deleterious variants such as mutations in BRCA1, BRCA2, TP53 must be studied in these types of patients' groups.

The above notion of Nagore et al. was confirmed by Monnerat and co-workers (Monnerat et al., 2007) who studied BRCA1, BRCA2, TP53 and CDKN2A genes in a group of female patients presenting both melanoma and breast cancer. The authors found that patients with a positive family history of both of these malignancies often carry variants of the aformentioned genes with a higher frequency than those without a family history. This study and all the above cited ones prompt us to draw two important conclusions: the co-occurrence of primary multi-organ malignancies are very often genetically determined but to reveal the exact pattern of genetic variants (the combination of high- and low-risk susceptibility factors), a well-defined set of genes must be studied in detail in large cohorts of patients. At the same time, we believe that single cases, for instance the one we present in this report, may add valuable data to the topic.

Until the mid-2000s, there was no opportunity to study the co-morbidities of familial melanoma in large cohorts of patients. The international GenoMEL Consortium, however, made it possible to perform large scale surveys in this topic and several hundreds of melanoma-prone families could be investigated both for their genetic predisposition and for their co-existing malignancies. Goldstein and the co-workers (Goldstein et al., 2007) of the GenoMEL Consortium published the results of their large scale survey in 2006. They studied 385 melanoma-prone families and out of them 39% carried one of the melanoma-predisposing CDKN2A mutations. The lowest ratio of such mutation carriers was identified in Australia, where the incidence of sporadic melanoma is higher than that of in Europe and in North America. This difference is also reflected in the relationship between pancreas cancer and CDKN2A mutations: while within the European and North American melanoma-prone families a clear connection could be identified between the mutation carrier status and pancreas carcinoma, no such relationship could be discovered in the

Australian patients. The authors hypothesize that the lack of pancreas cancer-CDKN2A mutation relationship in Australia reflects the divergent spectrum of CDKN2A mutations detected in Australian melanoma-prone families *versus* those from North America and Europe. In a follow-up paper (Goldstein et al., 2006), the authors extended their survey to neural system tumours and to uveal melanoma but found no association between CDKN2A mutations and these two malignancies either.

3. Conclusion

In this paper we presented the case of a 33-year-old female patient with the occurrence of three primary multi-organ malignancies, malignant melanoma, pancreas and breast carcinoma within a short period of time. The family history of the patient prompted us to perform a genetic study and we identified the melanoma-predisposing R24P CDKN2A germline mutation in her case as well as in her father, suffering from gastric and laryngeal carcinomas. Since the late aunt of the young female patient died of breast cancer at the age of her 20s several decades ago, we also surveyed the patient for the presence of BRCA1 and BRCA2 hotspot mutations but found no alterations in her case. Although we can not exclude the possibility that other predisposing gene variants may have contributed to the breast cancer of the patient, we suggest that the disclosed R24P CDKN2A mutation may have played a key role in the pathogenesis of her multi-organ primary malignancies.
Surveying the relevant literature clearly revealed that CDKN2A germline mutations are highly accepted as predisposing genetic factors for patients who suffer from co-existing pancreas carcinoma and malignant melanoma. However, no such consensus exists for the association of CDKN2A germline variants and the primary multiple occurrence of melanoma malignum and breast cancer. Studies performed in relatively small cohorts of patients resulted in contradictory data: some of them supporting while others rejecting the notion of the breast cancer-predisposing nature of CDKN2A germline mutations. To resolve this problem, extended studies on a wide range of low- and high-penetrance genetic predisposing factors must be examined on a multicentric base. We believe that single cases such as the one we presented in this paper may contribute to the understanding of the role of genetic susceptibility and environmental factors in the pathogenesis of multiple primary malignancies.

4. Acknowledgment

The work was supported by grants TÁMOP-4.2.1/B-09/1/KONV-2010-0005, TÁMOP-4.2.2-08/1-2008-0001, ETT-429-07 and OTKA 5K302.

5. References

Bohn, O.L., Fuertes-Camilo, M., Navarro, L., Saldivar, J., & Sanchez-Sosa, S. (2010). p16INK4a expression in basal-like breast carcinoma. *International Journal of Clinical and Experimental Pathology*, Vol.3, No.(6), pp. 600-607.

Borg, A., Sandberg, T., Nilsson, K., Johannsson, O., Klinker, M., Masback, A., Westerdahl, J., Olsson, H., & Ingvar, C. (2000). High frequency of multiple melanomas and breast and pancreas carcinomas in CDKN2A mutation-positive melanoma families. *Journal of the National Cancer Insitute.*, Vol.92, No.(15), pp. 1260-1266.

Ciotti, P., Struewing, J.P., Mantelli, M., Chompret, A., Avril, M.F., Santi, P.L., Tucker, M.A., Bianchi-Scarra, G., Bressac-de Paillerets, B., & Goldstein, A.M. (2000). A single genetic origin for the G101W CDKN2A mutation in 20 melanoma-prone families. *American Journal of Human Genetics*, Vol.67, No.(2), pp. 311-319.

Debniak, T., Gorski, B., Huzarski, T., Byrski, T., Cybulski, C., Mackiewicz, A., Gozdecka-Grodecka, S., Gronwald, J., Kowalska, E., Haus, O., Grzybowska, E., Stawicka, M., Swiec, M., Urbanski, K., Niepsuj, S., Wasko, B., Gozdz, S., Wandzel, P., Szczylik, C., Surdyka, D., Rozmiarek, A., Zambrano, O., Posmyk, M., Narod, S.A., & Lubinski, J. (2005a). A common variant of CDKN2A (p16) predisposes to breast cancer. *Journal of Medical Genetics*, Vol.42, No.(10), pp. 763-765.

Debniak, T., Scott, R.J., Huzarski, T., Byrski, T., Rozmiarek, A., Debniak, B., Gorski, B., Cybulski, C., Medrek, K., Mierzejewski, M., Masojc, B., Matyjasik, J., Zlowocka, E., Teodorczyk, U., Lener, M., Klujszo-Grabowska, E., Nej-Wolosiak, K., Jaworowska, E., Oszutowska, D., Szymanska, A., Szymanska, J., Castaneda, J., van de, W.T., Suchy, J., Kurzawski, G., Oszurek, O., Narod, S., & Lubinski, J. (2006). CDKN2A common variant and multi-organ cancer risk--a population-based study. *International Journal of Cancer*, Vol.118, No.(12), pp. 3180-3182.

Debniak, T., Scott, R.J., Huzarski, T., Byrski, T., Rozmiarek, A., Debniak, B., Zaluga, E., Maleszka, R., Kladny, J., Gorski, B., Cybulski, C., Gronwald, J., Kurzawski, G., & Lubinski, J. (2005b). CDKN2A common variants and their association with melanoma risk: a population-based study. *Cancer Research*, Vol.65, No.(3), pp. 835-839.

Ghiorzo, P., Ciotti, P., Mantelli, M., Heouaine, A., Queirolo, P., Rainero, M.L., Ferrari, C., Santi, P.L., De Marchi, R., Farris, A., Ajmar, F., Bruzzi, P., & Bianchi-Scarra, G. (1999). Characterization of ligurian melanoma families and risk of occurrence of other neoplasia. *International Journal of Cancer*, Vol.83, No.(4), pp. 441-448.

Goldstein, A.M., Chan, M., Harland, M., Gillanders, E.M., Hayward, N.K., Avril, M.F., Azizi, E., Bianchi-Scarra, G., Bishop, D.T., Bressac-de Paillerets, B., Bruno, W., Calista, D., Cannon Albright, L.A., Demenais, F., Elder, D.E., Ghiorzo, P., Gruis, N.A., Hansson, J., Hogg, D., Holland, E.A., Kanetsky, P.A., Kefford, R.F., Landi, M.T., Lang, J., Leachman, S.A., MacKie, R.M., Magnusson, V., Mann, G.J., Niendorf, K., Newton, B.J., Palmer, J.M., Puig, S., Puig-Butille, J.A., de Snoo, F.A., Stark, M., Tsao, H., Tucker, M.A., Whitaker, L., & Yakobson, E. (2006). High-risk melanoma susceptibility genes and pancreatic cancer, neural system tumors and uveal melanoma across GenoMEL. *Cancer Research*, Vol.66, No.(20), pp. 9818-9828.

Goldstein, A.M., Chan, M., Harland, M., Hayward, N.K., Demenais, F., Bishop, D.T., Azizi, E., Bergman, W., Bianchi-Scarra, G., Bruno, W., Calista, D., Albright, L.A., Chaudru, V., Chompret, A., Cuellar, F., Elder, D.E., Ghiorzo, P., Gillanders, E.M., Gruis, N.A., Hansson, J., Hogg, D., Holland, E.A., Kanetsky, P.A., Kefford, R.F., Landi, M.T., Lang, J., Leachman, S.A., MacKie, R.M., Magnusson, V., Mann, G.J., Bishop, J.N., Palmer, J.M., Puig, S., Puig-Butille, J.A., Stark, M., Tsao, H., Tucker, M.A., Whitaker, L., & Yakobson, E. (2007). Features associated with germline CDKN2A mutations: a GenoMEL study of melanoma-prone families from three continents. *Journal of Medical Genetics.*, Vol.44, No.(2), pp. 99-106.

Goldstein, A.M., Fraser, M.C., Struewing, J.P., Hussussian, C.J., Ranade, K., Zametkin, D.P., Fontaine, L.S., Organic, S.M., Dracopoli, N.C., Clark, W.H., Jr., & . (1995). Increased risk of pancreatic cancer in melanoma-prone kindreds with p16INK4 mutations. *New England Journal of Medicine*, Vol.333, No.(15), pp. 970-974.

Hashemi, J., Bendahl, P.O., Sandberg, T., Platz, A., Linder, S., Stierner, U., Olsson, H., Ingvar, C., Hansson, J., & Borg, A. (2001). Haplotype analysis and age estimation of the 113insR CDKN2A founder mutation in Swedish melanoma families. *Genes, Chromosomes & Cancer*, Vol.31, No.(2), pp. 107-116.

Holland, E.A., Beaton, S.C., Becker, T.M., Grulet, O.M., Peters, B.A., Rizos, H., Kefford, R.F., & Mann, G.J. (1995). Analysis of the p16 gene, CDKN2, in 17 Australian melanoma kindreds. *Oncogene*, Vol.11, No.(11), pp. 2289-2294.

Kopf, A.W., Hellman, L.J., Rogers, G.S., Gross, D.F., Rigel, D.S., Friedman, R.J., Levenstein, M., Brown, J., Golomb, F.M., Roses, D.F., & . (1986). Familial malignant melanoma. *Journal of the American Medical Association*, Vol.256, No.(14), pp. 1915-1919.

Lilischkis, R., Sarcevic, B., Kennedy, C., Warlters, A., & Sutherland, R.L. (1996). Cancer-associated mis-sense and deletion mutations impair p16INK4 CDK inhibitory activity. *International Journal of Cancer*, Vol.66, No.(2), pp. 249-254.

Lynch, H.T., Brand, R.E., Hogg, D., Deters, C.A., Fusaro, R.M., Lynch, J.F., Liu, L., Knezetic, J., Lassam, N.J., Goggins, M., & Kern, S. (2002). Phenotypic variation in eight extended CDKN2A germline mutation familial atypical multiple mole melanoma-pancreatic carcinoma-prone families: the familial atypical mole melanoma-pancreatic carcinoma syndrome. *Cancer*, Vol.94, No.(1), pp. 84-96.

MacKie, R.M. andrew, N., Lanyon, W.G., & Connor, J.M. (1998). CDKN2A germline mutations in U.K. patients with familial melanoma and multiple primary melanomas. *Journal of Investigative Dermatology*, Vol.111, No.(2), pp. 269-272.

Monnerat, C., Chompret, A., Kannengiesser, C., Avril, M.F., Janin, N., Spatz, A., Guinebretiere, J.M., Marian, C., Barrois, M., Boitier, F., Lenoir, G.M., & Bressac-de Paillerets, B. (2007). BRCA1, BRCA2, TP53 and CDKN2A germline mutations in patients with breast cancer and cutaneous melanoma. *Familial Cancer*, Vol.6, No.(4), pp. 453-461.

Monzon, J., Liu, L., Brill, H., Goldstein, A.M., Tucker, M.A., From, L., McLaughlin, J., Hogg, D., & Lassam, N.J. (1998). CDKN2A mutations in multiple primary melanomas. *New England Journal of Medicine*, Vol.338, No.(13), pp. 879-887.

Nagore, E., Montoro, A., Garcia-Casado, Z., Botella-Estrada, R., Insa, A., Lluch, A., Lopez-Guerrero, J.A., & Guillen, C. (2009). Germline mutations in CDKN2A are infrequent in female patients with melanoma and breast cancer. *Melanoma Research*, Vol.19, No.(4), pp. 211-214.

Prowse, A.H., Schultz, D.C., Guo, S., Vanderveer, L., Dangel, J., Bove, B., Cairns, P., Daly, M., & Godwin, A.K. (2003). Identification of a splice acceptor site mutation in p16INK4A/p14ARF within a breast cancer, melanoma, neurofibroma prone kindred. *Journal of Medical Genetics*, Vol.40, No.(8), pp. e102.

Ranade, K., Hussussian, C.J., Sikorski, R.S., Varmus, H.E., Goldstein, A.M., Tucker, M.A., Serrano, M., Hannon, G.J., Beach, D., & Dracopoli, N.C. (1995). Mutations associated with familial melanoma impair p16INK4 function. *Nature Genetics*, Vol.10, No.(1), pp. 114-116.

Soufir, N., Avril, M.F., Chompret, A., Demenais, F., Bombled, J., Spatz, A., Stoppa-Lyonnet, D., Benard, J., & Bressac-de Paillerets, B. (1998). Prevalence of p16 and CDK4 germline mutations in 48 melanoma-prone families in France. The French Familial Melanoma Study Group. *Human Molecular Genetics*, Vol.7, No.(2), pp. 209-216.

14

The Biology and Clinical Relevance of Sentinel Lymph Nodes in Melanoma

Brian Parrett, Lilly Fadaki, Jennifer Y. Rhee and Stanley P.L. Leong
Center for Melanoma Research & Treatment and Department of Surgery
California Pacific Medical Center and Research Institute
San Franciso, CA,
USA

1. Introduction

The initial route of metastases in most patients with melanoma is through lymphatics to the regional nodes (Morton et al., 1992) [Fig.1]. However, routine lymphadenectomy for patients with early stage melanoma is unwarranted because most of these patients (~80%) do not have nodal metastases, are unlikely to benefit from the operation, and may suffer complications including lymphedema, seroma, infection and wound breakdown. However, a significant portion of patients with melanoma, predicted by primary tumor factors, harbor clinically undetectable regionally lymph node metastases at time of presentation. Delay of elective lymph node dissection until the presence of palpable nodes may allow the spread of melanoma to other nodes and distant sites with a decrease in long-term survival (Morton et al., 2006). The key to solving this clinical dilemma is to provide a minimally invasive method to selecting the relevant "sentinel lymph node" (SLN) in a specific basin to determine nodal micrometastasis (Morton et al., 1992). The SLN is accordingly the first lymph node(s) receiving direct afferent drainage from the primary tumor and thus is most likely to contain metastatic disease if any regional lymph nodes are involved. The technique of SLN biopsy is best named selective sentinel lymph node dissection (SLND) and allows surgeons to determine the spread of melanoma through lymphatic channels from the primary tumor; it has substantially impacted the way cutaneous melanoma is staged and managed.

The relatively orderly fashion of melanoma metastasis from the primary site to the SLNs and then to the non-SLNs prior to systemic sites is supportive of the spectrum theory of cancer spread (Hellman, 1994; Leong, 2004) [Fig. 1]. This theory states that for a given malignant lesion, development of nodal and systemic metastasis from localized disease is a genetically driven process of progression within the tumor microenvironment to distant body sites, most often through the "gateway" of the SLN(s). Selective SLND is an ideal procedure because it is minimally invasive, yet powerful enough to select the relevant lymph node of the nodal basin, without a complete node dissection. It is now widely accepted that the SLN status is the most important factor in predicting outcomes and determining further treatment for melanoma and this is the focus of the chapter (Leong, 2004).

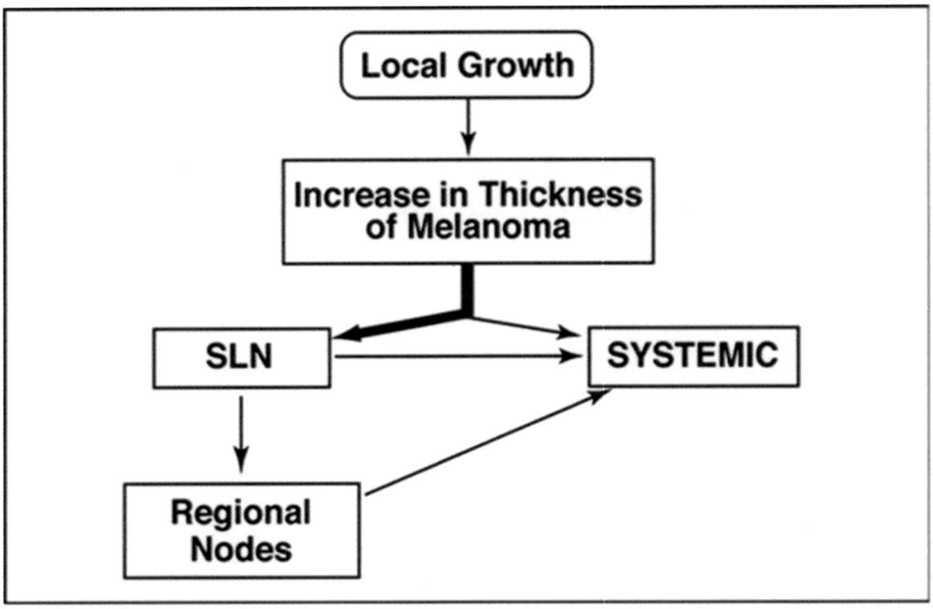

Fig. 1. The figure depicts progression of melanoma from the primary site to the SLN, then to non-SLN or regional nodes and distant sites. Occasionally, cancer cells may bypass the lymph nodes and spread to distant sites through vascular channels. In the majority of the cases (approximately 80%), the SLN is the gateway for cancer spread (bold arrow pathway in figure).

2. The sentinel lymph node in melanoma

2.1 History and rationale

In 1977, Cabanas described an approach to staging penile carcinoma after using lymphangiograms in patients to determine the lymphatic anatomy of the penis. He hypothesized that if penile carcinoma metastasized, it would do so to a node that was located medially and superiorly to the saphenofemoral junction in each groin (Cabanas, 1977). The term *sentinel node,* first coined by Gould in 1966 for parotid cancer (Gould et al., 1966), was used to describe the first node in this drainage pathway; if this was found to have metastatic disease, the patient required a lymphadenectomy. Conversely, when the SLN was negative for disease, the likelihood of metastatic disease in the groin was low and lymphadenectomy was unnecessary. The idea that a primary tumor would preferentially drain through the lymphatics to a *specific* lymph node, and that the status of that node would reflect the tumor status of the regional lymphatic basin, was revolutionary. However, the lymphatic drainage of solid tumors might vary from patient to patient and not necessarily be fixed to an anatomic location (Wong et al., 1991). To accurately identify the SLN, intraoperative techniques were needed to define the lymphatic drainage of a given primary tumor site rather than utilize an operative approach that was dependent upon the defined anatomy.

Thus, in 1992, Morton introduced the concept of identifying and selectively harvesting the SLN from the draining basin of a primary melanoma to identify patients with clinically occult lymph node disease (Morton et al., 1992). This was performed with intradermal

injection of vital blue dye around the primary melanoma and then exploration of the regional lymphatic basin to identify blue stained node(s). This technique was based on the observation that when a blue dye such as isosulfan blue is injected around the primary melanoma, it drains into the SLN. With meticulous dissection, the dermal lymphatics could be visualized and utilized to map the lymphatic drainage of the skin to a SLN. In this study, metastases were present in 18% of SLNs, while non-sentinel nodes were the sole site of metastases in only two of 3079 nodes from 194 lymphadenectomy specimens that had an identifiable SLN, resulting in a false-negative (FN) rate of less than 1% (Morton et al., 1992). Therefore, this technique identifies, with a high degree of accuracy, patients with early stage melanoma without nodal metastases who can be spared from a morbid radical lymphadenectomy. Several confirmatory studies, including prospective randomized trials, have provided a wealth of information regarding the SLN, including accuracy, prognostic value and candidate selection (Ross et al., 2011).
However, intraoperative lymphatic mapping with blue dye alone is technically difficult with prolonged learning curves to acquire satisfactory outcomes. Thus, radioguided techniques were sought to provide a simpler method to identify and harvest the SLN while minimizing the extent of the surgical dissection. In 1993, Alex and Krag reported on the use of an intra-operative hand-held gamma probe to identify regional nodes that had taken up technetium labeled sulfur colloid (Alex & Krag, 1993). Additionally, the development of a number of radiopharmaceuticals with appropriate particle size provided the opportunity for the development of cutaneous lymphoscintigraphy, developed by Robinson, Morton and associates in the 1970s (Robinson et al., 1977). Cutaneous lymphoscintigraphy was especially important given the recognition that the dermal lymphatics, particularly in trunk melanomas (Leong et al., 1999), could have substantial variability; this allowed surgeons to define the regional lymphatic basins that were at risk for harboring metastatic disease prior to selective SLND (Fig. 2). Preoperative lymphoscintigraphy to define the SLN from the primary site in combination with the gamma probe could direct the surgical incisions and make the procedure less invasive than the blue dye procedure. Also, selective SLND using lymphoscintigraphy allows the identification of affected lymph nodes that would not be routinely evaluated during an elective nodal dissection such as in-transit lymph nodes and lymph nodes in minor nodal basins (e.g., popliteal and epitrochlear regions) [Sumner et al., 2002]. Lymphoscintigraphy is also essential for selective SLND in head and neck melanomas as these have complex and less predictable lymphatic drainage patterns, resulting in lower SLN identification rates and higher FN rates (Klop et al., 2011; Leong et al., 1999). For these reasons, cutaneous lymphoscintigraphy has become a routine component of the management of most melanoma patients.

2.2 Accuracy and false-negative rate

The SLN concept has been supported by high accuracy rates and low false-negative (FN) rates in melanoma. The immediate FN rate, defined as the percentage of nodal basins that harbor nodal metastases in nodes other than the SLN as determined by synchronous elective lymph node dissection after a negative SLN biopsy, has been reported to be less than 5% in several studies (Gershenwald et al., 1999; Morton et al., 1992; Nowecki et al., 2003, 2006; Reintgen et al., 1994; Thompson et al., 1995; Uren et al., 1994). In the Multicenter Selective Lymphadenectomy Trial I (MSLT-I) [Morton et al., 2006], 2,001 patients with cutaneous melanoma were randomized to: (1) wide local excision alone with observation only and subsequent lymphadenectomy if nodal relapse occurred, or (2) wide local excision and selective SLND with lymphadenectomy if metastases were found in the SLN.

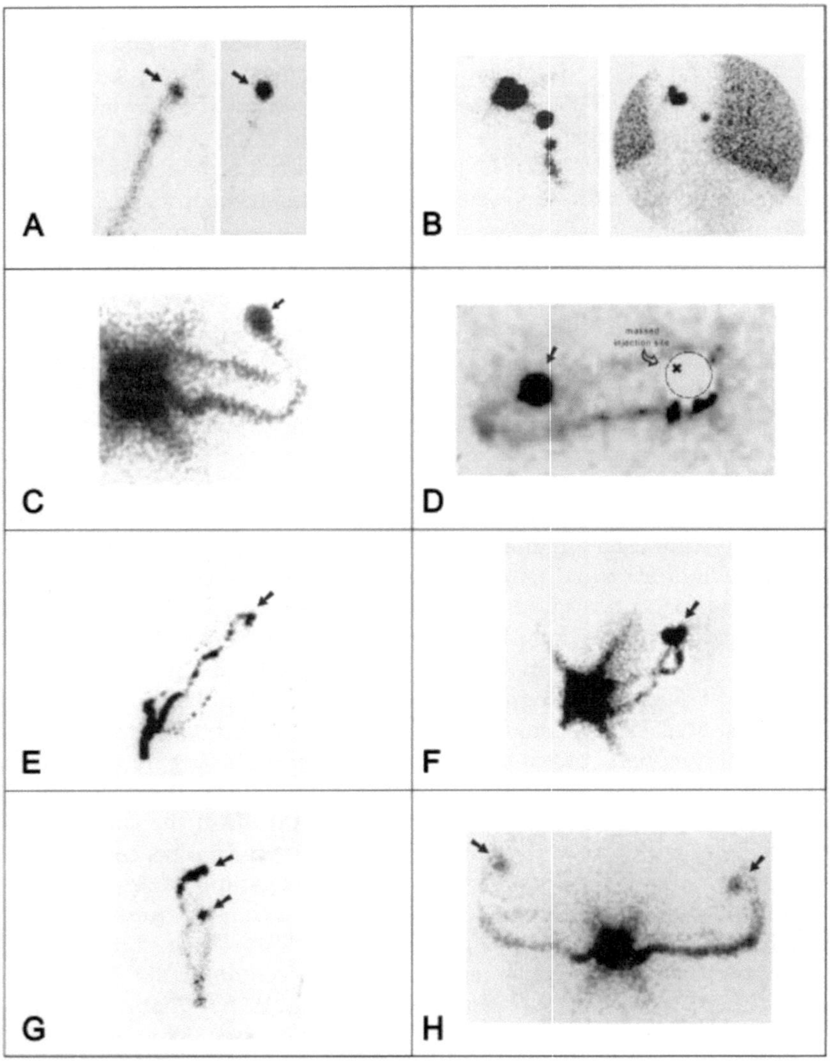

Fig. 2. Pre-operative lymphoscintigraphy demonstrates varying lymphatic channel patterns in patients with primary melanoma. (A) Drainage of a single channel from the right upper arm leading to one SLN in the right axilla. (B) Drainage of a single channel from a posterior midline neck lesion to multiple contiguous nodes in the right posterior neck. (C) Confluent channels drain from the upper back to a single SLN in the left axilla. (D) Multiple channels from the left upper back draining to a single SLN in the left axilla. (E) Single primary site drainage source from the right arm, diverting into several channels and leading to a single SLN in the right axilla. (F) Changing of drainage patterns from a lesion in the left anterior chest wall to one SLN in the left axilla. (G) Parallel simple channels from the right lower extremity, each draining to a single SLN, each in the same basin in the right groin. (H) Multiple channels from the midline back draining to multiple SLN(s) in different basins, the right and left axilla. This figure has been previously published by our group in *Clinical Nuclear Medicine* 30(3):150-158, 2005.

Results from 1,269 patients with intermediate-thickness primary melanoma (1.2 mm to 3.5 mm in this study) showed that 16% percent of SLNs had micrometastases, while 3.4% of those with "negative" SLNs developed nodal metastases, which is consistent with the accepted FN rates of the procedure.

Additional evidence that regional node metastasis constitutes an orderly, nonrandom event was provided from a study that examined 105 lymphadenectomy specimens in patients with at least one positive SLN (Gershenwald et al., 1998). They found that the SLN was the only node involved in 83 (79%) of the basins, with microscopic nodal metastasis identified in an additional 21% of the lymphadenectomy specimens. In 92% of patients who had at least one positive SLN and were mapped with blue dye and radiocolloid, lymphatic metastases were identified in the SLN that contained the greatest radiotracer uptake.

2.3 Current indications for selective SLND

In our practice, patients chosen for selective SLND have the following: (1) a Breslow thickness of 1 mm or greater; (2) a Breslow thickness less than 1 mm, but with high risk features such as lymphatic invasion, regression, ulceration, increased mitotic figures, or Clarks level IV; or (3) a shave biopsy that resulted in a Breslow thickness of less than 1 mm. Patients who are not recommended to undergo selective SLND have one of the following features: (1) known lymphatic or metastatic disease; (2) melanoma-in-situ; or (3) a Breslow thickness less than 1 mm with no high risk features. These are the most current indications for selective SLND and what most melanoma centers follow. Given this criteria, the positive SLN rate has been documented to be between 14-21% in most studies (Kapteijn et al., 1997; Leong et al., 2005; Morton et al., 1992, 2006; Thompson et al., 2005). Despite these guidelines, population based studies have shown that only 50% of patients with stage IB and II who met the criteria for selective SLND actually undergo selective SLND (Bilimoria et al., 2009; Cormier et al., 2005). The factors for this are likely multi-factorial including insurance, geographic area, socioeconomic factors, and age. This signifies the need for better education, access to health care, and melanoma multidisciplinary centers for patient referral.

3. Technique and evaluation of SLN

3.1 Pre-operative lymphatic mapping

The SLN is now reproducibly defined by lymphoscintigraphy and lymphatic mapping performed by the injection of Technetium-99m (Tc 99m) sulfur colloid radiotracer, a vital blue dye, or a combination of both around the melanoma site. Isosulfan blue (Lymphazurin 1%, Hirsch Industries, Inc., Richmond, VA) is the most commonly used blue dye in the United States and is the only dye approved by the Food and Drug Administration for lymphatic mapping. Regarding radiotracer, a more selective agent, Technetium-99m-labeled Tilmanocept, is a mannose receptor–targeted molecule that is being developed for identification of SLNs (Leong et al., 2011) and will likely be used in the near future.

A summary of the numerous studies using the blue dye technique, radiotracer mapping by a hand-held gamma probe, or a combination of both techniques is shown in Table 1. The success rate of harvesting the SLN by blue dye alone is less than that of radiotracer alone or the combination of blue dye and radiotracer, both of which now approach 100% (Table 1). Given this data, the use of radiotracer is the most commonly use technique now. With greater surgical experience, the use of blue dye is not essential as radiotracer has a higher sensitivity than blue dye alone and this can avoid reported allergic reactions seen with the injection of blue dye (Leong et al., 2000; Liu et al., 2011).

For this technique, filtered Tc99m sulfur colloid is injected intradermally at the primary melanoma site. Dynamic imaging is performed to follow the lymphatic collecting vessels until they reach the draining SLNs. An image should be acquired as the lymphatics reach the nodal basin so that SLN(s) directly receiving the channels can be identified and distinguished from any second tier nodes that may be seen. This phase of the study usually takes 10-20 minutes. Delayed scans are performed 2-2.5 hours later, at which time all regions that possibly drain the primary melanoma site are examined with 5-10 minute static images. The surface location of all SLN(s) is marked on the overlying skin. Close communication between the nuclear medicine physician and surgeon is invaluable, especially in cases where there are unusual draining patterns. Importantly, the SLN is not just the first node seen on dynamic imaging, since there may be multiple separate lymph channels that have different rates of lymph flow. If they drain to different nodes, these are all SLNs, regardless of the time taken for the lymph containing the radiocolloid to reach them (Fig. 2). The SLN is also not necessarily the closest node to the primary site. Lymphatic vessels can bypass many nodes and even whole node fields before reaching a SLN. Therefore, the best way to identify a SLN on lymphoscintigraphy is to see the lymphatic collecting vessel on dynamic imaging as it drains directly to the SLN (Fig. 2).

Author	Year	# of Patients	Blue Dye Alone	Radiotracer	Both
Morton et al.	1992	223	82% (basins)	-	-
Krag et al.	1995	121	91% (patients)	98% (patients)	-
Glass et al.	1996	148	60% (nodes)	80% (nodes)	97% (nodes)
Albertini et al.	1996	106	70% (nodes)	84% (nodes)	96% (basins)
Kapteijn et al.	1997	110	84% (nodes)	99.5% (nodes)	99.5% (nodes)
Leong et al.	1997	163	74%	98%	-
Pijpers et al.	1997	135	86% (nodes) 85% (basins)	100% (nodes) 100% (basins)	-
Gershenwald et al.	1998	626	87%	-	99%
Gennari et al.	2000	133	80.8% (nodes)	97.1%	99%
Nowecki et al.	2003	726	91.6%	-	97.3%

* Reporting of success rates is not standardized. Percentages are indicated in patients, nodal basins or SLNs.

Table 1. Success Rates of Melanoma Sentinel Lymph Node Identification Techniques in Studies with >100 patients*.

3.2 Intra-operative identification of the SLN(s)

After lymphoscintigraphy, the patient is transferred to the operating room and no further injection of radiotracer is necessary, but Lymphazurin (1-2 mL) may be injected intradermally prior to the procedure. The surgical sites are prepared and general anesthesia is most often used. Intraoperative mapping of the SLNs is achieved using a hand-held gamma probe (Neoprobe 2000, Neoprobe Corporation, Dublin, OH). A small incision is made over the marked area of greatest activity as detected by pre-operative lymphoscintigraphy and confirmed by the hand-held gamma probe. The incision is carried down through the subcutaneous fat and the fascia is incised as the lymph nodes usually reside beneath the fascia. Using the gamma probe, the SLNs can be located by detecting increased radioactivity in counts per second or blue dye within node. After the removal of the SLN, the gamma probe is used to search the resection bed to make sure that no residual elevated radioactivity remains. Theoretically, the single SLN with the highest radioactive count ("hottest" SLN) or the blue node is most likely to harbor tumor cells and is removed during biopsy. However, literature describes FN rates for SLN biopsy if only the single, "hottest" SLN is removed and the other nodes are left in place (McMasters et al., 2001). Thus, we and others use the 10% rule (Liu et al., 2011; McMasters et al., 2001): the gamma probe is applied and any SLNs that assessed ≥ 10% of the ex vivo radioactive count of "hottest" SLN are removed, including any blue nodes or suspicious nodes by digital palpation.

After selective SLND, the wound is closed in layers. On a side table we dissect the SLN(s) from the non-SLN(s) or lymphatic tissue within the resected specimen using the gamma probe so that each lymph node is correctly labeled with its respective radioactive counts for pathologic evaluation.

3.3 Pathologic assessment of the SLN

The standard histological technique for evaluating a nodal dissection specimen involves evaluating representative sections from each identified lymph node using hematoxylin and eosin (H&E). In actuality, given the large size of the nodal dissection specimen, <1% of the whole specimen is routinely evaluated (Ross et al., 2011; Sondak et al., 2007). With a smaller sample from a selective SLND, the SLN can be evaluated more intensively with multiple sections using a combination of H&E and immunohistochemistry (IHC) to stain for melanoma associated antigens such as S-100 and HMB-45 (Fig. 3).

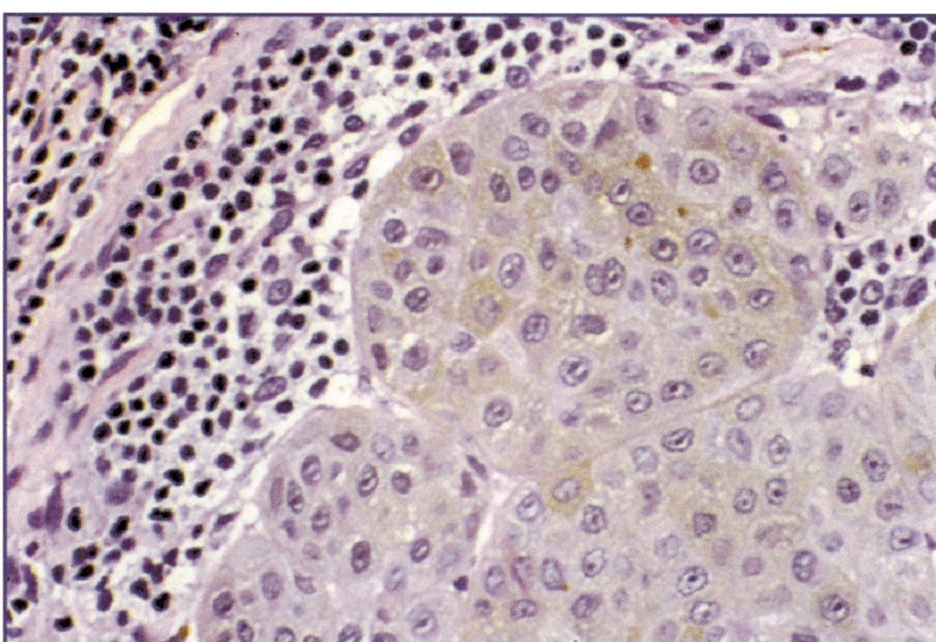

Fig. 3. Figure shows staining of melanoma micrometastasis within a SLN.

Therefore, despite the less invasive nature of selective SLND, the staging data is likely more accurate than an elective lymph node dissection.

4. Safety

Selective SLND is a safe procedure with a very low complication rate. Additionally, the risk of radiation has been studied in physicians injecting the radiotracer as well as the surgeons removing the nodes. The maximum recorded dose of radiation recorded was 1900 times smaller than the current 1 year dose limit recommended by the International Commission on Radiological Protection, and no limitations are needed in the number of surgical interventions performed yearly (Nejc et al., 2006; Sera et al, 2003).

There have been reports of adverse allergic reactions to blue dye (Leong et al., 2000) which can range from a mild allergic reaction to anaphylaxis associated with hypotension, pulmonary edema, and/or cardiovascular collapse. It is hypothesized that prior exposure to common household products is responsible for patient sensitization to blue dye. Single institution case studies quote allergic reaction rates of 0.7 to 2% for melanoma. A multi-institutional survey by our group of 14,800 melanoma patients treated with blue dye in over 185 institutions revealed a 0.4% rate of adverse blue dye reactions, most of which are mild. Despite this low rate, it is important to be aware of any adverse reactions such as urticaria, respiratory and hemodynamic changes which usually occur in the first 10 to 20 minutes. We recommend that the anesthesiologist and nursing team are made aware of the use of blue dye prior to its injection, an intravenous line always be inserted, and that the proper medications, including epinephrine and corticosteroids, be readily available. If blue dye is to be used, we suggest that the surgeon use as little blue dye as needed; we have found reliable results in head and neck melanoma using less than 1 cc per injection. Additionally, blue dye is not essential as we demonstrated in a recent study that using the 10% radioactivity rule (McMasters et al., 2001) with blue dye does not significantly decrease the Miss Rate when compared to the 10% radioactivity rule with technitium alone (Liu et al., 2011).

5. Clinical relevance of sentinel lymph node

Further support for the SLN concept stems from research that clearly shows that SLN status is the most significant prognostic factor with respect to disease-free and overall survival as shown in Table 2. Selective SLND is an excellent staging technique and can be used to identify patients who would or would not benefit from a complete lymphadenectomy and is also necessary for inclusion in clinical trials.

5.1 Positive node

As shown in Table 2, patients with a positive SLN have a significantly decreased overall 5-year survival compared to patients with a negative SLN. Therefore, for patients with a positive SLN, therapeutic decisions should be made and most often a regional lymphadenectomy is recommended. However, the survival benefit of selective SLND followed by completion lymph node dissection (CLND) is still controversial and many groups have attempted to study this by comparing melanoma patients after CLND after positive sentinel node biopsy and after therapeutic lymph node dissection for clinically detected regional lymph node metastases. In the MSLT-1 trial (Morton et al., 2006), among patients with nodal metastases (primary melanomas ranging from 1.2 to 3.5 mm), the 5-year melanoma specific survival rate of those who underwent selective SLND with immediate lymphadenectomy (72.3%) for a positive SLN was significantly higher than those in the observation group who had lymphadenectomy only when there was clinically evident nodal disease (52.4%; p = .004). However, no overall survival advantage was seen when comparing the entire cohort of patients randomized to selective SLND with those patients who had wide excision only and nodal observation. Other data from meta-analysis of 6 studies showed a significantly higher risk of death for patients who only underwent elective lymph node dissection after clinically evident nodal metastasis versus patients who underwent SLN-guided CLND (Pasquali et al., 2010). However, this is a complex topic and survival benefit is also likely related to other factors including age, primary tumor characteristics, and features of the nodal metastases. Additionally, these studies tend to be underpowered because of a low percentage of patients with positive SLN(s) who could potentially benefit from CLND (Ross et al., 2011).

5.2 Negative node

When SLNs are negative for micrometastasis, the remainder of the lymph node basin is usually negative (Morton et al., 1992; Reintgen et al., 1994; Albertini et al., 1996; Krag et al., 1995; Ross et al., 1993; Thompson et al., 1994) with FN rates under 5%. This is good evidence to conclude that melanoma metastases are most often spread in an orderly pattern (Fig.1). In general, if the SLNs are negative, there is no need to proceed with a more morbid regional lymph node dissection; selective SLN mapping replaces the more extensive lymph node dissection if SLNs are found to contain no metastasis.

Patients with a negative SLN have an overall 5 year survival of 84 to 92%, significantly better than positive node patients. Despite better survival results, a negative SLN is not an absolute predictor of survival. Recurrence and death in SLN negative patients may be related to FN SLN results or a pure hematogenous spread (Leong et al., 2004, 2011; Ross et al., 2011). In particular, head and neck melanomas have a higher FN rate, over 12% in some studies (Klop et al., 2011); this is likely due to a complex lymphatic drainage pattern with multiple basins in the head and neck (Leong, 2011). FN results for selective SLND may result from failed preoperative lymphoscintigraphy, including injection techniques and interpretation of the lymphoscintigraphy, failed intraoperative lymphatic mapping, failed pathologic identification of microscopic disease, and "skip" metastasis (Leong, 2004). Predictors of relapse and death in SLN negative patients include increasing tumor thickness and ulceration (Ross et al., 2011).

Author	Year	# of Patients	5-Year Overall Survival Negative Node	Positive Node	*p*-value
Nowecki ZI	2003	726	84%	40%	<0.001
Leong SP	2005	363	85.6%	61.5%	<0.0001
Morton DL	2006	1269	90%	72%	<0.001
Cascinelli N	2006	1108	90.6%	75.4%	<0.0001
Mandalà M	2009	1251	88.7%	42.9%	<.0001
Kunter C	2010	1049	90%	58%	<0.001
Ellis MC	2010	397	92%	73%	0.0001

Table 2. Overall Survival in Relation To Sentinel Lymph Node Status.

6. Biology and clinical impact of micrometastasis in SLN(s)

The dimensions and "amount" of micrometastasis in the SLN gives important prognostic data. According to the Rotterdam criteria for SLN tumor burden (van Akkooi et al., 2006, 2008), the maximum diameter of the largest focus of a positive SLN(s) is used as the measurement of record. There were 388 melanoma patients with positive SLNs from three European centers analyzed by this method with a median follow-up of 36 months. Three groups of patients were defined: (1) submicrometastasis with at least 10 cells but less than 0.1 mm (10%); (2) micrometastasis between 0.1 and 1.0 mm (35%); and (3) micrometastasis greater than 1.0 mm (55%). Patients with sub-micrometastasis (<0.1 mm) were identical to the SLN-negative group with an excellent survival rate. Tumor burden in SLNs increased with T-stage. Both T4 and SLN tumor burden were the most important factors for overall survival.

Similarly, 63 melanoma patients with positive SLNs from the UCSF melanoma SLN database with a median follow-up of 8 years were analyzed (Baehner et al., 2011). SLN micrometastasis was recorded for size, number of foci and anatomic location by H&E. Fourteen of 63 patients had positive non-SLNs. Using the log-rank test, maximum metastatic size and primary melanoma thickness were correlated with progression-free survival and overall survival. Neither number of metastatic foci nor microscopic location was statistically significant. Multivariate analysis showed that the maximum metastatic size and primary melanoma thickness were the most important prognostic factors for progression-free survival and overall survival. As a continuous variable, every 5.0 mm increase in maximum metastatic size was predictive of progression-free survival. The estimated 5-year overall survival rate was 90% in patients with maximum metastatic size <0.6 mm, 52% with maximum metastatic size from 0.6 to 5.5 mm, and 55% with maximum metastatic size >5.5 mm. When stratified by thickness, the estimated 5-year progression-free survival rates were 95% for patients with maximum metastatic size <1.6 mm, 70% between 1.6 and 4.5 mm, and 45% >4.5 mm; the overall survival were 82%, 52%, and 5%. Both primary melanoma thickness and maximum metastatic size were independently prognostic of progression-free survival and overall survival in melanoma patients (Baehner et al., 2011). Other studies have also demonstrated that the incidence of SLN metastases correlates directly with increasing tumor thickness (Gershenwald et al., 1998; Ross, 2011) as well as other factors including ulceration, lymphatic invasion, mitotic rate, Clark level, and anatomic site (Ross, 2011).

7. Conclusion

The overall challenge in melanoma is to identify patients with truly localized disease versus patients with metastasis to nodal and/or systemic sites, as early detection remains key to successful eradication. With this in mind, selective SLND was introduced 20 years ago and has become essential in the care of patients with cutaneous melanoma, with a multitude of publications validating the importance of the SLN. Selective SLND provides a minimally invasive standard of care (Morton et al, 2008), that allows accurate staging, gives significant prognostic information, facilitates therapeutic lymphadenectomy with regional disease control, avoids unnecessary elective lymph node dissection, and may improve survival in node-positive patients. However, in a minority situations (~20% of the time), cancer cells may spread through the vascular system to distant sites, bypassing the SLNs (Leong et al.,

2011). Therefore, it is important that all patients with melanoma be followed closely after their diagnosis.

8. References

Albertini, J.J., Cruse, C.W., Rapaport, D., Wells, K., Ross, M., DeConti, R., Berman, C.G., Jared, K., Messina, J., Lyman, G., Glass, F., Fenske, N. & Reintgen, DS. (1996). Intraoperative radiolymphoscintigraphy improves sentinel lymph node identification for patients with melanoma. *Ann Surg,* 223(2):217-224.

Alex, J.C. & Krag, D.N. (1993). Gamma-probe guided localization of lymph nodes. *Surg Oncol,* 2(3):137-143.

Baas, P.C., Schraffordt Koops, H., Hoekstra, H.J., van Bruggen, J.J., van der Weele, L.T. & Oldhoff, J. (1992). Groin dissection in the treatment of lower-extremity melanoma. Short term and long-term morbidity. *Arch Surg,* 127(3):281-286.

Baehner, F., Jenkins, T., Hwang, J. & Leong, S.P.L. (2011). Impact of microscopic tumor burden in sentinel lymph nodes on the outcome of melanoma patients. *Submitted for publication.*

Baldwin, B.T, Cherpelis, B.S., Sondak, V. & Fenske, N.A. (2010). Sentinel lymph node biopsy in melanoma: Facts and controversies. *Clin Dermatol,* 28(3):319-323.

Balch, C.M., Morton, D.L., Gershenwald, J.E., McMasters, K.M., Nieweg, O.E., Powell, B., Ross, M.I., Sondak, V.K. & Thompson, J.F. (2009). Sentinel node biopsy and standard of care for melanoma. *J Am Acad Dermatol,* 60(5):872-875.

Bilimoria, K.Y., Balch, C.M., Wayne, J.D., Chang, D.C., Palis, B.E., Dy, S.M. & Lange, J.R. (2009). Health care system and socioeconomic factors associated with variance in use of sentinel lymph node biopsy for melanoma in the United States. *J Clin Oncol,* 27(11):1857-1863.

Cabanas, R.M. (1977). An approach for the treatment of penile carcinoma. *Cancer,* 39(2):456-466.

Cormier, J.N., Xing, Y., Ding, M., Lee, J.E., Mansfield, P.F., Gershenwald, J.E., Ross, M.I. & Du, X.L. (2005). Population-based assessment of surgical treatment trends for patients with melanoma in the era of sentinel lymph node biopsy. *J Clin Oncol,* 23(25):6054-62.

Ellis, M.C., Weerasinghe, R., Corless, C.L. & Vetto, J.T. (2010). Sentinel lymph node staging of cutaneous melanoma: predictors and outcomes. *Am J Surg,* 199(5):663-668.

Glass, L.F., Messina, J.L., Cruse, W., Wells, K., Rapaport, D., Miliotes, G., Berman, C., Reintgen, D. & Fenske, N.A. (1996). The use of intraoperative radiolymphoscintigraphy for sentinel node biopsy in patients with malignant melanoma. *Dermatol Surg,* 22(8):715-270.

Gennari, R., Bartolomei, M., Testori, A., Zurrida, S., Stoldt, H.S., Audisio, R.A., Geraghty, J.G., Paganelli, G. & Veronesi, U. (2000). Sentinel node localization in primary melanoma: preoperative dynamic lymphoscintigraphy, intraoperative gamma probe, and vital dye guidance. *Surgery,* 127(1):19-25.

Gershenwald, J.E., Tseng, C.H., Thompson, W., Mansfield, P.F., Lee, J.E., Bouvet, M., Lee, J.J. & Ross, M.I. (1998). Improved sentinel lymph node localization in patients with primary melanoma with the use of radiolabeled colloid. *Surgery,* 124(2):203–1

Gershenwald, J.E., Thompson, W., Mansfield, P.F., Lee, J.E., Colome, M.I., Tseng, C.H., Lee, J.J., Balch, C.M., Reintgen, D.S. & Ross, M.I. (1999). Multi-institutional melanoma lymphatic mapping experience: The prognostic value of sentinel lymph node status in 612 stage I and II melanoma patients. *J Clin Oncol,* 17(3):976-983.

Gould, E.A., Winship, T., Philbin, P.H. & Kerr, H.H. (1960). Observations on a "sentinel node" in cancer of the parotid. *Cancer,* 13:77-78.

Hellman, S. (1994) Natural history of small breast cancers. JCO Karnofsky Memorial Lecture 12, 2229-2234.

Kapteijn, B.A, Nieweg, O.E., Liem, I., Mooi, W.J., Balm, A.J., Muller, S.H., Peterse, J.L., Valdés Olmos, R.A., Hoefnagel, C.A. & Kroon, B.B. (1997). Localizing the sentinel node in cutaneous melanoma: gamma probe detection versus blue dye. *Ann Surg Oncol,* 4(2):156-160.

Klop, W.M., Veenstra, H.J., Vermeeren, L., Nieweg, O.E., Balm, A.J. & Lohuis, P.J. (2011). Assessment of lymphatic drainage patterns and implications for the extent of neck dissection in head and neck melanoma patients. *J Surg Oncol,* Jan 31.

Leong, S.P., Achtem, T.A., Habib, F.A., Steinmetz, I., Morita, E., Allen, R.E., Kashani-Sabet, M. & Sagebiel, R. (1999). Discordancy between clinical predictions vs lymphoscintigraphic and intraoperative mapping of sentinel lymph node drainage of primary melanoma. *Arch Dermatol,* 135(12):1472-1476.

Leong, S.P., Donegan, E., Heffernon, W., Dean, S. & Katz, J.A. (2000). Adverse reactions to isosulfan blue during selective sentinel lymph node dissection in melanoma. *Ann Surg Oncol,* 7(5):361-6

Leong, S.P. (2004), Sentinel lymph node mapping and selective lymphadenectomy: the standard of care for melanoma. *Curr Treat Options Oncol,* 5(3):185-194

Leong, S.P., Kashani-Sabet, M., Desmond, R.A., Kim, R.P., Nguyen, D.H., Iwanaga, K., Treseler, P.A., Allen, R.E. Jr, Morita, E.T., Zhang, Y., Sagebiel, R.W. & Soong, S.J. (2005). Clinical significance of occult metastatic melanoma in sentinel lymph nodes and other high-risk factors based on long-term follow-up. *World J Surg,* 29(6):683-691.

Leong, S.P., Kim, J., Ross, M., Faries, M., Scoggins, C.R., Rich Metz, W.L., Cope, F.O. & Orahood, R.C. (2011). A Phase 2 Study of 99mTc-Tilmanocept in the Detection of Sentinel Lymph Nodes in Melanoma and Breast Cancer. *Ann Surg Oncol,* 18:961–969.

Leong, S.P. (2011). Role of selective sentinel lymph node dissection in head and neck melanoma. *J Surg Oncol,* in press.

Leong, S.P., Zuber, M., Ferris, R.L., et al. (2011). Impact of nodal status and tumor burden in sentinel lymph nodes on the clinical outcomes of cancer patients. *J Surg Oncol,* in press.

Liu, L.C., Parrett, B.M., Jenkins, T., et al. (2011). Selective Sentinel Lymph Node Dissection for Melanoma: Importance of Harvesting Nodes with Lower Radioactive Counts without the Need for Blue Dye. *Ann Surg Oncol,* in press.

McMasters, K.M., Reintgen, D.S., Ross, M.I., Wong, S.L., Gershenwald, J.E., Krag, D.N., Noyes, R.D., Viar, V., Cerrito, P.B. & Edwards, M.J. (2001). Sentinel Lymph Node Biopsy for Melanoma: How Many Radioactive Nodes Should Be Removed? *Ann Surg Oncol,* 8(3):192-197.

Morton, D.L., Wen, D.R., Wong, J.H., Economou ,J.S., Cagle, L.A., Storm, F.K., Foshag, L.J. & Cochran, A.J. (1992). Technical details of intraoperative lymphatic mapping for early stage melanoma. *Arch Surg,* 127(4):392-399.

Morton, D.L., Thompson, J.F., Essner, R., Elashoff, R., Stern, S.L., Nieweg, O.E., Roses, D.F., Karakousis, C.P., Mozzillo, N., Reintgen, D., Wang, H.J., Glass, E.C. & Cochran, A.J. (1999). Validation of the accuracy of intraoperative lymphatic mapping and sentinel lymphadenectomy for earlystage melanoma: a multicenter trial. Multicenter Selective Lymphadenectomy Trial Group. *Ann Surg,* 230(4):453-463.

Morton, D.L., Thompson, J.F., Cochran, A.J., Mozzillo, N., Elashoff, R., Essner, R., Nieweg, O.E., Roses, D.F., Hoekstra, H.J., Karakousis, C.P., Reintgen, D.S., Coventry, B.J., Glass, E.C. & Wang, H.J.; MSLT Group. (2006). Sentinel-node biopsy or nodal observation in melanoma. *N Engl J Med,* 355(13):1307-1317.

Morton, D.L., Cochran, A.J. & Thompson, J.F. (2008). The rationale for sentinel-node biopsy in primary melanoma. *Nat Clin Pract Oncol,* 5(9):510-511.

Nejc, D., Wrzesień, M., Piekarski, J., Olszewski, J., Pluta, P., Kuśmierek, J. & Jeziorski, A. (2006). Sentinel node biopsy in skin melanoma patients--measurements of absorbed doses of radiation to the hands of medical staff. *J Surg Oncol,* 93(5):355-361.

Nowecki, Z.I., Rutkowski, P., Nasierowska-Guttmejer, A. & Ruka, W. (2003). Sentinel lymph node biopsy in melanoma patients with clinically negative regional lymph nodes--one institution's experience. *Melanoma Res,* 13(1):35-43.

Pasquali, S., Mocellin, S., Campana, L.G., Bonandini, E., Montesco, M.C., Tregnaghi, A., Del Fiore, P., Nitti, D. & Rossi, C.R. (2010). Early (sentinel lymph node biopsy-guided) versus delayed lymphadenectomy in melanoma patients with lymph node metastases : personal experience and literature meta-analysis. *Cancer,* 116(5):1201-1209.

Reintgen, D., Cruse, C.W., Wells, K., Berman, C., Fenske, N., Glass, F., Schroer, K., Heller, R., Ross, M. & Lyman, G. (1994). The orderly progression of melanoma nodal metastases. *Ann Surg,* 220(6):759-767.

Robinson, D.S., Sample, W.F., Fee, H.J., Holmes, C. & Morton, D.L. (1977). Regional lymphatic drainage in primary malignant melanoma of the trunk determined by colloidal gold scanning. *Surg Forum,* 28:147-148.

Ross, M.I., Thompson, J.F. & Gershenwald, J.E. (2011) Sentinel lymph node biopsy for melanoma: critical assessment at its twentieth anniversary. *Surg Oncol Clin N Am,* 20:57-78.

Sera, T., Mohos, G., Papos, M., Osvay, M., Varga, J., Lazar, M., Kiss, E., Kapitany, K., Dobozy, A., Csernay, L. & Pavics, L. (2003). Sentinel node detection in malignant melanoma patients: radiation safety considerations. *Dermatol Surg,* 29(2):141-145.

Sondak, V.K., Zager, J.S. & Messina, J.L. (2007). Sentinel lymph node biopsy as the standard of care for cutaneous melanoma. *Clin Adv Hematol Oncol,* 5(6):483-490.

Stebbins, W.G., Garibyan, L. & Sober, A.J. (2010). Sentinel lymph node biopsy and melanoma: 2010 update Part I. *J Am Acad Dermatol,* 62(5):723-734.

Sumner, W.E. 3rd, Ross, M.I., Mansfield, P.F., Lee, J.E., Prieto, V.G., Schacherer, C.W. & Gershenwald, J.E. (2002). Implications of lymphatic drainage to unusual sentinel lymph node sites in patients with primary cutaneous melanoma. *Cancer,* 95(2):354-360.

Thompson, J.F., McCarthy, W.H., Bosch, C.M.J., O'Brien, C.J., Quinn, M.J., Paramaesvaran, S., Crotty, K., McCarthy, S.W., Uren, R.F. & Howman-Giles, R. (1995). Sentinel lymph node status as an indicator of the presence of metastatic melanoma in regional lymph nodes. *Melanoma Res,* 5(4):255-260.

Uren, R.F., Howman-Giles, R., Thompson, J.F., Shaw, H.M., Quinn, M.J., O'Brien, C.J., McCarthy, W.H. (1994). Lymphoscintigraphy to identify sentinel lymph nodes in patients with melanoma. *Melanoma Res,* 4(6):395-399.

van Akkooi, A., de Wilt, J., Verhoef, C., Schäfer-Hesterberg, G., Michej, W., de Wilt, J.H., Rutkowski P, Verhoef, C. & Eggermont, A.M. (2006) Clinical relevance of melanoma micrometastases (< 0.1 mm) in sentinel nodes: Are these nodes to be considered negative? *Ann Oncol,* 17:1578–1585.

van Akkooi, A.C., Nowecki, Z.I., Voit, C., Schäfer-Hesterberg, G., Michej, W., de Wilt, J.H., Rutkowski, P., Verhoef, C. & Eggermont, A.M. (2008) Sentinel node tumor burden according to the Rotterdam criteria is the most important prognostic factor for survival in melanoma patients: A multicenter study in 388 patients with positive sentinel nodes. *Ann Surg,* 248(6):949–955.

Wong, J.H., Cagle, L.A. & Morton, D.L. (1991). Lymphatic drainage of skin to a sentinel lymph node in a feline model. *Ann Surg,* 214(5):637-641.

Wrightson, W.R., Wong, S.L., Edwards, M.J., Chao, C., Reintgen, D.S., Ross, M.I., Noyes, R.D., Viar, V., Cerrito, P.B. & McMasters, K.M.; Sunbelt Melanoma Trial Study Group. (2003). Complications associated with sentinel lymph node biopsy for melanoma. *Ann Surg Oncol,* 10(6):676-680.

Part 4

Melanoma Complications and Rare Types of Disease

15

Melanoma and Pregnancy

C. Pagès and M. Viguier
Université Paris7 Denis Diderot, Saint Louis Hospital
France

1. Introduction

Melanoma is one of the most commonly diagnosed cancer during the childbearing age and during pregnancy. It is also the malignancy that is most often reported in the literature in association with placental and/or foetal metastasis (Alexander et al., 2003).
The coexistence of melanoma and pregnancy is therefore not an exceptional situation, difficult to manage, raising numerous questions in terms of prognosis, feasibility of the different imaging and radio-diagnostic investigations, and of the various modes of treatment. On the other hand, when melanoma is diagnosed during the childbearing age, out of the immediate context of pregnancy, several questions are raised regarding the potential consequences on the evolution of melanoma of being pregnant later on.

2. Epidemiological data

Cancer is now among the leading causes of non-accidental death in women of child-bearing age. In the USA, malignancy accounts for about 19% of mortality in women aged between 15 and 34 years (Pavlidis, 2002). The most frequently observed cancers among young women of child-bearing age are breast cancer, cervical cancer, malignant haemopathies (Hodgkin's disease and leukaemia) and melanoma (Langagergaard, 2011).
In France, between 1980 and 2000, the standardized worldwide population incidence rate of melanoma increased from 3,9 to 9,5/100,000 persons/year among women. In 2000, the estimated number of new cases of skin melanoma was 7,231, with 58% diagnosed in women. The incidence increased by a factor of 3,2 among men and by a factor of 2,4 among women. Despite this greater increase among men, incidence remained higher among women across the whole period (Grange, 2005). In Denmark, for instance, the incidence of melanoma among women between the ages of 15 and 34 increased by 4,3% per year on average from 1970 to 1999 (Van der Horst et al., 2006). Altogether, it is estimated that about one third of all melanomas in women is diagnosed during their childbearing years (Langagergaard, 2001).
In Western countries, women often postpone childbearing for different reasons (Langagergaard, 2011) and because the incidence rates of most cancers increases with advancing age, more women can therefore be expected to be diagnosed with cancer before childbearing or during pregnancy. Although the exact incidence and prevalence are unknown, estimates suggest one to two new cases of cancer in every 1,000 pregnancies (Alexander, 2003). The most frequently encountered cancers during pregnancy are in line with those the most frequently described among young women of childbearing age: for breast and cervical cancer, the incidences estimated per number of pregnancies are of the

order of 1/2,000 to 1/10,000; for lymphomas, the incidence is estimated at 1/1,000 to 1/6,000. The incidence of melanomas in pregnancy is estimated at 1/1,000 to 1/10,000, and melanoma is thought to amount to around 8% of cancers diagnosed during pregnancy (Oduncu et al., 2003).
However, the real incidence of cutaneous melanoma occurring in pregnancy is still not known. Lens et al., 2004 examining the data from the Swedish National and Regional Cancer and Mortality Registries found that, among 19,337 women diagnosed with cutaneous melanoma in the period from 1958 to 1999, 28,6% were diagnosed with melanoma during their reproductive period, while only 0,9% of the women were diagnosed with melanoma during pregnancy. Stensheim et al., 2009 used the Cancer and Medical Birth Registry of Norway to assess 42,511 women (516 pregnant) aged to 16 to 49 with various cancers. The most commonly diagnosed cancer during pregnancy was melanoma.

3. Melanoma and influence of hormonal factors

For many years, there have been concerns that hormonal and immunological changes occurring during pregnancy may be important in the development of melanoma. Changes in pigmentation are associated with pregnancy, oral contraceptives and hormone replacement therapy. These observations have led to speculation concerning a relationship between hormones and melanoma.

3.1 Exogenous female hormones

Numerous epidemiological studies have questioned whether the use of oral contraceptives (OCs) or hormone replacement therapy (HRT) could increase a woman's risk for melanoma. Risk is expressed as an estimate of relative risk (RR) or odds ratio (OR). OR is the odds of melanoma occurring in women exposed to OCs/ odds of melanoma occurring in those not exposed to OCs. These studies showed conflicting results: a recent case-control study of OCs and risk of melanoma (Koomen et al., 2009) suggests a cumulative dose-dependent increased risk of melanoma with the use of OCs: 778 cases and 4,072 controls were included; melanoma risk was significantly associated with estrogen use (≥ 0.5 year; adjusted OR= 1,42, 95% CI 1,19-1,69). The major limitation of this study was the lack of information concerning sun exposure, skin type, sunburn history which are important potential confounders. However, in their review of the literature, Gupta et al. (Gupta δ Driscoll, 2010) identify 22 studies that have explored whether or not OCs enhance a woman's risk for melanoma, and most have not shown an effect of use of OCs at some time in life compared with women who never used OCs. No studies have specifically reported the impact of OCs on prognosis for women diagnosed with melanoma. The data concerning HRT and melanoma risk are more limited than for OCs, but most of these studies have shown no effect of HRT (Gupta δ Driscoll, 2010).
In summary, current clinical evidence does not suggest that exogenous female hormones contribute significantly to increased risk of melanoma.

3.2 Endogenous female hormones

The effects of high concentrations of oestrogen as a result of pregnancy on melanogenesis have long been debated, leading to different questions: is there an influence on melanoma prognosis if a woman is diagnosed with it during pregnancy? Should women with a previous history of melanoma avoid subsequent pregnancies in order to limit the risks of local or systemic recurrences?

3.2.1 Prognosis of melanoma diagnosed during pregnancy

Many studies since the 1980s have investigated whether survival was impacted in women diagnosed during pregnancy with melanoma classified as localized stage I or II according to the American Joint Committee on Cancer, AJCC (Balch et al., 2001). Randomized or non randomized clinical trials to assess the implication of pregnancy in women with cutaneous melanoma do not exist. In the literature, there is population-based studies or consecutive or non-consecutive case series ; these studies assess survival rates between pregnant women with melanoma compared to age adjusted non pregnant women. Two recent population - based studies addressed the question of whether pregnancy adversely affects survival in melanoma patients. Lens et al., 2004 reported on 185 patients from the Swedish Cancer registry who were pregnant at the time of diagnosis of localized melanoma. The outcome of these patients was compared with 5,348 non-pregnant age- and gender-matched controls. Multivariate regression analysis showed that pregnancy at the time of melanoma diagnosis was not a significant variable in relation to overall survival. Authors noted that pregnant melanoma patients had somewhat thicker melanomas, with a mean Breslow thickness of 1,28 mm versus 1,07 mm in controls.

A second population-based study (O'Meara et al., 2005) used the database from the California Cancer Center to evaluate "pregnancy-associated melanoma", specified as a woman diagnosed with melanoma during pregnancy or within 1 year after delivery (post partum group). The control group was an age-matched group of patients who were not pregnant at the time of diagnosis. The median Breslow thickness was 0,77 mm in pregnant patients, 0,9 mm in post partum patients and 0,81 mm in the controls. O'Meara et al., 2005 found no evidence of a decrease in survival of patients who were pregnant (HR=0,79;P=0.570) or post partum compared to controls. The size of the study population is a strength, but one limitation is that approximately 20% of the Breslow thickness data were missing for both the study and the control group and we cannot extrapolate therefore whether the groups were well balanced or not regarding this important prognosis marker.

In the most recent population-based study, Stensheim et al., 2009 used the Cancer and Medical Birth Registry of Norway to assess 42,511 women (516 pregnant) aged to 16 to 49 with various cancers. The cancer most commonly diagnosed during pregnancy was melanoma. When compared to age- and gender-matched non pregnant controls, there was a slightly increased cause-specific death rate if melanoma was diagnosed during pregnancy. No difference in Breslow index was found between the two groups; however the Breslow thickness was collected for only 55% of the pregnant patients.

The details of the other studies and the results are presented in Table 1. Altogether, no statistically significant difference in survival rates between women diagnosed with melanoma during pregnancy and women diagnosed with melanoma out of pregnancy was established, suggesting that pregnancy does not favour the development of more aggressive melanoma.

There are little data to address the question of whether pregnancy has a negative effect on survival in patients with more advanced disease. In a study reported by Shiu et al., 1976, 14 patients with regional stage III AJCC melanoma diagnosed during pregnancy were found to have an important decrease in survival compared with 11 regional stage III AJCC melanoma nulliparous patients. The 5-year survival was 29% for the pregnant patients and 55% for the control group, not statistically different, but very small numbers of patients were involved. We recently observed that the 2-year survival rate in 16 AJCC stage III patients diagnosed during pregnancy was 56% (Pagès et al., 2010), which is close to that reported in the literature for those not pregnant (Balch et al., 2001); the AJCC stage IV (6 patients) 2-year survival rate was 17% which was shorter than that reported in the literature (Balch et al., 2001). Nevertheless, this data does not make it possible to draw definitive conclusions, on account of the small sample number and the absence of a control group in our study.

Authors	Number of patients diagnosed with melanoma during pregnancy (Group 1)	Number of patients diagnosed with melanoma out of pregnancy (Group 2)	Breslow thickness (mm) Group 1/ Group 2	Survival rates between groups	Follow-up time
Reintgen et al. 1985	58	585	1,90/ 1,51	NS	5 y (mean)
McManammy et al. 1989	23	243	1,62/ 1,72	NS	2 mo-20 y
Wong et al. 1989	66	619	1,24/ 1,28	NS	NR
Slingluff et al. 1990	100	86	2,17/ 1,52	NS	6 y (mean)
MacKie et al. 1991	92	143	2,38/ 1,96	NA	NA
Daryanani et al. 2003	46	368	2/ 1,70	NS	106 mo (median)
Lens et al. 2004	185	5348	1,28/ 1,07	NS	11,6 y (median)
O'Meara et al. 2005	149	Within 1 year postpartum: 263 Non pregnant: 2,451	0,77/0,90/ 0,81	NS	2-10 y

Abbreviations: Mo: months; y: years; NA: not available, NS: statistically non-significant difference in survival rates between groups.

Table 1. Controlled studies evaluating the impact of pregnancy on survival in women with AJCC stage I/II melanoma.

3.2.2 Impact of subsequent pregnancy on melanoma prognosis

A small number of studies have addressed the impact of pregnancy after a diagnosis of melanoma. One of them (Lens et al., 2004) was a secondary analysis within a large retrospective cohort study of Swedish patients: 966 women who became pregnant after melanoma diagnosis were compared with 4,567 women without pregnancies subsequent to the melanoma diagnosis. A multivariable Cox regression model showed that pregnancy after melanoma diagnosis was not related to survival (Hazard Ratio for death in women who had pregnancy subsequent to the diagnosis of melanoma: 0.58, 95% CI= 0.32-1.05). Based on the current evidence, there is no reason to recommend deferral of subsequent pregnancy in women diagnosed with localized melanoma. Counselling women on subsequent pregnancies should be based upon well-known prognostic factors, such as Breslow thickness and ulceration (Balch et al., 2001). In women with thick tumours (over 1.5 mm), it may be recommended to discuss with the patient the fact that if melanoma recurs it is more likely to do so in the first 2 years; physicians can thus advise these women to delay pregnancy for 2 to 3 years.

Altogether, the issue of whether hormones influence malignant melanoma has been controversial for many years. There is no evidence that pregnancy adversely affects outcome in melanoma patients who have clinically localized disease. Continuing to recommend a postponement of childbearing for these patients is not supported by available clinical evidence suggesting an increased risk of cancer progression due to pregnancy itself. For more advanced disease, recommendations must be based on individual patients and their wishes.

4. Maternal-foetal transmission of melanoma during pregnancy

Only disseminating, metastatic cancers appear to be liable to produce placental and foetal metastasis, in an haematogenic way. The real incidence rates for placental and foetal metastasis, and the natural history of cancers during pregnancy, are still little known. In France, for instance, there are no epidemiological surveillance tools for cancers among pregnant women. In the literature, irrespective of type of cancer, about a hundred cases of placental metastasis (excluding cases of foetal origin and trophoblastic disease) have been described since 1866 (Dessolle et al., 2007). Alexander et al. in a literature review reported 87 cases of placental metastasis secondary to maternal cancer. In this study, melanoma was the cancer the most frequently responsible for this type of development: 27 cases out of 87 (31%). Given the possibility of placental metastasis, the placenta should be very carefully examined, both macroscopically and microscopically in case of metastatic melanoma in the mother.

Furthermore, the placenta represents an ideal site for metastases during gestation, because of its vascularisation, its large surface area and its biological environment and also because of its hyperkinetic state associated with pregnancy.

Table 2 sums up the cases of placental and/or foetal metastasis in connection with melanoma described in the literature and is an actualisation of the table presented in the paper of Alexander et al. Of the 27 placentas subjected to anatomo-pathological investigation, 17 cases of microscopic placental metastasis are reported, without any anomaly being macroscopically visible. The microscopic examination of the placenta should be as thorough as possible: in the case reported by Baergen et al, the placental metastatic localisations were visible on only 3 of the 50 sections performed, in the case reported by

Valenzano Menada et al. the microscopic examination with normal staining of the placenta showed no particular anomaly and the micro-metastases were only visualised by the mean of immuno-histo-chemical analyses (PS100).

Considering now the problematic of foetal metastasis secondary to maternal cancer, according to the review of the literature by Dessolle et al, 15 cases have been published since 1866. Several types of cancer have been incriminated: among the 15 cases, 5 foetal metastasis were secondary to maternal melanoma, 5 to acute leukaemia or lymphoma, 2 to bronchial cancer, 2 to sarcomas and one to a non-specified maternal cancer. Thus, although foetal metastasis in case of disseminated cancer in the mother is an exceptional situation, melanoma does appear as the most frequent cause. The study by Alexander et al. collates 6 reports of foetal metastasis secondary to maternal metastatic melanoma. Two further cases of foetal metastasis (Trumble et al., 2005 and Valenzano Menada et al., 2010) have been further reported. Among these 8 cases (Weber et al., 1930 Holland et al., 1949 Gottron et al., 1940 Dargeon et al., 1950 Aronsson Cavel et al., 1963 Brodsky et al., 1965 Ferreira et al., 1998 Trumble et al., 2005 Valenzano Menada et al., 2010), tumoral encroachment on the placenta was observed for 4. The 4 remaining cases were not examined in this respect. These 8 observations, although some are incomplete, enable the following characteristics:

- Melanoma metastasis appearance occurring shortly after birth, with a mean time lapse of around 3 months (age at diagnosis ranging from 1 day to 9 months, missing data for 1 case).
- Relatively homogeneous clinical presentation of metastatic proliferation to the child: the neonatal metastases were for the most part in the form of subcutaneous metastatic nodules, or intra-abdominal tumoral masses; there are exceptions for the cases published by Trumble et al. and Valenzano et al, where intracranial proliferations were diagnosed at 7 and 3 months after birth, respectively.
- Extremely poor prognosis, as the large majority of the infants died before the age of 1 year, with the exception of two cases (Aronsson, Cavell et al., 1963 and Valenzano Menada et al., 2010) of secondary regression of the metastatic disease in the children. In the case published by Aronsson and Cavell, spontaneous resolution of pulmonary and subcutaneous metastases occurred at 13 weeks after birth; the remission was secondarily confirmed during follow-up, with the child presenting no particular heath problem at the age of 14 years. Valenzano Menada et al. reported the case of a regression of intracranial and pulmonary metastases at 5 months after birth following initial failure of chemotherapy associating ifosfamide and adriamycine (1 month after discontinuation of chemotherapy). Complete remission of the disease was later confirmed when the child was seen at 24 months, with no residual signs of disease.
- Predominance of male children: 6 cases out of 8, one girl and one stillborn child whose gender was not reported.

5. Management of melanoma in a pregnant woman

Diagnosing melanoma during pregnancy will raise several questions, depending notably of the stage of malignancy (primary melanoma, lymph node metastasis, visceral metastasis, type of visceral metastasis) and of the gestational age. One of the first step will be the evaluation of the extent of the cancer and will raise the question of the feasibility of some radiological diagnosis procedures and another step will be the feasibility of the oncologic treatment (surgery, adjuvant therapy with immunotherapy, radiotherapy, chemotherapy…).

Authors	Placental Findings: Macroscopic involvement/ Microscopic involvement	Post delivery maternal survival	Existence of fetal metastases/ age at diagnosis	Infant outcomes/ follow -up
Weber et al., 1930, Holland et al. 1949	+/+	2 m	+/ 8 m	Death 10.5mo
Gottron et al., 1940	NE	2 m	+/ NR	Death 5 mo
Dargeon et al., 1950	NE	4 d	+/ 9 m	Death 10 mo
Aronsson et al. , Cavell et al., 1963	NE	4 d	+/ 2 m	Melanoma Regression, Alive (14 years follow up)
Brodsky et al., 1965	+/+	17 d	+/ 11 j	Death 48 d
Ferreira et al., 1998	+/+	2 d	+/ 1 j	Stillbirth
Trumble et al., 2005	NE	NR	+/ 7 m	Death 25 mo
Valenzano Menada et al., 2010	-/+	15 d	+/ 3 m	Melanoma Regression Alive (24 mo follow up)
Markus et al., 1918	+/+	5 h	No	Death 1 d*
Byrd et al., 1954	-/+	21 d	No	Death j*
Reynolds et al., 1955	-/+	1 m	No	Alive/ 10mo
Freedman et al., 1960	+/+	1.5 m	No	Alive/ 24mo
Stephenson et al., 1971	-/+	3m	No	Alive/ 24mo
Holcomb et al., 1975	-/+	18 d	No	Alive/ 3mo
Sokol et al., 1976	+/+	54 d	No	Death 2 d*
Smythe et al., 1976	-/+	20 d	No	Alive/ 9mo
Gillis et al., 1976	+/+	7.5 m	No	Alive/ 24mo
Russel et al., 1977	+/+	15 d	No	Alive/ 5mo
Looi et al., 1979	-/+	48 d	No	Alive/ 1mo
Moller et al., 1986	+/+	30 d	No	Alive/ 6mo
Anderson δ Machin 1989	-/+	6 m	No	Alive/ 12mo

Authors	Placental Findings: Macroscopic involvement/ Microscopic involvement	Post delivery maternal survival	Existence of fetal metastases/ age at diagnosis	Infant outcomes/ follow -up
Brossard et al. 1994	-/+	4 d	No	Alive/ 12mo
Marsh et al., 1996	-/+	21 d	No	Lost to follow up
Dillman et al.,	-/+	5 m	No	Lost to follow up
Baergen et al. 1997	-/+	7 d	No	Alive/ 7mo
Dipaola et al., 1997	-/+	1 m	No	Alive/ 17mo
Jonhston et al., 1998	-/+	4 d	No	Alive/ 12mo
Merkus et al., 1998	-/+	2 m	No	Alive/ 48mo
Altman et al., 2003	-/+	19 m	No	Alive/ 19mo
Alexander et al., 2004	-/+	56 d	No	Alive/ 10mo
Pagès et al., 2010	+/+	3,5 m	No	Alive/ 56mo

Abbreviations : NE: not examined, NR : not reported, d: days, mo: months ,
* : cause of death = prematurity.

Table 2. Placental and/or foetal melanoma metastases.

The question of the maternal prognosis will be central and the opportunity of pursuing or not the pregnancy will be asked by the patient, her family and the medical staff.

5.1 Radiological diagnosis in pregnant women

A recent review (Lazarus E. et al., 2007) pointed out a 121% increase over 10 years in the use of imagery investigations requiring ionizing radiation during pregnancy, with computed tomography (CT) increasing by 25% per year. In pregnancy, the use of the irradiating techniques of classic radiology should be strictly evaluated. The French *Institut de Protection et de Sûreté Nucléaire* recalls some principles:

- In almost all cases, if a radiological diagnostic examination is considered medically necessary, the risk incurred by the mother of failure to perform such examination should be greater than the risk potentially incurred by the foetus.
- The radiation doses resulting from most diagnostic procedures usually do not present serious risk of death, malformation or altered mental development of the foetus. If the foetus is in the direct radiation beam, the procedure can often be adapted so as to reduce the foetal dose.

- When an ionizing examination is indicated in the course of which the fœtus is to be in the direct beam, and when this examination cannot be postponed until after parturition, the dose delivered to the foetus should be minimised as far as possible.
- In diagnostic radiology, the estimation of the radiation dose to the fœtus is generally not required, except when the fœtus is in the direct beam.

Thus, in most cases, irradiating radiological procedures are feasible for diagnosis or assessment of the extent of a maternal cancer (Chen et al., 2008). It is considered that the threshold fœtal irradiation dose that is potentially teratogenic is of the order of 0,1 to 0,2 Gray, Gy (Kal et al., 2005)). The radiation dose to the foetus from a typical CT study of the maternal pelvis is variable and depends on the gestational age and scanning parameters. The estimated dose of an investigation of this sort ranges from 0,024 Gy in the first trimester to 0,046 Gy in the third trimester (Pentheroudakis et al., 2006). Therefore, the radiation dose of the pelvis is likely to be below the estimated threshold level for inducing congenital malformations. Likewise, as mentioned by the International Radioprotection Commission, a foetal dose of 0,1 Gy is probably reached neither from 3 pelvic tomodensitometry examinations, nor from 20 conventional diagnostic radiographic examinations of the abdomen or pelvic area. In a review of the literature published by Pentheroudakis et al, the foetal doses received according to one or another type of ionising radiological examination performed on the mother are given, and estimated to be on average at 0,0004 mGy for chest radiography, 0,17mGy for chest tomodensitometry, and 18 to 25 mGy for abdominal-pelvic tomodensitometry. This information can be used to counsel pregnant patients who require investigation involving ionizing radiation. Nevertheless, a risk of carcinogenesis in the foetus after *in utero* irradiation always still, regardless of the dose. The baseline risk of fatal childhood cancer is 5 in 10.000 and the relative risk after exposure to 0,05 Gy is 2 (Chen et al., 2008); this relative risk may appear substantial but it should be remembered that the baseline risk is very low and that the 2004 Guidelines of the American College of Obstetricians and Gynecologists do not precisely indicate the estimated carcinogenic risk in case of irradiation *in utero,* describing it as "very small" and it is concluded that it is exceptionally unlikely that any single diagnostic radiological examination would deliver a radiation dose sufficient to justify pregnancy termination. Numerous authors agree that it can be thought that radio-diagnostic examinations in pregnant women can be performed after appropriate evaluation of the risk/benefit ratio; however, it is generally the "substitution" rule that predominates, by way of endeavours either to delay the investigation to the post-partum period, or to obtain the information required by other means, avoiding ionisation. For instance, Nicklas et al., 2000 suggest a certain number of alternatives to the standard radiographic procedures in the context of metastatic cancer in pregnant women: the use of non ionising examinations such as chest and abdominal Magnetic Resonance Imaging (MRI), to look for deep nodal involvement and evaluation of the pulmonary and liver parenchyma as an alternative to chest and abdominal tomodensitometries, and cerebral MRI for the evaluation of the central nervous system.
However, concerning MRI, the current guidelines of the U.S. Food and Drug Administration indicate that the safety of MRI with respect to the foetus « has not been established ». The risk incurred by the foetus during MRI examination without injection is on the one hand related to teratogenic effects, and on the other to the possible occurrence of damage to hearing. In view of the theoretical risk of foetal overheating/cavitation, first trimester MRI should be avoided (Chen et al., 2008) ; damaging effects could indeed arise from different

mechanisms, among which the thermal effect of magnetic resonance gradient changes and direct non-thermal interaction of the electromagnetic field with biological structures (Campbell FA et al., 2006). It should be noted that the 2007 American College of Radiology guidance document for safe MRI practices does not differentiate among the pregnancy trimesters and states that all pregnant patients can receive MRI as long as the "risk- benefit ratio to the patient warrants that the study be performed" (Kanal et al., 2007): MRI, thus, seems safe to use among pregnant women in the second and third trimesters.
The injection of contrasting substances (iodine or gadolinium) for imagery investigations is also questionable during pregnancy. Iodine-based substances belong to FDA category B. This category includes molecules for which animal studies do not show any foetal risk but for which human studies are lacking, or molecules for which animal studies have shown damaging effects on the foetus but where this effect has not been confirmed by studies among pregnant women in the first trimester of pregnancy. In animals, regarding the use of iodine-based contrast substances, no teratogenic, abortive or mutagenic effect has been reported (Webb et al., 2005). However the agents pass through the placental barrier, allowing a risk of neonatal hypothyroidism (Webb et al., 2005). This risk is only really present from the 20th week of gestation, at the time when the thyroid starts to be functional. The screening for neonatal hypothyroidism is in practice an examination that is carried out systematically by paediatric teams, but the importance of ensuring that this is indeed carried out among infants exposed *in utero* to iodine-based contrast substances should be emphasised (Chen et al., 2008).
Regarding the injection of gadolinium chelate, this is not at present authorised during pregnancy; intravenous gadolinium is teratogenic in animal studies, albeit at high and repeated doses (Chen et al., 2008). Gadolinium is classified as a category C drug by the U.S Food and Drug Administration but can be used if considered critical. In humans, knowledge on this subject relies on isolated clinical cases or small series showing no teratogenic effect (Lin et al., 2007). For instance, Marcos et al., 1997, report a series of 11 pregnant patients at terms ranging from 16 to 37 gestation weeks, who underwent MRI with gadolinium injection (gadopentatate dimeglumine: 0.1mmol/kg) for the purpose of evaluating a placental pathology, and no adverse effect was reported among the neonates. Likewise, in a prospective series of 26 pregnant patients exposed in the first trimester of pregnancy to MRI with gadolinium injection, de Santis et al., 2007, observed no abnormalities among the neonates overall. However, data is as yet insufficient in humans to justify concluding to the fact that the use of gadolinium among pregnant women is without risk for the foetus.
In practice, when there is an issue regarding whether or not investigations can be carried out for tumoral extension in pregnant women, the indications for the different examinations should be discussed one by one, taking into account the gestational stage, the anatomical area to be explored and the sensitivity of the considered radiodiagnosis tests. For instance, MRI, after injection of gadolinium chelate, is the most sensitive method for the detection of intracranial metastasis (Naggara et al., 2006)). However, as previously mentioned, the use of this contrast agent is not authorised in pregnant women. Therefore, in order to decrease the risk of false negatives, a brain scan with injection will have to be preferred to cerebral MRI without injection to look for cerebral metastases during pregnancy. Regarding the exploration of the chest, it was seen above that some authors recommend thoracic MRI. This technique is very sensitive for the exploration of the mediastinum, the heart or the rachis (Thompson et al., 2000)) but for the exploration of the pulmonary parenchyma, thoracic CT remains the first-line examination, even among pregnant women (Pentheroudakis et al.,

2006). This can be backed up if necessary, beyond the first trimester of pregnancy, by abdominal-pelvic non-injected MRI.

Therefore, although there is no general agreement regarding the initial investigations for metastatic melanoma during pregnancy, in terms of the risk / benefit balance, the association of contrast-enhanced brain and chest CT scan with abdominal ultrasonography can be proposed (Pagès et al., 2010).

5.2 Sentinel lymph node procedure and pregnancy

The sentinel node is the first lymph drainage node invaded from the primary tumour. Sentinel lymph node biopsy (SLNB) is carried out in order to determine the presence or absence of lymph-node micro-metastases in a patient without clinical adenomegalia. For melanoma, SLNB is currently considered as a staging procedure, that can be offered to the patient. In practice, the detection of sentinel node encroachment is performed by injection of a Technetium-labelled radiocolloid (isotopic method) in the area of the excision of the primary melanoma, generally the day before surgery. This injection can be coupled with a vital blue staining (colorimetric method). If the sentinel node shows micro metastasis, lymph node dissection is at present recommended.

In the literature, some publications have attempted to assess the foetal dose received during SLNB in non-pregnant women, using devices so as to mimic the different stages of pregnancy as close as possible. Thus, Gentilini et al., 2004 report a series of 26 non-pregnant patients with breast cancer and candidates for SLNB. This consisted in peri-tumoral injection of about 12 Mbq of nanocolloid ^{99m} Tc-HAS before surgery; thermoluminescent dosimeters were positioned at the injection site, between the injection site and the epigastrium, and in three other locations mimicking the position of the foetus in the different trimesters of pregnancy: epigastrium, umbilicum, and hypogastrium. The scintigraphic images showed no diffusion of the radiographic marker except at the injection point and in the sentinel node. In 23 of the 26 patients, all the measures of absorbed doses were below the dosimeter detection thresholds. For 3 patients, the doses absorbed in the epigastric, umbilical and hypogastric areas were within the following ranges: 40-320; 120-250; 30-140 µGy. The authors concluded that the foetal doses absorbed during the SLNB were negligible and that this procedure could therefore be used in pregnant women, on condition that a standardised protocol was developed. In a retrospective series of 9 patients (3 breast cancers, 6 melanomas) in whom the sentinel node procedure was performed in the course of pregnancy, Mondi et al. 2007 observed no neonatal abnormality among the newborns, while in 22% of the cases the procedure occurred in the first trimester of pregnancy. Thus the SLNB appears feasible in pregnant women, exposing the foetus to a negligible level of irradiation and hence to minimum risk. However, the concomitant use of methylene blue is still the subject of controversy in the literature, counter-indicated for some authors (Pentheroudakis et al., 2010), and envisaged for others (Pruthi et al., 2011). On the other hand, since SLNB can not currently be considered as a standard of care, except for accurate staging purpose, its realization in melanoma pregnant patient should be carefully questioned, with clear information delivered to the patient.

5.3 Treatment of melanoma during pregnancy

The optimal therapeutic strategy should be jointly discussed by the medical team, the patient and her family and will depend on gestational age, stage of cancer, treatment options and patient wishes. It ideally requires a multidisciplinary approach with an obstetrician, a neonatologist, a medical oncologist, a surgeon and a psychologist. We will expose below the feasibility of the different therapeutical approaches usually used in melanoma during pregnancy: surgery, radiotherapy, immunotherapy and chemotherapy.

5.3.1 Surgery

Surgery in the course of pregnancy is not an exceptional occurrence. It is estimated that in the USA 1 to 2% of pregnancies will entail surgical intervention for non-obstetric purposes at some time in gestation (Kuczkowski et al., 2004). Risks to the foetus during surgery are not only anaesthesis-related, they also include intraoperative complications such as hypoxia and hypotension (Moran et al., 2007). Furthermore, decreased placental perfusion secondary to long-term positioning of the mother in the supine position is a mechanical problem in late pregnancy. Some physiological changes occurring in pregnancy have a direct impact on anaesthesic procedures, for instance :

- the total body water and plasma volume increase by about 50%, resulting in an increase in the distribution volume of hydrosoluble drugs, thus modifying their pharmaco-kinetic,
- with the increase in volume of the uterus during pregnancy, there is a decrease in the return of blood via the lower vena cava, and a risk of aortic-caval syndrome, depending on the patient's position during surgery (dorsal decubitus) which can lead to severe maternal hypotension with serious consequences on the foetus,
- gastro-intestinal motility is classically reduced during gestation with a relaxing of the lower oesophagal sphincter, presenting increased risk of inhaling gastric fluid during intubation under general anaesthetic.

The surgeon and the anaesthetist should take into account all these alterations at the time of surgery in order to avoid secondary effects on mother or foetus as far as possible. Maternal and foetal monitoring should be set up as early a possible by a trained team. Mazze δ Kallen, 1989 examined adverse outcomes after non-obstetric operations during pregnancy (data from 3 Swedish health care registries from 1973 to 1981); there were 5,405 operations in the population of 720,000 pregnant women. The incidences of congenital malformations and stillbirths were not increased in the offspring of women having an operation. However, the incidences of very- low and low- birth weight were higher in the population having surgery and attributed to the underlying cause of the emergency of surgery during pregnancy. Commonly-used anaesthetics, including nitrous oxide, enflurane and narcotics, have been extensively used safely in pregnancy (Rosen, 1999). Most authors agree that anaesthesia (general, regional or local) can be administered to pregnant women without damaging effects on the development of the embryo or fœtus. (Moran et al., 2007) With modern surgical and anaesthesia techniques, the maternal death rate is negligible and surgery during the first trimester does not appear to increase the incidence of major birth defects.

For localized melanoma, as in non pregnant patient, surgery is the mainstay of treatment for pregnant patients. With local anesthesia, local resection can occur whatever the trimester without increased risk (Richards δ Statsko, 2002). Concerning teratogenicity of local anesthesia, when administered to pregnant rats, it did not result an increased incidence of congenital malformations or adverse outcomes (Fujinaga δ Mazze, 1986). In a study of 34 pregnant women having cutaneous surgery, Gormley et al., 1990 found no maternal or neonatal adverse events in 23 mothers who were available for follow up. However, in view of the absence of adequate clinical studies in humans, it is classically recommended (when possible and excluding emergencies) to avoid surgical interventions in the first trimester of pregnancy, or even to postpone it until after childbirth, in accordance with risk-benefit trade-off and precautionary principles, assessed for each individual case. In regard to melanoma during pregnancy, cautious but definitive treatment is recommended.

5.3.2 Adjuvant therapy with Interferon α

Patients who are at higher risk for recurrence after definitive surgery (those with thicker primary tumors and/or with primary tumor ulceration and those with lymph node involvement) should be considered for adjuvant therapy (Kirkwood et al., 1996). Interferon -α-2b (IFNα2b) is the only effective adjuvant therapy for these patients that has been approved by regulatory authorities worldwide. The safety of IFNα2b during pregnancy has not been studied formally, however low to moderate doses of interferon alpha have been safely administered in pregnant patients with chronic myeloid leukemia, CML (Regierer et al., 2006; Mesquita et al., 2005). In their review of literature, Azim et al., 2010, reported 26 CML patients exposed to IFN α during the course of pregnancy (one third during the first trimester). No congenital abnormalities were reported. Authors suggest that is probably due to IFNα high molecular weight, making it unlikely to cross the placenta. Egberts et al., 2006 reported no specific birth defects in children born to mothers receiving IFNα 2b for melanoma. It seems that IFN α can be safely administered throughout the course of pregnancy, however the potential for severe toxicity and the marginal improvement with this regimen for melanoma make its administration during pregnancy inadvisable.

5.3.3 Radiation therapy

Exposure to ionising radiation *in utero* entails a certain number of risks, and these latter vary according to the foetal dose received and the gestational age at the time of irradiation of the mother. The real dose received by the foetus depends on the size of the field irradiated, the anatomical irradiated site, the distance of the embryo or foetus from the irradiated site and the total dose prescribed. Regarding the gestational age, classically, three periods are distinguished:

- the so-called implantation period corresponding to the first 10 days after conception. During this phase, the "all or nothing" rule applies, terminating either in the loss of the embryo, or in the absence of any damage. Doses ranging from 0,05 to 0,15 Gy have been reported to increase the death rate *in utero* in studies on rats and mice (Roux et al., 1983).
- the embryogenesis or the organogenesis phase, from the 9th day to the 8th week, which involves risk of foetal malformation. These risks are related to a threshold dose of irradiation (Kal et al., 2005). Before the explosion of the atomic bomb, knowledge of radiation risks in humans relied on cases reported of pelvic irradiation in pregnant women. Thus Dekaban et al., 1968 conducted a review of the literature of published cases between 1921 and 1956 of pelvic irradiation among pregnant women, covering different terms in pregnancy (ranging from the 4th to the 25th week of amenorrhea (WA)). Twenty-six cases were analysed, with a wide variety of received doses, but, for the most part, above 2,5 Gy. Twenty children aged 3 months to 16 years were alive at the time of the last clinical examination. After exposure between the 4th and the 11th WA, numerous congenital abnormalities were reported: microcephaly, skeletal malformations, malformation of the genital organs, of the eyes (cataract,

microphthalmia, pigmentary degeneration of the retina) and damage to the central nervous system (severe mental retardation). The most frequent malformations observed among children exposed *in utero* in Hiroshima and Nagasaki was microcephaly (Stovall et al. 1995).

- the period of foetal maturation and growth, from the 8th week to the end of gestation. At this stage, the organogenesis process is complete, but the CNS and the gonads continue to differentiate and are therefore more vulnerable to irradiation. During this period, the main ionising radiation risks *in utero* are intrauterine growth delays and severe mental retardation (Otake et al., 1996).

It is however important to note that for foetal doses of 0,1 Gy, the spontaneous incidence of mental retardation, which is basically estimated to be 3%, is greater than the potential effect of radiation on the decrease in Intelligence Quotient (Streffer et al., 2003). In contrast, for foetal doses of 1 Gy, between the 8th and 15th WA, the probability of *radio-induced* decrease in IQ and mental retardation resulting from this, could be around 40%, thus superior to the spontaneous incidence (Kal et al., 2005).

In practice, after consideration of all the potentially deleterious effects for the foetus, it is at present agreed that the maximum dose should not exceed 0,1 Gy on a gravid uterus (Kal et al., 2005). Pregnancy termination in case of doses received below 0,1 Gy is therefore not justified on the basis of the irradiation risk (Pentheroudakis et al., 2010)

The other risk from irradiation *in utero*, independently of the term of pregnancy, is the one of development of solid cancers and leukaemia among children born to irradiated mothers. The spontaneous incidence of cancers and leukaemia in children aged 0 to 15 is estimated at 2-3/1,000 (Kal et al., 2005). The scale of the risk after low dose radiation and the variation of this risk according to pregnancy stage, have been the subject of numerous publications, but the interpretation of the data is still a subject of controversy. Most authors agree that prenatal exposure to ionising radiation at a dose of 0,01 Gy could increase the incidence by 40% (to reach 3-4 per 1,000) (Kal et al., 2005). It is however possible to envisage medical radiotherapy procedures in pregnant women, on condition that the foetal dose is kept to a minimum. The following recommendations should be applied:

- First, conduct an *in vitro* evaluation of the dose received by the foetus. This modelling process is based on the use of phantoms and, for data collection, on the use of thermoluminescence dosimeters.
- Secondly, depending on these latter results, set up the devices aiming to minimise the foetal dose. Useful techniques for the minimisation of foetal radiation exposure include the use of lead shielding and modification of radiotherapy techniques, including the use of multileaf collimators reducing the field size and modifying the beam energy.
- Thirdly, perform *in vivo* dosimetry.

Thus, numerous authors consider that radiotherapy can be envisaged in the course of pregnancy, in particular in certain situations such a breast cancer, supra-diaphragm Hodgkin's disease, some primary and secondary cerebral tumours, and some head and neck tumours. Indeed, as an example, the irradiation of the breast in the course of pregnancy exposes the fœtus to around 0,1 to 0,3% of the total dose (total dose estimated: 50 Gy) (Antypas et al., 1998). Luis et al. published in 2009 a review of the literature on radiotherapy administered during pregnancy, grouping their series of 9 patients with 100 cases described in the literature, irrespective of cancer type, since 1950 (sources Cochrane, Medline, PubMed). These cases excluded radiotherapy for tumour in the pelvic area, and cases of combined chemo-radiotherapy during pregnancy. Among these 109 cases, there were 13

adverse outcomes: 2 spontaneous abortions, 5 perinatal deaths, 1 stillbirth, 1 sensorineural hearing loss, 1 case of undescended testis and ventricular septal defect, 1 case of learning difficulties, 1 case of hypospadias and 1 case of delayed development. The estimated fœtal dose was reported for only 4 cases, and was below 0,1 Gy, the threshold dose thought to apply for the appearance of radio-induced fœtal malformation. The authors underline that at doses estimated to be under 0,1 Gy for *in utero* foetal exposure, the occurrence of fœtal malformations cannot be distinguished from the background rate of spontaneous congenital abnormalities. When possible, an extended follow-up of patients and their offspring should be undertaken ; in the same review of the literature, Luis SA et al. report a median duration of follow-up of 37 months (maximum follow-up : 372 months).
Although the important role of radiotherapy in achieving locoregional control and palliation in oncology is well recognised, this approach is not always incorporated into the management of melanoma. In general, patients with stage I-III melanoma (confined to the primary site and regional lymph nodes) are treated surgically with curative intent; in most cases, no further local treatment is needed. For stage IV melanoma, radiotherapy has an important role in the palliation of many symptoms (bleeding, pain, spinal cord compression from vertebral metastasis…) caused by recurrence or metastasis. Furthermore, for a few brain metastases, patients can be treated by neurosurgical resection or stereotactic irradiation. Whole brain radiotherapy after either stereotactic radiosurgery or surgical excision remains controversial (Patel et al., 2010). In most of cases, brain melanoma metastases are multiple and in this setting, high dose steroids and whole brain radiotherapy are frequently associated and provide temporary relief of symptoms (Cranmer et al., 2010). We reported 2 cases of radiotherapy during pregnancy for cerebral metastases of melanoma (Pagès et al., 2010). In the first case, a whole brain radiotherapy was associated with chemotherapy (fotemustin) during the second and third trimesters; in the second case, brain gamma knife stereotactic radiosurgery was performed as a single treatment at 23 WA for 3 cerebral metastases. The fetal dose was estimated for only the 2^{nth} case with thermoluminescent dosimeters put on epigastrium and in vagina and was between 0,02 and 0,04 Gy for a maximum tumour dose of 20 Gy; the fetal exposure was less than 0,1 Gy, a dose below the deterministic threshold. No morphological abnormalities were observed in the two newborns with a follow-up of respectively 23 and 2 months. Several case series (Yu et al., 2003; Magné et al., 2001) have reported the birth of healthy babies from mothers who received radiotherapy for cerebral metastases.

5.3.4 Chemotherapy

Malignancy during pregnancy poses special challenges because of the conflict between the need to optimally treat the mother, while minimising risk to both mother and fœtus. The mother should be properly counselled so that she can reach an informed decision. The risks incurred by the foetus differ according to the moment of the exposure: indeed, the instatement of chemotherapy in the first trimester of pregnancy entails the risk of foetal death *in utero*, spontaneous miscarriage and congenital malformation (teratogenicity). In the course of the second and third trimesters, the risks are different, mainly prematurity and intra-uterine growth retardation. The risk incurred also varies with the molecule used. Fotemustine and dacarbazine are two molecules belonging to the alkylating agent group, frequently used in the treatment of metastatic melanoma. Their use in pregnant women has been the subject of only a few publications in the literature. Since the 1960s, 37 cases of administration of dacarbazine to pregnant women have been reported, of which 8 concerned the first trimester (Table 3). Two neonates exposed during the first trimester presented congenital malformations: hypoplasia of the left thumb and bilateral agenesis of the metacarpals in the case reported by Dilek et al; microphthalmia and severe hypermetropia in the case reported by Li et al. (Table 3). The imputability of dacarbazine in these malformations was nevertheless hypothetical, since the drug had been administered in both cases in association with other cytotoxic agents. Among the 29 infants exposed *in utero* to dacarbazine in the second and third trimesters of pregnancy (Table 4), no congenital malformation was noted and nearly 50% were born prematurely, which is a significantly high proportion in comparison to prematurity rates in France in 2003, of the order of 7% (Bourillon, 2005). Nevertheless, we can not exclude that the alterated general health status of the mother take an important part in the high rate of prematurity observed. Likewise, in the general population, spontaneous abortion ranges from 10 to 20% while 3-4% of live birth suffers congenital anomalies (New York State Department of Health. Congenital Malformation Registry 1995 - annual Report); it is important to consider this information in the interpretation of the outcome of pregnant cancer patients treated during gestation.

Authors	**Number of cases reported**	**Type of maternal cancer**	**Chemo-therapy**	**Term at delivery (WA)**	**Existence of congenital malformation**	**Infant outcome (follow-up)**
Zemlickis et al., 1992	1	Melanoma	Dacarbazine	TA	NA	NA
Avilès et al., 1991	4	Hodgkin's disease	ABVD	37 38 40 40	No	All alive (4-14 years)
Dilek et al., 2006	2	Hodgkin's disease	ABVD	NR	Yes, 1 case hypoplasia of the left thumb and bilateral agenesis of the metacarpals	NR
Li et al., 2007	1	Melanoma	Cisplatin, carmustin, dacarbazine, tamoxifen	34	Micro-phthalmia, hypermetropia	Alive (1 year)

Abbreviations : ABVD : adriamycin, bleomycin, vinblastine, dacarbazine, WA : weeks of amenorrhea, TA: therapeutic abortion, NA: not applicable, NR: not reported

Table 3. Cases reported of administration of Dacarbazine during the first trimester of pregnancy.

The series published by Avilès et al. provides a relatively long follow-up of children exposed *in utero* to dacarbazine administered with other chemotherapy agents: the median follow-up was 9 years (range 3-16 years). The development of these 10 children, in terms of stature and weight, was considered normal in comparison with a control group of the same age and from the same socio-cultural environment. Likewise, no case of delayed psycho-motor development was observed: all the children entered normal schooling when the time came; the results of IQ tests showed no significant differences with the control group.

Authors	Number of cases reported	Type of maternal cancer	Chemotherapy received	Term at delivery (WA)	IUGR	Infant outcome (follow-up)
Avilès et al., 1991	6	Hodgkin's disease	ABVD	38 34 35 37 38 36	No	All healthy. (median follow-up: 9 y)
Cardonick et al., 2004	9	Hodgkin's disease	ABVD	NR	No	Healthy (median follow-up:5 y)
Lishner et al.1992	4	Hodgkin's disease	ABVD	NR	No	NR
Hill et al., 1974	1	Melanoma	Dacarbazine	NR	No	Healthy (3 y)
Toussi et al., 1974	1	Melanoma	Dacarbazine	32	No	Healthy (3 y)
Harkin et al.,1990	1	Melanoma	Dacarbazine	38	No	Healthy (4 y)
DiPaola et al.,1997	1	Melanoma	Cisplatin, dacarbazine, carmustin, tamoxifen	30	No	Healthy (1 y)
Dilek et al., 2006	1	Hodgkin's disease	ABVD	IUFD (36)	NR	NA
Jonsthon et al., 1998	1	Melanoma	Dacarbazine	31	No	Healthy (1 y)
Pagès et al., 2010	3	Melanoma	Dacarbazine	36 37 26	Yes (n=1)	Healthy (median follow-up: 8 m)
Gottschalk et al., 2009	1	Melanoma	Dacarbazine, cisplatin	28	Yes	NR

Abbreviations: ABVD: adriamycin, bleomycin, vinblastine, dacarbazine, IUFD : intra-uterine foetal death, IUGR : intra-uterine growth retardation, NR : not reported, NA : not applicable, Y: years, M: months

Table 4. Cases reported of administration of Dacarbazine during second and third trimesters of pregnancy.

Thus, present knowledge concerning the use of dacarbazine in pregnant women is sparse, based on isolated clinical cases or small series, and in the majority of cases dacarbazine was administered as part of poly-chemotherapy. All these elements make it difficult to determine the risk associated specifically with the use of this molecule.

Regarding fotemustin, we reported a case of administration in the second and third trimesters of pregnancy in a patient aged 28 followed for a stage IVM1C melanoma, together with whole brain radiotherapy. On account of a marked degradation in the general

condition of the mother and significant intra-uterine growth retardation, the delivery was induced at 30 WA, giving birth to a female child weighing 820 grammes, with no notable malformation or sign suggesting metastatic localisations; the placenta was free of metastases; at 23 months, the child was alive and well.
In conclusion, dacarbazine and fotemustin should not be electively started during the first trimester of pregnancy, but these drugs can be administered during the second and third trimesters with reasonable safety, although there is an increased risk of stillbirth, growth retardation and premature delivery. The follow-up of these children is an important issue. Indeed, in the literature, the follow-up of children exposed *in utero* to chemotherapy is often too short and therefore the risk of secondary malignancy is likely to be underestimated.

6. Conclusion

The diagnosis of melanoma in the course of pregnancy is not an exceptional situation, and the provision of treatment in the case of advanced melanoma in pregnant women raises certain issues that are at once medical, ethical and philosophical. While in previous decades, pregnancy in patients with cancer was discouraged, currently such pregnancies are treated with more optimism; however, a right balance has to be found between the risks for the mother and those for the foetus. This particular situation requires a multidisciplinary approach involving, among others, surgeons, oncologists, paediatricians, gynaecologists, obstetrician and radiotherapists. Despite the lack of published guidelines, most of the conventional treatment strategies appear to be feasible in the second and third trimesters of pregnancy with appropriate protection measures. International collaboration is required in order to collect data on a sufficient numbers of births among women with cancer in order to obtain more precise risk estimates for adverse infant outcomes. A long-term follow-up of these children born to women with cancer should also be established and documented.
The information given to the mother and her family should be clear and honest, and in line with present scientific knowledge, not only concerning the possible damaging effects on the fœtus of any given substance, but also on the possible transmission of cancer to the child, in particular in case of advanced maternal melanoma. The prognosis of the disease, and the possibility that the child might have to grow up without his mother, should also be brought up.
The arrival of innovatory therapies in the area of advanced melanoma, such as immunotherapy with anti-CTLA4 antibodies (ipilimumab) or targeted therapies (anti BRAF, anti MEK) constitute a revolution in the care of these patients and raise genuine hopes in terms of prognosis. If these hopes are confirmed, dealing with these drugs during pregnancy will be our tomorrow challenge.

7. References

Alexander A, Samlowski W, Grossman D, *et al*: Metastatic melanoma in pregnancy: risk of transplacental metastases in the infant. *J Clin Oncol*, 2003, vol. 21, pp. 2179-2186
Alexander A. Vulvar melanoma: diffuse melanosis and metastasis to the placenta. *J Am Acad Dermatol*, 2004, vol. 50, n° 2, pp. 293-298
Altman JF, Lowe L, Redman B, *et al.* Placental metastasis of maternal melanoma. *J Am Acad Dermatol*, 2003, vol. 49, n°6, pp. 1150-1153

Anderson JF, Kent S, Machin GA. Maternal malignant melanoma with placental metastasis: a case report with literature review. *Pediatr Pathol*, 1989, vol. 9, pp. 35-42

Antypas C, Sandilos P, Kouvaris J, *et al.* Fetal dose evaluation during breast cancer radiotherapy. *Int J Radiat Oncol Biol Phys*, 1998, vol.40, n°4, pp. 995-999

Aronsson S: A case of transplacental tumor metastasis. *Acta Pediatr Scand*, 1963, vol. 52, pp. 123-134

Arora R, Robinson WA. Breast metastases from malignant melanoma. *J Surg Oncol*, 1992, vol. 50, n°1, pp. 27-29

Avilès A, Diaz-Maqueo JC, Talavera A, *et al.* Growth and development of children of mothers treated with chemotherapy during pregnancy: current status of 43 children. *Am J Hematol*, 1991, vol. 36, pp. 243-248

Azim HA, Pavlidis N, Peccatori FA. Treatment of tye pregnant mother with cancer : a systematic review on the use of cytotixic, endocrine, targeted agents and immunotherapy during pregnancy. Part II: Hematological tumors. *Cancer Treat Rev* 2010, vol 36, pp. 110-121

Baergen R, Johnson D, Moore T, *et al:* Maternal melanoma metastatic to the placenta. *Arch Pathol Lab Med*, 1997, vol. 121, pp. 508-511

Balch CM, Buzaid AC, Soong SJ, *et al.* Final version of the American Joint Committee on Cancer staging system for cutaneous melanoma. *J Clin Oncol*, 2001, vol. 19, pp. 3635-3648

Bourrillon A. Pédiatrie. 3e éd. Paris : Masson, 2005. 880p. 978-2-294-01947-0

Brodsky I, Baren M, Kahn SB, et al: Metastatic melanoma malignant from mother to the fetus. *Cancer*, 1965, vol. 18, pp. 1048-1054

Brossard J, Abish S, Bernstein ML *et al.* Maternal malignancy involving the products of conception. *Am J Pediatr Hematol Oncol*, 1994, vol. 16, pp. 380-383

Byrd BF, McGanity WJ. The effect of pregnancy on the clinical course of malignant melanoma. *South Med J*, 1954, vol. 47, pp. 196-200

Campbell FA: Magnetic resonance imaging for stage IV melanoma during pregnancy. *Arch Dermatol*, 2006, vol. 142, pp. 393

Cardonick E, Iacobucci A. Use of chemotherapy during human pregnancy. *Lancet Oncol*, 2004, vol. 5, pp. 283-291

Cavell B: Transplacental metastasis of malignant melanoma: Report of a case. *Acta Paediatr Suppl*, 1963, vol. 146, pp. 37-40

Chen M.M, Coakley F.V, Kaimal A, Laros Jr R.K. Guidelines for Computed Tomography and Magnetic Resonance Imaging use during pregnancy and lactation. *Obstet Gynecol* 2008, vol 112, pp. 333-40

Cranmer LD, Jeter JM, Morgan SS et al. Whole brain radiotherapy in melanoma: an open question. *Lancet Oncol* 2010, vol 11, n°1, pp. 13

Dargeon HW, Eversole JW, Del Duca V: Malignant melanoma in an infant. *Cancer*, 1950, vol. 3, pp. 299-306

Daryanani D, Plukker JT, De Hullu JA, *et al.* Pregnancy and early stage melanoma. *Cancer*, 2003, vol.97, pp.2248-2253

Dekaban S. Abnormalities in children exposed to X-radiation during human various stages of gestation. I. Tentative timetable of radiation injury to the human fetus. *Int J Nucl Med*, 1968, vol. 9, pp. 471-477

De Santis M, Straface G, Cavaliere AF *et al.* Gadolinium periconceptionnal exposure: pregnancy and neonatal outcome. *Acta Obstet Gynecol Scand*, 2007, vol. 86, n°1, pp. 99-101

Dessolle L, Dalmon C, Roche B, et al: Métastases placentaires de cancers maternels: revue de la littérature. *J Gynecol Obstet Biol Reprod*, 2007, vol. 36, pp. 344-353

Dilek I, Topcu N, Demir C, *et al.* Hematological malignancy and pregnancy: a single-institution experience of 21 cases. *Clin Lab. Haem*, 2006, vol. 28, pp. 170-176

Dillman RO, Vandermolen LA, Barth NM *et al.* Malignant melanoma and pregnancy: ten questions. *West J Med*, 1996, vol. 164, pp. 156-161

Dipaola RS, Goodin S, Ratzell M *et al.* Chemotherapy for metastatic melanoma during pregnancy. *Gynecol Oncol*, 1997, vol. 66, pp. 526-530

Egberts F, Lischner S, Russo P et al. Diagnostic and management procedures for management of melanoma during pregnancy; risk for the fetus? *J Dtsch Dermatol Ges.*2006, vol 4, pp. 717-720

Ferreira CM, Maceira JM, Coelho JM: Melanoma and pregnancy with placental metastases: Report of a case. *Am J Dermatopathol*, 1998, vol. 20, pp. 403-407

Freedman WL, McMahon FJ. Placental metastasis: review of the literature and report of a case of malignant melanoma. *Obstet Gynecol*, 1960, vol. 16, pp. 550-560

Fujinaga M, Mazze RI. Reproductive and teratogenic effects of lidocaine in Sprague-Dawley rats. *Anesthesiology* 1986, vol 65, pp. 626-32

Gentilini O, Cremonesi M, Trifiro G *et al.* Safety of sentinel node biopsy in pregnant patients with breast cancer. *Ann Oncol*, 2004, vol. 15, pp. 1348-1351

Gillis H, Mortel R, McGavran MH. Maternal malignant melanoma metastatic to the product of conception. *Gynecol Oncol*, 1976, vol. 4, pp. 38-42

Gormley DE. Cutaneous surgery and the pregnant patient. *J Am Acad Dermatol* 1990, vol 23, pp. 269-79

Gottschalk N, Jacobs V.R, Hein R et al. Advanced metastatic melanoma during pregnancy: a multidisciplinary challenge. *Onkologie* 2009, vol 32, pp 748-751

Gottron H, Gertler W: Zur frage des ubertritts von melanogen der mutter au den saugling uber die muttermilch. *Arch Dermatol Syph*, 1940, vol. 181, pp. 91-98

Grange F. Epidémiologie du mélanome cutané: données descriptives en France et en Europe. *Ann Dermatol Venereol*, 2005, vol. 132, pp. 975-982

Guidelines for diagnostic imaging during pregnancy. ACOG Committee Opinion No. 299. American College of Obstetricians and Gynecologists. *Obstet Gynecol* 2004, vol 104, pp. 647-651

Gupta A, Driscoll MS. Do hormones influence melanoma? Facts and controversies. *Clin Dermatol* 2010, vol 28, pp.287-292

Harkin KP, Drumm JE, O'Brien P, *et al.* Metastatic melanoma in pregnancy. *Ir Med J*, 1990, vol. 83, n° 3, pp. 116-117

Hill GJ, Ruess R, Berris R *et al.* Chemotherapy of malignant melanoma with dimethyl triazeno imidazole carboxamide and nitrosourea derivatives. *Ann Surg*, 1974, vol. 180, n° 2, pp. 167-174

Holcomb BW, Thigpen JT, Puckett JF *et al.* Generalized melanosis complicating disseminated malignant melanoma in pregnancy: a case report. *Cancer*, 1975, vol. 35, pp. 1459-1464

Holland E: A case of transplacental metastasis of malignant melanoma from mother to foetus. *J Obstet Gynaecol Br Emp*, 1949, vol. 56, pp. 529-536

Jonsthon SR, Broadley K, Henson G *et al.* Management of metastatic melanoma during pregnancy. *Br Med J*, 1998, vol. 316, pp. 848-849

Kal HB, Struikmans H: Radiotherapy during pregnancy: fact and fiction. *Lancet Oncol*, 2005, vol. 6, pp. 328-333

Kanal E, Barkovich AJ, Bell C et al. ACR guidance document for safe MR pratices: 2007. *Am J Roentgenol* 2007, vol 188, pp. 1447-74

Kirkwood JM, Strawderman MH, Ernstoff MS et al. Interferon alfa-2b adjuvant therapy of high risk resected cutaneous melanoma: the Eastern Cooperative Oncology Group Trial EST 1684. *J Clin Oncol*.1996, vol 14, n°7, pp.17-

Koomen ER, Joosse A, Herings R.M.C, Casparie M.K, Guchelaar H.J δ Nijsten T. Estrogens, oral contraceptives and hormonal replacement therapy increase the incidence of cutaneous melanoma: a population-based case-control study. *Ann Oncol* 2009, vol 20, pp. 358-364

Kuczkowski KM. Nonobstetric surgery during pregnancy: what are the risks of anesthesia? *Obstet Gynecol Surv*, 2004, vol. 59, n° 1, pp. 52-56

Langagergaard V. Birth outcome in women with breast cancer, cutaneous malignant melanoma, or Hodgkin's disease: a review. *Clinical Epidemiology*, 2011, vol.3, pp. 7-19

Lazarus E. 2007 Use of radiological examinations in pregnant women: a ten-year review 1997-2006. Radiological Society of North America Scientific Assembly and Annual Meeting p. 436 Chicago

Lens MB, Rosdahl I, Ahlbom A, *et al.* Effect of pregnancy on survival in women with cutaneous malignant melanoma. *J Clin Oncol*, 2004, vol. 22, pp.4369-4375

Li RHW, Tam WH, Cheung PN, *et al.* Microphtalmos associated with Darmouth combination chemotherapy in pregnancy. *J Reprod Med*, 2007, vol.52, pp. 575-576

Lin SP, Brown JJ. MR Contrast Agents: physical and pharmacologic basics. *J Magn Reson Imaging*, 2007, vol. 25, pp. 884-899

Lishner M, Zemlickis P, Degendorfer T, *et al.* Maternal and foetal outcome following Hodgkin's disease in pregnancy. *Br. J Cancer*, 1992, vol. 65, pp. 114-117

Looi LM, Wang F; Malignant melanoma metastases in chorionic villi: a case report. *Malays J Pathol*, 1979, vol. 2, p. 73-75

Luis SA, Christie DRH, Kaminski A, Kenny L, Peres MH. Pregnancy and radiotherapy : management options for minimising risk, case series and comprehensive literature review. *J Med Imaging Radiat Oncol* 2009, vol 53, pp. 559-568

MacKie RM, Bufalino R, Morabito A, *et al.* Lack of effect of pregnancy on outcome of melanoma. *Lancet*, 1991, vol.337, pp.653-655

Magné M, Marcié S, Pignol JP, *et al.* Radiotherapy for a solitary brain metastasis during pregnancy: a method for reducing fetal dose. *Br J Radiol*, 2001, vol.74, n°883, pp.638-641

Marcos HB, Semelka RC *et al.* Normal placenta: gadolinium-enhanced dynamic MR imaging. *Radiology*, 1997, vol. 205, pp. 493-496

Markus N. Gleichzeitige entwicklung melanosarcoma ovarii und carcinoma hep der schwangerschaft, eklampsie, placentarmetastazen. *Arch F Gynakol*, 1918, vol.92, pp.659-678

Marsh RD, Chu NM. Placental metastasis from primary ocular melanoma: a case report. *Am J Obstet Gynecol*, 1996, vol. 174, pp. 1654-1655

Mazze RI, Kallen B. Reproductive outcome after anesthesia and operation during pregnancy: a registry study of 5405 cases. *Am J Obstet Gynecol*, 1989, vol. 161, n° 5, pp. 1178-85

McManammy DS, Moss ALH, Pocock PV, *et al.* Melanoma and pregnancy: a long- term follow-up. *Br J Obstet Gynecol*, 1989, vol.96, pp.1419-1423

Merkus JM, Teepen JL. The indispensable anamnesis: in-vitro fertilization in a woman under treatment for melanoma. *Ned Tijdschr Geneeskd*, 1998, vol. 142, pp. 2073-2075

Mesquita MM, Pestana A, Mota A. Successful pregnany occurring with interferon alpha therapy in chronic myleoid leukemia; *Acta Obstet Gynecol Scand* 2005, vol 84, pp. 300-1

Moller D, Ipsen L, Asschendeldt P. Fatal course of malignant melanoma during pregnancy with dissemination to the product of conception. *Acta Obstet Gynecol Scand,* 1986, vol. 65, pp. 501-502

Mondi MM, Cuenca RE, Ollila DW, *et al.* Sentinel lymph node biopsy during pregnancy: initial clinical experience. *Ann Surg Oncol*, 2007, vol. 14, n°1, pp. 218-221

Moran B.J, Yano H, Zahir N, Farquaharson M. Conflicting priorities in surgical intervention for cancer in pregnancy. *Lancet Oncol* 2007, vol 8, pp. 536-44

Naggara O, Brami-Zylberberg F, Rodrigo S, *et al.* Imaging of intracranial metastases in adults. *J Radiol*, 2006, vol. 87, pp. 792-806

New York State Department of Health. Congenital Malformation Registry 1995- annual report.

Nicklas AH, Baker ME: Imaging strategies in the pregnant cancer patient. *Semin Oncol*, 2000, vol. 27, n°6, pp. 623-32

Oduncu F.S, Phil M.A, Kimmig R, *et al:* Cancer in pregnancy: maternal-fetal conflict. *J Cancer Res Clin Oncol*, 2003, vol. 129, pp.133-146

O'Meara AT, Cress R, Xing G, *et al.* Malignant melanoma in pregnancy: a population- based evaluation. *Cancer, 2005,* vol.103, pp.1217-1226

Otake M, Schull WJ, Lee S. Treshold for radiation related severe mental retardation in prenatally exposed A bomb survivors: a re-analysis. *Int J Radiat Biol,* 1996, vol. 70, n° 6, pp. 755-763

Otake M, Schull W. Radiation-related small head sizes among prenatally exposed A-bomb survivors. *Int J Radiat Oncol Biol Phys*, 1992, vol. 63, pp. 255-270

Pagès C, Robert C, Thomas L, et al.. Management and outcome of metastatic melanoma during pregnancy.*Br J Dermatol;* 2010, vol 162, pp.274-281

Patel AJ, Suki D, Hatoboqu MA et al. Factors influencing the risk of local recurrence after resection of a single brain metastasis. *J Neurosurg* 2010, vol 113, n°2, pp. 181-9

Pavlidis NA. Coexistence of pregnancy and malignancy. *Oncologist* 2002, vol 7, pp. 279-87

Pennoyer JW, Grin CM, Driscoll *et al.* Changes in size of melanocytic nevi during pregnancy. *J Am Acad Dermatol*, 1997, vol. 36, pp.378-82

Pentheroudakis G, Pavlidis N. Cancer and pregnancy: poena magna, not anymore. *Eur J Cancer,* 2006, vol.42, pp. 126-140

Pentheroudakis et al. Cancer, fertility and pregnancy : ESMO clinical practice guidelines fir diagnosis, treatment and follow-up. *Ann Oncol* 2010, vol 21, n°5, pp. 266-273

Pruthi S, Haakenson C, Brost B;C et al. Pharmacokinetics of methylene blue dye for lymphatic mapping in breast cancer - implications for use in pregnancy. *Am J Surg* 2011, vol 201, n°1, pp.70-5

Regierer AC, Schulz CO, Kuehnhardt D et al. Interferon alpha therapy for chronic myeloid leukemia during pregnancy. *Am J Hematol* 2006, vol 81, pp. 149-150

Reintgen DS, McCarty KS, Vollmer R, *et al.* Malignant melanoma and pregnancy. *Cancer,* 1985, vol.55, pp.1340-1344

Reynolds AG. Placental metastasis from malignant melanoma: report of a case. *Obstet gynecol,* 1955, vol. 6, pp. 205-209

Richards K.A, Stastko T. Dermatologic surgery and the pregnant patient. *Dermatol Surg* 2002, vol 28, n°3, pp. 248-56

Rosen MA. Management of anesthesia for the pregnant surgical patient. *Anesthesiology,* 1999, vol. 91, n° 4, pp. 1159-63

Roux C, Horvath C, Dupuis R. Effects of pre-implantation lowdose radiation on rat embryos. *Health Phys,* 1983, vol. 45, n°5, pp.993-999

Russell P, Laverty CR. Malignant melanoma metastases in the placenta: a case report. *Pathology,* 1977, vol. 9, pp. 251-255

Shiu MH, Schottenfeld D, Maclean B, Fortner JG. Adverse effect of pregnancy on melanoma: a reappraisal. *Cancer,* 1976, vol 37, n°1, pp. 181-187

Slingluff CL, Reintgen DS, Vollmer RT, *et al.* Malignant melanoma arising during pregnancy: a study of 100 patients. *Ann Surg,* 1990, vol.211, pp.552-559

Smythe AR, Underwood PB, Kreutner A. Metastatic placental tumors. *Am J Obstet Gynecol,* 1976, vol. 125, pp. 1149-1151

Sokol RJ, Hutchinson P, Cowan D *et al.* Amelanotic melanoma metastatic to the placenta. *Am J Obstet Gynecol,* 1976, vol. 124, pp. 431-432

Stensheim H, Moller B, Van Dijk T, Fossa SD. Cause-specific survival for women diagnosed with cancer during pregnancy or lactation: a registry-based cohort study, *J Clin Oncol,* 2009, vol 27, n°1, pp. 45-51

Stephenson HE Jr, Terry CW, Lukens JN *et al.* Immunologic factors in human melanoma "metastatic" to the products of gestation. *Surgery,* 1971, vol. 69, pp. 515-522

Stovall M, Blackwell R.C, Cundiff J et al. Fetal dose from radiotherapy with photon beams: report of AAPM Radiation Therapy Committee Task Group. *Med Phys,* 1995, vol. 22, n° 1, pp. 63-82

Streffer C, Shore R, Konermann G, *et al.* Biological effects after prenatal irradiation (embryo and fetus). A report of the International Commission on Radiological Protection. *Ann ICRP,* 2003, vol. 33, n°1-2, pp. 5-206

Thompson BH, Stanford W. MR imaging of pulmonary and mediastinal malignancies. *Magn Reson Imaging Clin N Am,* 2000, vol. 8, pp. 729-739

Toussi T, Blais M, Langevin P, et al. Mélanome métastatique traité chez une femme enceinte : implications pré et postnatales. *Union Med Can,* 1974, vol. 103, pp. 1968-1973

Trumble ER, Smith RM, Pearl G, et al: Transplacental transmission of metastatic melanoma to the posterior fossa. *J Neurosurg (Pediatrics 2),* 2005, vol. 103, pp.191-193

Valenzano Menada M, Moioli M, Garaventa A, Nozza P, Foppiano M, Trimarchi N, Fulcheri E. Spontaneous regression of transplacental metastases from maternal melanoma in a newborn: case report and review of the literature. *Melanoma Research* 2010, vol 20, pp. 443-449

Van der Horst M, Winther JF, Olsen JH. Cancer incidence in the age range 0-34 years: historical and natural status in Denmark. *International Journal of Cancer*, 2006, vol 118, n°11, pp. 2816-2826

Webb JA, Thomsen H, Morcos SK *et al.* The use of iodinated and gadolinium contrast media during pregnancy and lactation. *Eur Radiol*, 2005, vol. 15, pp. 1234-1240

Weber FP, Schwarz E, Hellenschmied R: Spontaneous inoculation of melanotic sarcoma from mother to foetus. *Br Med J*, 1930, vol. 1, pp.537-539

Wong JH, Styerns EE, Kopald KH, *et al.* Prognostic significance of pregnancy in stage I melanoma. *Arch Surg*, 1989, vol.124, pp.1227-1231

Yu C, Jozsef G, Apuzzo ML, *et al.* Fetal radiation doses for model C gamma knife radiosurgery. *Neurosurgery*, 2003, vol. 52, n°3, pp. 687-693

Zemlickis D, Lishner M, Degendorfer P, *et al.* Fetal outcome after in utero exposure to cancer chemotherapy. *Arch Intern Med*, 1992, vol. 152, pp. 573-576

16

Malignant Melanoma in Genito-Urinary Tract

Abdulkadir Tepeler, Mehmet Remzi Erdem, Sinasi Yavuz Onol,
Abdullah Armagan and Alpaslan Akbas
Bezmialem Vakif University
Istanbul
Turkey

1. Introduction

1.1 Adrenal melanoma

Adrenal melanoma- first reported by Kniseley et al in 1946 is a relatively aggressive tumor affecting the middle-aged adults.[1] The longest postoperative survival reported is 46 months.[2] In cases with adrenal metastases originating from a primary melanoma source, prognosis is worse with a median overall survival of 6 months.[3] Adrenal glands are the sixth most common site of distant metastases from melanoma (after lymph nodes (73.6%), lungs (71.3%), liver (58.3%), brain (54.6%) and bone (48.6%)).[4]

It manifests itself with flank pain and usually renal involvement is detected at the time of diagnosis. Additionally, distant lymph node metastasis could also be detected. Absence of previous unilateral adrenal gland involvement, presence of pigmented lesions without any signs of endocrine disorder, and negative immunohistochemical endocrine markers are typical characteristics of primary malignant melanoma of the adrenal gland. Presence of an occult primary lesion should also be excluded by autopsy.

Pluripotent neural crest cells are localized within adrenal gland medulla. They are precursors of melanocytes, neurons, glial cells of the peripheral nervous system, and adrenal chromaffin cells. Under the influence of microenvironment, and various growth factors, these multipotent cells might transform into different cell types.[5]

Differential diagnosis is difficult to establish based on the radiological criteria. Melanomas do not usually display disease- specific signs. Computerized tomography has been the preferred diagnostic tool for the evaluation of adrenal glands. Rajaratnam et al concluded that an adrenal mass greater than 5 cm in diameter, with central or irregular areas of necrosis/hemorrhage (and no lipomatous component) is a characteristic metastasic focus from malignant melanoma.[4] ^{18}F-FDG PET is a well-established diagnostic tool for restaging.[6]

Histopathologically, it is very hard to discriminate adrenal melanoma and pheochromocytoma. Melanin and melanin-like pigment can be detected in pheochromocytomas.[7] Some authors suggest that adrenal melanoma takes origin from pheochromocytoma, and thus it should be termed as melanotic malignant pheochromocytoma.[8] However, some others do not agree this opinion, and suggest that these tumors should have diverse origins.[9] Differential diagnosis between adrenal melanoma and pheochromocytoma could be established using immunohistochemical staining. Neuroendocrine markers including synaptophysin, chromographin and neuron-specific enolase and neurosecretory granules (under electron microscopy) are detected only in pheochromocytomas.[2,9,10]

Since these tumors adhere to the adjacent kidney, nephroadrenelectomy is the preferred surgical treatment modality. Liatsikos et al performed the first laparoscopic adrenalectomy in a patient with primary adrenal malignant melanoma.[10] Because of its rare occurrence, a consensus has not yet been established with respect to adjuvant therapies such as radiotherapy[1] or chemotherapy with dacarbazine.[11] Adrenal metastases of melanoma provide additional evidence of systemic disease with an overall poor prognosis. For these patients, systemic therapy is usually preferred. Mittendorf et al suggested the option of adrenalectomy for those patients with no or limited extra-adrenal disease.[12]

1.2 Renal melanoma

Melanoma formed by melanin producing cells accounts for 68,000 newly reported cases, and is responsible for 8600 deaths annually in the United States.[13] It ranks sixth among the most frequently encountered malignancies in the UK, and malignant melanoma is most often encountered between the ages of 15 and 34 years.[14] Its incidence over the last decade has increased faster than the other types of malignancies.[15]

Renal metastasis of melanoma is rarely seen entity among the renal metastatic tumors. Accordingly, it is reported that kidney involvement in patients with malignant melanoma was around 24% to 50% of the cases.[16] In a series-consisting of 142 cases of metastatic genitourinary tract melanomas reported by Abeshouse, the primary cancer source was skin in 80 % of the cases.[17] However, renal involvement unrelated to any primary pigmented skin lesion was also reported.[18] Levin et al. reported a case of an isolated renal metastasis- 20 years after initial diagnosis and treatment secondary to an ocular melanoma occurring.[19]

Renal metastases secondary to cutaneous melanomas have been detected as multiple microscopic or millimetric foci. They usually progress insidiously and tend to invade adjacent perirenal space. They are highly vascularized. Boughan reported a metastatic case of melanoma localized in the upper renal pole and infiltrated the inferior vena cava (IVC).[18] Anecdotal reports of renal vein invasion by the tumor thrombi arising from secondary metastatic renal tumors have been encountered in the literature. Indeed, Klatte presented a case of renal metastasis of a malignant melanoma in which renal vein had been occluded by a tumor thrombus.[20] It was also underlined that renal metastases of malignant melanoma usually reflect end-stage renal disease.[20]

Transmission of donor malignancies to organ transplant recipients is a rare complication of transplantation. Malignant melanoma is one of the most commonly reported donor-derived malignancies. The mechanism of transmission of melanoma from the donor to recipient is unknown. Circulating tumor cells or dormant micro metastases residing in the organ parenchyma has been blamed for this transmisssion.[14] In the literature, there are 15 case-reports of melanoma transferred from donor organs to 28 recipients. The organs were transplanted in the range of six months to 16 years after the donors had undergone melanoma surgery.[21-24] MacKie et al had underlined that none of the patients with invasive melanoma should ever be an organ donor because of the possibility of the late and ultra-late recurrences in melanoma.[21] It has been estimated that between 0.98% to 6.7% of melanomas recur 10 years after the initial treatment.[25] Its ulcerated nature and depth of cutaneous infiltration are risk factors in favor of recurrences and also the distant recurrences were mostly encountered type of recurrence pattern (60%).[26]

Biological behavior of malignant melanoma is quite complex. Recurrences might be seen years after remission and it is believed that recurrences have been associated with re-activation of dormant cells. The maintenance of dormancy is hypothesized to be the result of a proficient immune system. Therefore, tumor cells remain dormant in an immunocompetent host. However immunosuppressed status of the patient as seen after transplantation serves as an ideal environment for the re-activation of the dormant cells.[27]

Radiological differentiation of renal metastases from renal cell carcinoma (RCC) is quite a complicated issue. The sensitivity of ^{18}F-FDG PET that is routinely used for the diagnosis of advanced disease, visceral, deep soft-tissue and lymph node involvement is quite low for the detection of early-stage malignant melanoma.[28] PET which uses a new analogue of fluoronicotinamide i.e. ^{18}F-MEL050 has a higher specificity, and sensitivity.[29] Definitive diagnosis of melanoma is established through cytological examination of the renal biopsy specimen. In malignant melanoma, cellular shapes and patterns might show variations depending of the originator tissue. Cytological features of a melanoma resemble those of the other poorly differentiated neoplasms like carcinomas, lymphomas, and sarcomas.[30] For diagnostic purposes immunocytochemical staining is used. In clinical practice, mostly S100 protein, and HMB-45 antibodies, and recently found MART-1 melanocyte antigens have been used.[30,31]

S100 protein is a calcium binding protein which had been isolated from brain tissue, and it is 90% sensitive for melanoma. However its sensitivity might drop to 70 % with respect to its discriminative potential between malignant melanomas, and spindle cell lesions with similar cytomorphologic features. In addition, primary renal tumors also stain with melanocytic markers. As previously demonstrated by Lin et al, 14.8 % of primary RCC's were stained positively with S100 protein.[32]

HMB-45 staining is relatively more specific for melanoma, and it is positive in 96.8 % of the cases. However its sensitivity decreases in spindle-cell and desmoplastic variants of melanomas, because of their lack of reactivity to HMB-45 staining. This phenomenon has led to the development of a more sensitive, and specific novel monoclonal antibody. MART-1 is a melanocytic antigen encoding gene which is only expressed in skin, retina, and melanocytic cells. MART-1 possesses 95 % sensitivity, and 97 % specificity for the detection of melanomas. However sensitivity of MART-1 reportedly decreases in the detection of spindle-cell, and desmoplastic variants of melanoma.

Angiomyolipomas originating from blood vessels, smooth muscle, and adipose tissue, and primary renal tumors carrying a translocation domain on t(6;11)(p21.1;q12) chromosome of TFEB ALPHA gene may also stain positively for melanin proteins. Epithelioid and spindle cell angiomyolipomas have a staining pattern for melanoma-specific, HMB-45 marker.[33] Translocation of ALPHA gene on chromosome on to intron 1 on TEFB located chromosome 6 is related to a RCC subgroup with pleomorphic histological characteristics, and they stain positively for melanocytic markers such as HMB-45, and Melan-A.[34]

Malignant melanoma is an immunologically active disease. Various forms of systemic immunotherapy such as Bacille Calmette Guerin (BCG), interferon-alpha and allogenic tumor vaccines have demonstrated significant improvements in overall and disease-free survival rates.[35-38] Currently, recommended treatment modalities for donor-related melanoma transmission consist of cessation of immunosuppressive therapy, achievement of rejection, and removal of the donor organ. In addition adjuvant chemotherapy or interferon-alpha therapy are also recommended to achieve complete resection of the tumoral mass.[21,39]

1.3 Malignant melanoma of the ureter

Ureteral malignant melanoma is a rarely seen entity. Generally it emerges as a metastatic focus. In the English medical literature limited numbers of ureteral malignant melanomas have been reported. Clinically, it manifests itself with symptoms of colicky pain. Radiologically, hydronephrosis, hydroureteonephrosis, and filling defects are seen in the upper urinary tract depending on the level of ureteral involvement. Ureteral mass lesion is verified by ureteroscopic examination.

Definitive diagnosis is established after immunohistochemical examination of the biopsy material. A clear-cut consensus on its management is lacking due to its rarity. Tumor can spread to all parts of the urinary tract after URS or DJ stenting. In their case-presentation, Gakis et al. proposed a management protocol for ureteral malignant melanoma in consideration of literature findings.[40-43] Accordingly, they recommended nephroureterectomy and regional lymphadenectomy for unilateral upper urinary tract involvement. Positive surgical margins, positive lymph nodes or depth of primary cutaneous tumor exceeding 1.5mm necessitate administration of adjuvant chemotherapy (dacarbazine). Local recurrences could be managed with resection and chemotherapy. In the presence of bilateral resectable lymphometastatic lesions, partial ureterectomy, and bilateral regional lymphadenectomy should be employed. Besides, adjuvant chemotherapy is recommended. For non-resectable lesions, radiation therapy and chemotherapy are among the treatment alternatives.

2. Malignant melanoma of the lower urinary tract

Lower urinary system contains bladder, urethra, and prostate gland in men. Symptoms of lower urinary tract diseases generally mimic each other. In older men, benign prostatic hyperplasia triggers symptoms such as dysuria, urgency, frequency, nocturia. On the other hand, over-active bladder is another frequently seen entity in women. Melanoma also mimics lower urinary tract symptoms during involvement of these areas.

2.1 Malignant melanoma of the bladder

Despite rarity of primary malignant melanoma of the bladder, genitourinary system metastases of the bladder melanoma have a relatively higher incidence. Renal (45 %), and vesical (18 %) metastases had been found in patients deceased because of melanoma.[44] Therefore, discrimination between primary and metastatic melanomas of the bladder is crucial. Stein[45] and Ainsworth[46] established some diagnostic criteria for primary bladder tumors: (1) absence of any previous skin lesion (2) or cutaneous malignant melanoma (3) or primary visceral malignant melanoma (4) recurrence pattern showing consistency with the primary tumor diagnosis (5) atypical melanocytes at the tumor margin on microscopic examination. In the literature including the most recent case- reported by Siroy AE et al. the number of cases with primary melanoma of the bladder amounts to 20.[44,47] However all the cases reported in the literature as primary melanoma of the bladder do not fit in these criteria of primary vesical melanoma.

Its initial clinical presentation is hematuria, as seen in other types of bladder carcinomas. However hematuria is a clinical sign of locally advanced disease.[1]Some patients present with lower urinary tract symptoms. During advanced stages of the disease, clinical symptoms peculiar to metastatic disease can be observed.

Cystoscopy is the primary diagnostic modality. Cystoscopy usually reveals a dark pigmented mass with varying dimensions. Mucosal layer surrounding the tumoral mass has a dark brown appearance, while the mucosa distant from the lesion has a pinkish white color.[46] Diagnosis is made with histopathological examination of the biopsy material. Immunohistochemical studies shorten and facilitate diagnostic work-up.

Despite treatment alternatives including transurethral resection, partial and radical cystectomy, radiotherapy, immunotherapy, and chemotherapy, overall it has a poor prognosis. Transurethral resection is curative for lesions restricted to epithelium, and actually the definitive cure could be achieved by radical cystectomy.[44,47] In cases where surgery is contraindicated or chemotherapy is not tolerated because of its side effects, radiation therapy and immunotherapy with interferon-alpha can be applied.[47] Despite all these treatment alternatives, the prognosis is poor and the patients are generally lost within 3 years because of metastatic complications.

2.2 Prostatic malignant melanoma

In general, prostatic melanoma symptomatically resembles benign prostatic hyperplasia. First, obstructive signs and symptoms are detected in these patients. Sometimes irritating symptoms might be more prominent and they may mimic urinary tract infections or overactive bladder. This symptomatic ambiguity may lead to misdiagnosis and delay correct therapy. Therefore, patients with refractory symptoms to treatments or improper features of patients for suspected diseases such as young patient with BPH symptoms must warn us to overlook another extraordinary disease.[48] Prostatic melanoma is a rare neoplasm of prostate and must be kept in mind in the differential diagnosis after a thorough evaluation. Rare incidence of primary prostatic malignant melanoma in clinical practice, early diagnosis and differentiation of primary malignant melanoma from epithelial cancer are extremely important considerations, because while prostate cancer can be treated as a chronic disease for years, malignant melanoma of the prostate can rapidly progress to terminal stage with a high mortality.[49-51]

If one suspects malignancy after digital rectal examination, computerized tomography and/or transrectal ultrasound as well as radical prostatectomy and if needed lymph node dissection should be added to the diagnostic work-up. Alternatively, transurethral resection or transrectal ultrasound guided prostate biopsy could be performed to establish a diagnosis. Notably, not only surgical approach but also chemotherapeutic treatment plays a major role in the management of prostatic melanoma.[48]

2.3 Urethral malignant melanoma

Primary malignant melanoma of urethra is a rare entity, representing less than 1% of all melanoma and 4% of urethral cancers.[52] Rarity and difficulty in diagnosis results in a fairly late detection and poor prognosis. Noteworthy, urethral malignant melanomas are generally associated with immuno-compromised conditions including alcoholism, dialysis, and poor self-care.

Patients with urethral malignant melanoma admit to the clinics with various complaints. Protruding mass is s one of the most common clinically observed because distal urethra is involved more frequently than the other parts.[53,54] Lower urinary system complaints sometimes mask melanoma mass-related symptoms particularly in males. Symptoms may sometimes mimic benign prostatic hyperplasia or chronic prostatitis. Unfortunately, only after medical treatment fails in these patients, cancer diagnosis could be established with a significant delay.[55] Additionally, hematuria and urethral discharge are other complaints in patients with urethral melanoma.

Routine physical examination of urogenital system and inguinal region must be performed meticulously as well since a complete examination may sometimes provide crucial clues to reach final diagnosis. Direct visual detection of tumor mass in females is frequently easy and straightforward because of shorter length of female urethra. Likewise, most of the urethral tumor mass located in the distal part with protrusion could easily be detected.

Unfortunately, at the time of admission of the patients, there is no available specific serum tumor markers like- 5-S-cysteinyl-dopa, an intermediate metabolite of melanin biosynthesis which is used in postoperative melanoma follow-up, high in chronic renal failure- no urine tests or imaging methods to detect the exact nature of the lesion and neoplastic features in early period. After the diagnosis is verified, evaluation of recurrence, lymph node and other organ involvement must be investigated using ultrasound, computerized tomography, magnetic resonance imaging or PET scan.

Although atypical pigmented melanocytic cells might be seen in cytological examination, this clue should increase the suspicion of melanoma and lead to a more meticulous cancer work-up at this point. Unfortunately, cytology sometimes could not provide any evidence of cancer. However, even in cases of inconclusive cytology, false negativity must always be kept in mind. Histopathological examination of specimens is performed based on the cellular differentiation, pleomorphism, solidity and grade of tumor according to WHO's schema. Additionally, diagnosis is supported by immunostainings with a specific marker for melanoma (anti-Vimentin +, Protein S-100 +, HMB - 45 +, Melan A +; AE1/AE3 +, CD 20 +).

Although the optimum therapy has not yet been established, considering the rarity of the urethral melanoma, surgical intervention plays the major role in first line therapy. Melanoma spreads to the other organs via the lymphatic drainage. The urethra, particularly the distal urethra including fossa navicularis and urethral meatus are the most common locations and about 30% of patients already harbor metastasis at the time of diagnosis with dangerous boundaries with regards to the depth of invasion and size of the tumor mass.[57,58] While cancers of the anterior urethra preferentially infiltrate into superficial inguinal lymph nodes, those involving the posterior urethra generally infiltrate into pelvic lymphatic channels.[57] However, the presence or absence of lymph node metastasis is the most significant prognostic factor for survival, as survival rates are approximately halved by the presence of nodal metastasis. Consequently, melanoma's aggressiveness, higher stage, and palpable lymphadenopathy require lymphadenectomy. However, unnecessary lymphadenectomy may result in lymphedema, pain, infections and other complication. For this reason, lymphadenectomy must be standardized especially for those patients with:

1. Palpable adenopathy (extended lymphadenectomy superficial and deep inguinal LND)
2. Lesions more than 1 cm in size
3. Presence of ulceration
4. Clark's level IV-V

Modified lymphadenectomy must be performed for all anterior urethral lesions other than Tis.[59] Local relapses and systemic metastases frequently develop in the early postoperative period following the removal of primary urethral malignant melanoma. Therefore, surgery alone is not adequate to control local relapses and systemic metastases, thus adequate postoperative adjuvant therapy is required to prevent the relapse and progression of the disease. Combined use of multiple chemotherapeutic agents such as cisplatin, dacarbazine, carmustine and tamoxifen has been recommended in lieu of monotherapy.[60] However; even combination regimens do not satisfactorily increase the survival rates of patients with metastatic melanoma. Immunotherapy based on α-interferon and tumor vaccines has also been suggested in recent studies.[61]

2.4 Penile, scrotal and testicular malignant melanoma

These organs are external organs of male genital system. Primary malignant melanoma of these organs will be presented together with the metastatic ones under the same title because of their close relation.

Penile melanomas usually present as pigmented macule, papule, or ulcerations with an irregular border; however, it might be unpigmented as well. It is typically found on the glans penis and less often on the prepuce. The American Joint Committee on Cancer system classifies cutaneous melanomas based on the depth of invasion (Clark staging) and tumor thickness (Breslow level, direct measurement). Hematogenous metastases occur through the vascular structures of the corporal bodies; and lymphatic spread to the regional lymphatic ilioinguinal nodes occurs by lymphatic flow.[62] Scrotal melanoma has also been detected with similar appearance of penile melanoma. Testicular, epididymis and seminal vesicle malignant melanomas are metastatic and display no symptoms until before reaching sizeable masses so as to be detected during physical examination, and are mostly detected at autopsies.[63]

Definitive diagnosis of penile, scrotal and testicular melanoma could only be established histopathologically. However, imaging methods such as CT or MRI may help to delineate the boundaries of the lesion and macroscopical invasion to neighboring structures. After treatment, nuclear scintigraphy is useful for whole body scanning. Starting from early 1990s- as an adjunct to follow-up scanning protocol, sentinel lymphadenectomy using radio colloid mapping and dye localization for melanoma has been described. This technique is minimally invasive and sensitive enough to detect the relevant nodes in the correct nodal location without complete dissection. When the sentinel node is negative for metastatic disease the incidence of micro metastases in the remaining structure is less than 1% to 2%.[64]

In patients with penile lesions less than 1.5 mm deep, less aggressive treatment with local excision has been effective.[65-67] However, the risk of metastasis to regional lymph nodes with a resultant poor outcome is high. Considering the rarity of the disease, aggressive treatment in selected patients with penectomy or partial penectomy of the primary tumor with bilateral lymph node dissection has been recommended.[65] Despite aggressive surgical treatment and chemotherapy, patients with metastatic disease have a poor prognosis.

Patients with penile melanoma of stage III or more have an extremely poor prognosis; the 5-year and 10-year survival rates of Japanese patients with stage IIIB melanoma are 40% and 38%, respectively.[68] Penile malignant melanoma patients with positive lymph nodes carry a poor prognosis of less than 2 years of mean survival.[65] According to the guidelines for treatment of patients in each stage, in addition to radical dissection of regional lymph nodes, DAV-Feron therapy is recommended as a postoperative adjuvant chemotherapy for patients with stage III melanoma. 5DAV-Feron therapy dacarbazine, ACNU (nimustine hydrochloride), VCR (vincristine sulfate), plus interferon-b is recommended as a postoperative adjuvant therapy for patients with stage IIIB melanoma. Therapy can significantly improve the 5-year survival rate of patients with malignant melanoma compared to the DAV therapy alone.[69] The Feron therapy, in which interferon-b (300 ¥ 104 IU) is locally injected into the wound area for 10 days, is recommended as an adjuvant therapy for patients with stage I–II melanoma. Scrotal melanoma is treated with orchiectomy and lymphadenectomy; and additional chemotherapy must also be planned.[70]

3. References

[1] Kniseley RM, Baggenstoss AH. Primary melanoma of the adrenal gland. Arch Pathol (Chic). 1946; 42: 345-9.
[2] Amérigo J, Roig J, Pulido F, Belda R, Vázquez-Ramírez FJ, González-Cámpora R. Primary malignant melanoma of the adrenal gland. Surgery. 2000; 127(1): 107-11.
[3] Mittendorf EA, Lim SJ, Schacherer CW, Lucci A, Cormier JN, Mansfield PF, et al. Melanoma adrenal metastasis: natural history and surgical management. Am J Surg. 2008; 195(3): 363-8; discussion 368-9
[4] Rajaratnam A, Waugh J. Adrenal metastases of malignant melanoma: characteristic computed tomography appearances. Australas Radiol. 200; 49(4): 325-9.
[5] Lallier TE. Cell lineage and cell migration in the neural crest. Ann N Y Acad Sci. 1991; 615: 158-71.
[6] Kumar R, Mavi A, Bural G, Alavi A. Fluorodeoxyglucose-PET in the management of malignant melanoma. Radiol Clin North Am. 2005; 43(1):23-33.
[7] Landas SK, Leigh C, Bonsib SM, Layne K. Occurrence of melanin in pheochromocytoma. Mod Pathol. 1993; 6(2): 175-8.
[8] Dao AH, Page DL, Reynolds VH, Adkins RB Jr. Primary malignant melanoma of the adrenal gland. A report of two cases and review of the literature. Am Surg. 1990; 56(4): 199-203.
[9] Zalatnai A, Szende B, Tóth M, Rácz K. Primary malignant melanoma of adrenal gland in a 41-yr-old woman. Endocr Pathol. 2003; 14(1): 101-5.
[10] Granero LE, Al-Lawati T, Bobin JY. Primary melanoma of the adrenal gland, a continuous dilemma: report of a case. Surg Today. 2004; 34(6): 554-6.
[11] Liatsikos EN, Papathanassiou Z, Voudoukis T, Repanti M, Sklavou C, Filos KS, et al. Case report: laparoscopic adrenalectomy in a patient with primary adrenal malignant melanoma. J Endourol. 2006; 20(2): 123-6.
[12] Bastide C, Arroua F, Carcenac A, Anfossi E, Ragni E, Rossi D. Primary malignant melanoma of the adrenal gland. Int J Urol. 2006; 13(5): 608-10.
[13] Jemal A, Siegel R, Ward E, Hao Y, Xu J, Thun MJ. Cancer statistics, 2009. CA Cancer J Clin. 2009; 59(4): 225-49.
[14] Strauss DC, Thomas JM. Transmission of donor melanoma by organ transplantation. Lancet Oncol. 2010; 11(8):790-6.

[15] Cancer Research UK. Skin cancer-UK incidence statistics (June 2, 2009) http://info.cancerresearchuk.org/cancerstats/types/skin/incidence/#source11 (accessed Sept 3, 2009)

[16] Stein BS, Kendall AR. Malignant melanoma of the genitourinary tract. J Urol. 1984; 132(5): 859-68.

[17] Abeshouse BS. Primary and secondary melanoma of the genitourinary tract. South Med J. 1958; 51(8): 994-1005; discussion 1005-6.

[18] Boughan KM, Setrakian S, Lee CH, Spiro TP, Daw HA. A renal mass in a patient with melanoma. Clin Genitourin Cancer. 2009; 7(3): E98-E100.

[19] Levin BM, Boulos FI, Herrell SD. Metastatic ocular melanoma to the kidney 20 years after initial diagnosis. Urology. 2005; 66(3): 658.

[20] Klatte T, Rao JY, Ribas A, Pantuck AJ. Metastatic melanoma to the kidney presenting with renal vein tumor thrombus. Urology. 2007; 69(5): 982.e7-9

[21] MacKie RM, Reid R, Junor B. Fatal melanoma transferred in a donated kidney 16 years after melanoma surgery. N Engl J Med. 2003; 6; 348(6): 567-8.

[22] Penn I. Malignant melanoma in organ allograft recipients. Transplantation. 1996; 27; 61(2): 274-8

[23] Elder GJ, Hersey P, Branley P. Remission of transplanted melanoma--clinical course and tumour cell characterisation. Clin Transplant. 1997; 11(6): 565-8.

[24] Suranyi MG, Hogan PG, Falk MC, Axelsen RA, Rigby R, Hawley C, at al. Advanced donor-origin melanoma in a renal transplant recipient: immunotherapy, cure, and retransplantation. Transplantation. 1998; 15; 66(5): 655-61.

[25] Crowley NJ, Seigler HF. Late recurrence of malignant melanoma. Analysis of 168 patients. Ann Surg. 1990; 212(2): 173-7.

[26] Brauer JA, Wriston CC, Troxel AB, Elenitsas R, Shin DB, Guerry D, et al. Characteristics associated with early and late melanoma metastases. Cancer. 2010; 15; 116(2): 415-23.

[27] Sidky YA, Borden EC. Inhibition of angiogenesis by interferon's: effects on tumor- and lymphocyte-induced vascular responses. Cancer Res. 1987; 1; 47(19): 5155-61.

[28] Krug B, Crott R, Lonneux M, Baurain JF, Pirson AS, Vander Borght T. Role of PET in the initial staging of cutaneous malignant melanoma: systematic review. Radiology. 2008; 249(3): 836-44.

[29] Denoyer D, Greguric I, Roselt P, Neels OC, Aide N, Taylor SR, et al. High-contrast PET of melanoma using (18)F-MEL050, a selective probe for melanin with predominantly renal clearance. J Nucl Med. 2010; 51(3):441-7.

[30] Sheffield MV, Yee H, Dorvault CC, Weilbaecher KN, Eltoum IA, Siegal GP, et al. Comparison of five antibodies as markers in the diagnosis of melanoma in cytologic preparations. Am J Clin Pathol. 2002; 118(6): 930-6.

[31] Ordóñez NG, Ji XL, Hickey RC. Comparison of HMB-45 monoclonal antibody and S-100 protein in the immunohistochemical diagnosis of melanoma. Am J Clin Pathol. 1988; 90(4): 385-90.

[32] Lin F, Yang W, Betten M, Teh BT, Yang XJ; French Kidney Cancer Study Group. Expression of S-100 protein in renal cell neoplasms. Hum Pathol. 2006; 37(4): 462-70.

[33] Stone CH, Lee MW, Amin MB, Yaziji H, Gown AM, Ro JY, et al. Renal angiomyolipoma: further immunophenotypic characterization of an expanding morphologic spectrum. Arch Pathol Lab Med. 2001; 125(6): 751-8.

[34] Davis IJ, Hsi BL, Arroyo JD, Vargas SO, Yeh YA, Motyckova G, et al. Cloning of an Alpha-TFEB fusion in renal tumors harboring the t(6;11)(p21;q13) chromosome translocation. Proc Natl Acad Sci U S A. 2003; 13; 100(10): 6051-6.

[35] Veronesi U, Adamus J, Aubert C, Bajetta E, Beretta G, Bonadonna G, et al. A randomized trial of adjuvant chemotherapy and immunotherapy in cutaneous melanoma. N Engl J Med. 1982; 7; 307(15): 913-6.

[36] Kirkwood JM, Strawderman MH, Ernstoff MS, Smith TJ, Borden EC, Blum RH. Interferon alfa-2b adjuvant therapy of high-risk resected cutaneous melanoma: the Eastern Cooperative Oncology Group Trial EST 1684. J Clin Oncol. 1996; 14(1): 7-17.

[37] Hsueh EC, Gupta RK, Qi K, Morton DL. Correlation of specific immune responses with survival in melanoma patients with distant metastases receiving polyvalent melanoma cell vaccine. J Clin Oncol. 1998; 16(9): 2913-20.

[38] Morton DL, Ollila DW, Hsueh EC, Essner R, Gupta RK. Cytoreductive surgery and adjuvant immunotherapy: a new management paradigm for metastatic melanoma. CA Cancer J Clin. 1999; 49(2): 101-16, 65.

[39] Zavos G, Papaconstantinou I, Chrisostomidis C, Kostakis A. Metastatic melanoma within a transplanted kidney: a case report. Transplant Proc. 2004; 36(5): 1411-2.

[40] Gakis G, Merseburger AS, Sotlar K, Kuczyk MA, Sievert KD, Stenzl A. Metastasis of malignant melanoma in the ureter: possible algorithms for a therapeutic approach. Int J Urol. 2009; 16(4): 407-9.

[41] Török P, Kiss T. Multiple metastases of a malignant cutaneous melanoma in the cavitary system of the upper urinary tract. Int Urol Nephrol. 1997; 29(1): 19-24.

[42] Leo F, Cagini L, Rocmans P, Cappello M, Geel AN, Maggi G, et al. Lung metastases from melanoma: when is surgical treatment warranted? Br J Cancer. 2000; 83(5): 569-72.

[43] Berger AC, Buell JF, Venzon D, Baker AR, Libutti SK. Management of symptomatic malignant melanoma of the gastrointestinal tract. Ann Surg Oncol. 1999; 6(2): 155-60.

[44] Pacella M, Gallo F, Gastaldi C, Ambruosi C, Carmignani G. Primary malignant melanoma of the bladder. Int J Urol. 2006; 13(5): 635-7.

[45] Stein BS, Kendall AR. Malignant melanoma of the genitourinary tract. J Urol. 1984; 132(5): 859-68.

[46] Ainsworth AM, Clark WH, Mastrangelo M, Conger KB. Primary malignant melanoma of the urinary bladder. Cancer. 1976; 37(4): 1928-36.

[47] Siroy AE, MacLennan GT. Primary melanoma of the bladder. J Urol. 2011; 185(3): 1096-7.

[48] Li Ma, Wenying Liu and Fa Sun. Primary malignant melanoma of the prostate. Int J Urol. 2010; 17, 94–95.

[49] Nguyen AT, Kavolius JP, Russo P, Grimaldi G, Katz J, Brady MS. Primary genitourinary melanoma. Urology. 2001; 57: 633–8.

[50] Wong J, Wise GJ, Clark B. Malignant melanoma of the prostate: a case report. Can J Urol. 2008; 15(2): 4027-9.

[51] Hubler J, Pajor L, Kincses I. Primary malignant melanoma of the prostate. Acta Chir. Acad. Sci. Hung. 1980; 21: 239–43.

[52] Robutti F, Betta PG, Bellingeri M, Bellingeri D. Primary malignant melanoma of the female urethral meatus. Eur Urol. 1986; 12: 62–3.

[53] Ander H, Esen T, Tellaloglu S, Uysal V. Successful management of malignant melanoma of male urethra with local excision and adjuvant radiochemotherapy. Prog ClinBiol Res. 1991; 370:379–83.

[54] Akbas A, Akman T, Erdem MR, Antar B, Kilicarslan I, Onol SY. Female urethral malignant melanoma with vesical invasion: Case report. Kaohsiung J Med Sci. 2010;
26: 96-8.

[55] Comploj E, Palermo S, Trenti E, Lodde M, Mian C, Carella R, et al. Unexpected long survival in primary malignant melanoma of the male urethra. Case Rep Dermatol. 2009; 1: 93-9.

[56] Gupta R, Bhatti SS, Dinda AK et al. Primary melanoma of the urethra: a rare neoplasm of the urinary tract. Int Urol Nephrol. 2007; 39: 833–6.

[57] Carroll PR, Dixon CM. Surgical anatomy of the male and female urethra. Urol Clin North Am. 1992; 19: 339–46.

[58] Batsakis JG, Suarey P. Mucosal melanomas: a review. Adv Anat Pathol. 2000; 7: 167-80.

[59] Sánchez-Ortiz R, Huang SF, Tamboli P, Prieto VG, Hester G, Pettaway CA. Melanoma of the penis, scrotum and male urethra: a 40-year single institution experience. J Urol. 2005; 173(6): 1958-65.

[60] McClay EF, McClay ME. Tamoxifen: is it useful in the treatment of patients with metastatic melanoma? J Clin Oncol. 1994; 12: 617–26.

[61] Kubo H, Miyawaki I, Kawagoe M, et al. Primary malignant melanoma of the male urethra. Int J Urol. 2002; 9: 268-71.

[62] Pettaway C, Lynch D, and Davis J: Tumors of the Penis, in Wein A, Kavoussi L, Novick A, Partin A, and Peters C (Eds): Campbell- Walsh Urology, 9th ed. New York, Elsevier, 2007, 967.

[63] Benjamin S, Abeshouse. Primary and secondary melanoma of genitourinary tract. South Med J. 1958: 994-1006.

[64] Morton DL, Wen DR, Wong JH, Economou JS, Cagle LA, Storm FK, et al. Technical details of intraoperative lymphatic mapping for early stage melanoma. Arch Surg. 1992; 127(4): 392-9.

[65] Stillwell TJ, Zincke H, Gaffey TA, Woods JE. Malignant melanoma of the penis. J. Urol. 1988; 140: 72–5.

[66] Sánchez-Ortiz R, Huang SF, Tamboli P, Prieto VG, Hester G and A. Petteway C. Melanoma of the penis, scrotum and male urethra: a 40-year single institution experience. J Urol. 2005; 173: 1958-65.

[67] Orlandini V, Kolb F, Spatz A, et al. Melanoma of the penis: 6 cases. Ann Dermatol Venereol. 2004; 131: 541-4.

[68] The Japanese Skin Cancer Society. General Rules for Clinical and Pathological Studies on Malignant Neoplasms of the Skin. The Japanese Skin Cancer Society, Kanehara & Co. Ltd., 2002.

[69] Yamamoto A. Clinical study of DAV+IFN-beta therapy for malignant melanoma. Int. J. Immunotherapy. 1996; XII: 73–8.

[70] Berkmen F, Tandogdu R, and Ardjcoglu A. Primary scrotal malignant melanoma: report of 2 cases and review of the literature. J Exp Clin Cancer Res 1998; 17: 91-93.

17

The Stage of Melanogenesis in Amelanotic Melanoma

Naoki Oiso and Akira Kawada
Department of Dermatology, Kinki University Faculty of Medicine
Japan

1. Introduction

Malignant melanoma is a tumor arising from epidermal melanocytes. It is one of the most frequently occurring malignant tumors in Caucasians. Melanoma is classified into four major primary types, superficial spreading melanoma, nodular melanoma, lentigo maligna melanoma, and acral lentiginous melanoma (palmoplantar malignant melanoma) and four minor types - subungual melanoma, mucosal melanoma, secondary melanoma from an occult primary site, and multiple primary malignant melanomas. The highly undifferentiated melanoma may produce no melanin granules. The term, amelanotic melanoma, is used loosely for both true amelanotic lesions with no pigmentation and melanomas with minimal residual pigmentation. Most cases of amelanotic melamona are metastatic, but cases of primary amelanotic melanoma have been reported.
This chapter defines amelanotic melanoma and reviews the clinical and histopathological features. This chapter also provides a basic review of melanogenesis in melanosomes in the melanocytes as well as describes the uses of immunohistochemical staining for not only diagnosing melanomas but also determining the degree of differentiation of melanoma cells. As the production of melanin granules in melanosomes is distinctly regulated from stages I to IV, immunohistochemical staining may identify the damaged step in melanogenesis, which would indicate the degree of differentiation of melanoma cells in amelanotic melanoma. This chapter is designed to improve understanding of the pathogenesis of amelanotic melanoma, which is not monogeneous but heterogenous.

2. The stage of melanogenesis in amelanotic melanoma

2.1 Amelanotic melanoma

2.1.1 The definition of amelanotic melanoma

Amelanotic melanoma is used for both true amelanotic lesions with no pigmentation and melanomas with minimal residual pigmentation (Wain et al., 2008). Recently, the term "hypomelanotic melanma" is used for melanomas with faint pigmentation (Piccolo et al., 2010; Menzies et al., 2008). The melanoma cells in amelanotic melanoma cannot produce mature melanin granules, resulting in the absence of melanin granules.

2.1.2 The clinical features of amelanotic melanoma

The absence of pigmentation is the main difficulty encountered when clinically diagnosing amelanotic melanoma (Piccolo et. al., 2008). In amelanotic melanoma, the most prevalent clinical and histopathological type is nodular melanoma (Gualandri et al., 2009). The higher Breslow thickness of amelanotic melanoma may be associated with a worse prognosis (Gualandri et al., 2009). Amelanotic melanoma can develop from any type of melanoma, including superficial spreading melanoma (Holder et al., 1996), nodular melanoma (Kanoh et al., 2010; Oiso et al., 2010), lentigo maligna melanoma (Martires et al., 2010), acral lentiginous melanoma (Yasuoka et al., 1999), subungual melanoma (Gosselink et al., 2009; Matsuta et al., 2000), and mucosal melanoma (Khaled et al., 2009; Notani et al., 2002), as well as from primary amelanotic melanoma of the esophagus (Terada, 2009; Wang et al., 2008), cervix (Duggal & Srinivasan, 2010), and colon (Sashiyama et al., 2010).

Common clinical differential diagnoses of amelanotic or hypomelanotic melanoma may include hypomelanotic nevus, Spitz nevus, basal cell carcinoma, seborrhoeic keratosis, dermatofibroma, keratoacanthoma, pyogenic granuloma, haemangioma and Bowen's disease (Piccolo et al., 2008; Zalaudek et al., 2005; Blum et al., 2004; Ferrari et al., 2004; Zalaudek et al., 2004; Holder et al., 1996; Elmets & Ceilley, 1980).

Most reported cases of amelanotic melanoma are metastatic, but cases of primary lesions also have been described (Wain et al., 2008; Yanagi et al., 2005; Gupta & Lallu, 1997; Holder et al., 1996). Most primary cases are melanomas with minimal residual pigmentation or hypomelanotic melanoma. The depicted figure is a typical case; an 80-year-old Japanese woman having an asymptomatic bulky ulcerated nodule 20 mm in size, with slight pigmentation located peripherally on the left vulva (Oiso et al., 2010) (Fig. 1).

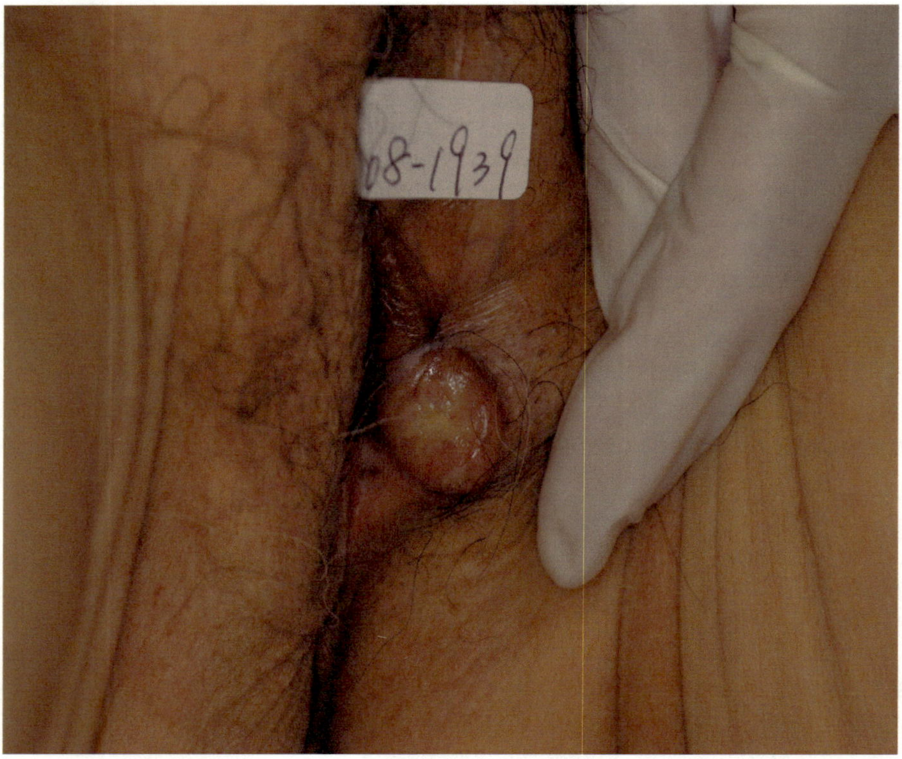

Fig. 1. An 80-year-old Japanese woman having an asymptomatic bulky ulcerated nodule 20 mm in size, with slight pigmentation located peripherally on the left vulva.

2.1.3 The histopathological features of amelanotic melanoma

Amelanotic melanoma is undifferentiated melanoma with no or few melanin granules. True amelanotic melanomas produce no melanin granules, resulting in no pigmentation, while amelanotic melanomas with minimal residual pigmentation or hypomelanotic melanomas produce a few melanin granules, resulting in some pigmentation in some part of the tumor. The histopathology of the case in Fig. 1 showed amelanotic melanomas with minimal residual pigmentation. One of the specimens had melanoma cells in the epidermis and upper dermis, with infiltration of mononuclear cells as the initial developmental lesion on the left side (Hematoxylin and eosin (HE) staining, ×100) (Fig. 2a) (Oiso et al., 2010). Massively proliferated melanoma cells were present in the dermis on the right side (Fig. 2a) (Oiso et al., 2010). The melanoma cells from the left side of the specimen had irregular shapes and large hyperchromatic nuclei with melanin granules in the upper dermis (HE, ×400) (Fig. 2b) (Oiso et al., 2010). The massively proliferated cells produced no melanin granules in the dermis on the right side (Fig. 2b) (Oiso et al., 2010). As shown here, amelanotic melanomas with minimal residual pigmentation have few melanin granules inside the tumor. However, true amelanotic melanomas have no melanin granules. The identification of melanin granules is necessary for a histopathological diagnosis of malignant melanoma other than true amelanotic melanoma.

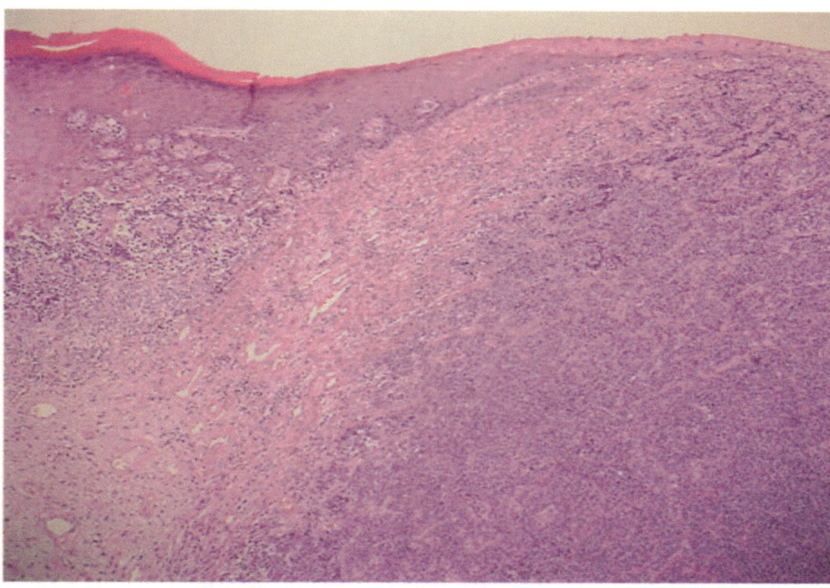

Fig. 2a. One of the specimens showed melanoma cells in the epidermis and upper dermis with infiltration of mononuclear cells as the initial developmental lesion on the left side, and massively proliferative melanoma cells in the dermis on the right side (Hematoxylin and eosinstaining (HE), ×100).

2.2 Melanogenesis in melanosomes

2.2.1The stages of melanosomes in melanocytes

Melanin granules are produced in the melanosomes in melanocytes. Each melanosome moves from the perinuclear area towards the dendrites and changes its shape from stage I to stages II, III, and IV. Stage I melanosomes (also called premelanosomes) are relatively

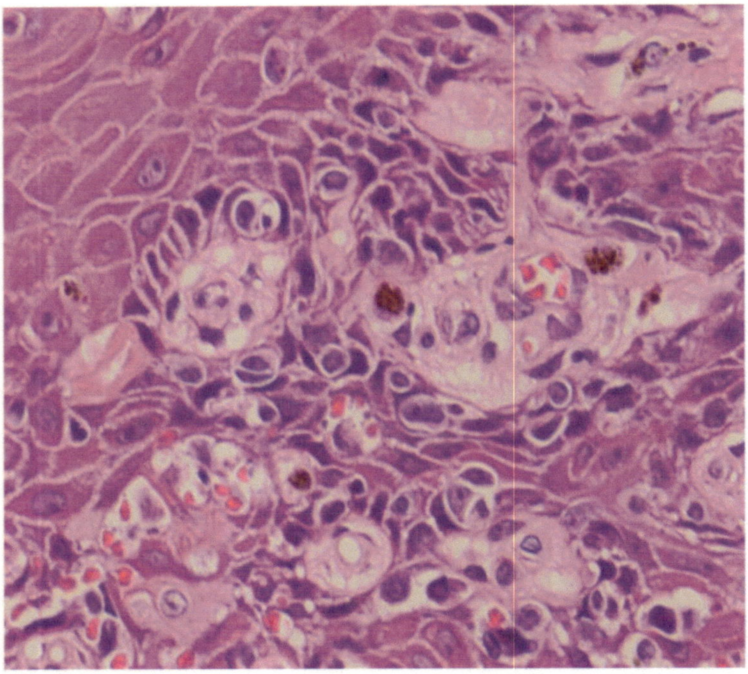

Fig. 2b. The melanoma cells from the left side of the specimen had irregular shapes and large hyperchromatic nuclei with melanin granules in the upper dermis. The massively proliferated cells in the dermis on the right side produced no melanin granules (HE, ×400).

spherical organelles with matrix material (i.e. filaments) that is beginning to assemble; stage II melanosomes are oval-shaped organelles with an organized internal matrix that does not contain melanin; stage III melanosomes are organelles with a matrix that contains deposits of melanin; and stage IV melanosomes are organelles completely filled with melanin (Boissy et al., 2006). Therefore, true amelanotic melanoma may contain stage I and/or II melanosomes, but not stage III and IV melanosomes.

2.3 Immunohistochemical staining

2.3.1 Immunohistochemical staining for diagnosis

Amelanotic melanoma is diagnosed by means of immunohistochemical staining, especially using a panel of melan-A/melanoma antigen recognized by T cells-1 (MART-1), S-100, and HMB-45 (Oiso et al, 2010). In the case shown in Fig. 1, the tumor was immunohistochemically stained with melan-A/MART-1, HMB-45, and S-100. Immunohistochemical staining with melan A/MART-1 was positive for the melanoma cells of the initially developed lesion and massively proliferated lesion (Figs. 2c, 2d) (c, ×100; d, ×400) (Oiso et al., 2010). Immunohistochemical staining with S-100 was positive for the melanoma cells of the initially developed lesion, but neative for the massively proliferated lesion except in one spot (Figs. 2e, 2f) (e, ×100; f, ×400) (Oiso et al., 2010). Immunohistochemical staining with HMB-45 was positive of for the melanoma cells of the initially developed lesion, but negative for the massively proliferated lesion (Figs. 2g, 2h) (g, ×100; h, ×400) (Oiso et al., 2010). Immunohistochemical staining is required for precisely diagnosing amelanotic melanoma.

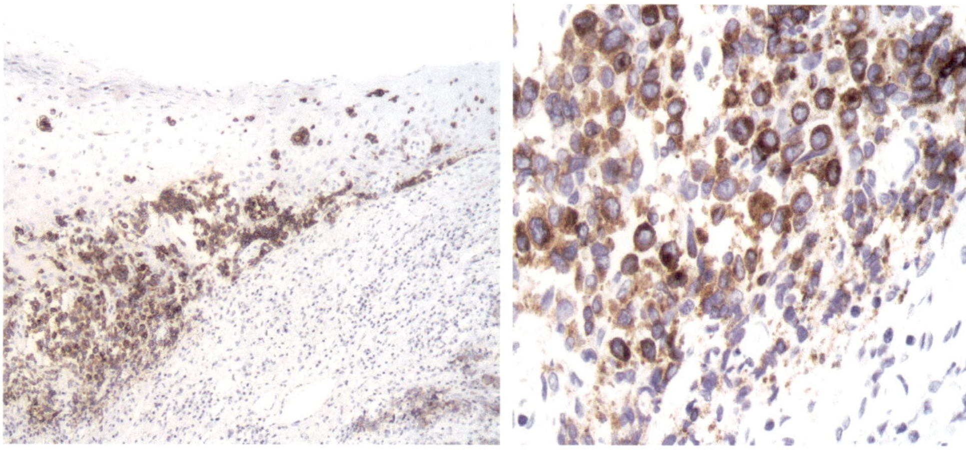

Fig. 2c-d. Immunohistochemical staining with melan A/MART-1 was positive for the melanoma cells of the initially developed lesion and the massively proliferated lesion (c, ×100, d, ×400).

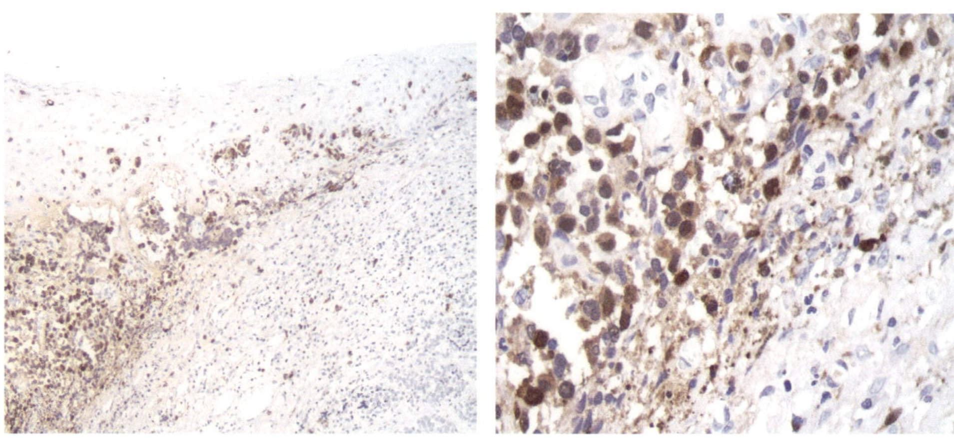

Fig. 2e-f. Immunohistochemical staining of the melanoma cells with S-100 was positive for the initially developed lesion, but negative for the massively proliferated lesion except in one spot (e, ×100, f, ×400).

Blessing *et al.* summarized the sensitivity and specificity of immunohistochemical staining using three markers for malignant melanoma: melan A/MART-1, S-100, and HMB-45 (Blessing et al., 1998). They concluded that S100 was the most sensitive marker for all primary and secondary malignant lesions and the least specific marker, that melan-A/MART-1 and HMB-45 were both highly specific, and that HMB-45 was the least sensitive of the three (Blessing et al., 1998). Several other studies have reported a similar tendency in melanin granule-producing malignant melanoma (Ohsie et al., 2008; Karimipour et al., 2004; Zubovits et al., 2003). The sensitivity of S-100, Melan-A/MART-1, and HMB-45 were 97-100%, 75-92%, and 69-93% (77-100% for primary melanomas and 56-83% for metastatic melanomas), respectively (Ohsie et al., 2008). The specificity of S-100, Melan-A/MART-1, and HMB-45 were 75-87%, 95-100%, and almost 100%, respectively (Ohsie et al., 2008).

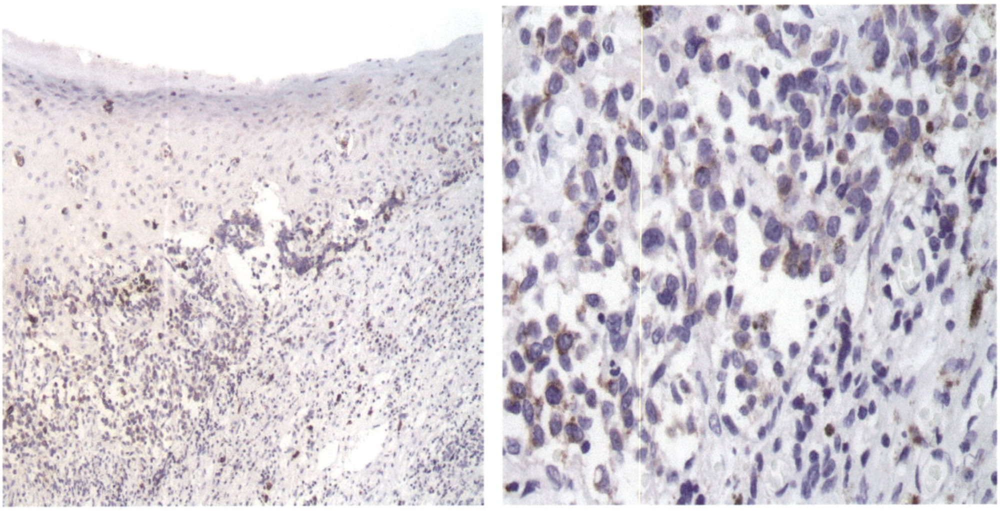

Fig. 2g-h. Immunohistochemical staining with HMB-45 was positive for the melanoma cells of the initially developed lesion, but negative for the massively proliferated lesion (g, ×100, h, ×400).

Additional candidate markers for malignant melanoma are derived from melanocytic differentiation markers, proliferation markers, immunomodulatory markers, signaling molecules, and nerve growth factors and receptors (Ohsie et al., 2008). We recommend that a tumor or a macule suspected of being a malignant melanoma be initially stained with melan-A/MART-1, HMB-45 and S-100, and, for a more precise diagnosis, secondarily stained with various markers, including microphthalmia transcription factor (MITF), tyrosine hydroxylase, tyrosinase, and tyrosinase-related proteins 1 (TRP-1) and 2 (TRP-2).

2.3.2 Immunohistochemical staining to identify the damaged step in amelanotic melanoma

Immunohistochemical stains react with the expressing and specifically modified proteins. Staining may indicate the damaged step of melanogenesis. Fig. 3 illustrates the relationship of early melanogenesis and the proteins targeted for immunohistochemical staining.

Melan-A/MART-1 is a membrane protein localized in the endoplasmic reticulum, *trans*-Golgi network, and melanosomes, especially in early melanosomes (stage I and II melanosomes) (Kawakami et al., 1994). HMB-45 specifically reacts with sialylated PMEL17/GP100 in the fibrillar matrix in the stage II melanosomes (Hoashi et al., 1996). The production of internal matrix fibers depends on the maturation and trafficking of PMEL17/GP100 (Kushimoto et. al., 2001; Hoashi et. al., 1996; Hoashi et al., 1995). In the presence of Melan-A/MART-1, PMEL17/GP100 produces melanosomal matrix fibers in melanocytes (Hoashi et al., 1995). In amelanotic melanoma, a positive reaction to both Melan-A/MART-1 and HMB-45 indicates the presence of stage I and II melanosomes; a positive reaction to only Melan-A/MART-1 indicates the presence of only stage I melanosomes. In the case shown in Fig. 1, immunohistochemical staining showed only a positive reaction to Melan-A/MART-1, indicating immature differentiation of melanosomes prior to stage II (Oiso et al., 2010).

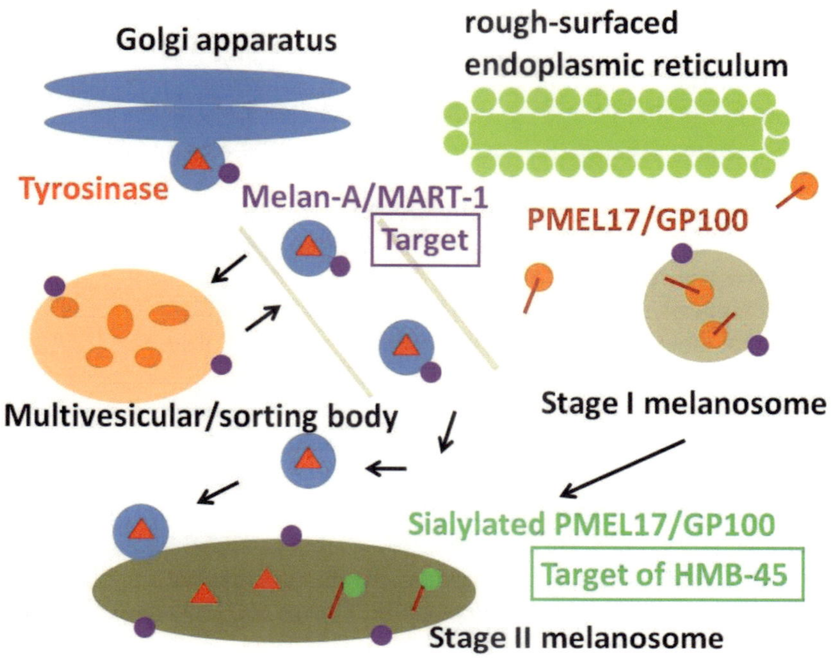

Fig. 3. The early melanogenesis in the melanocytes.

3. Conclusion

This chapter summarizes the features of amelanotic melanoma on the basis of immunohistochemical staining with melanocyte-specific proteins as targets. The results show that the damaged step in melanogenesis in amelanotic melanoma can be evaluated histopathologically. The histopathological method is useful for at least two reasons: it describes the precise pathogenesis of amelanotic melanoma with intratumor heterogeneity, and it allows the sub-classification of the damaged step in melanogenesis to be determined.

4. Acknowledgment

We thank the patient and her daughter for signing the informed consent form allowing us to describe the patient's case for scientific purposes.

5. References

Boissy, R. E., Huizing, M. & Gahl, W. A. (2006) Biogenesis of melanosomes.*in* Nordlund JJ, Boissy RE, Hearing VJ, King RA, Oetting WS, Ortonne J-P, eds: *The pigmentary system: physiology and pathophysiology*. 2nd edn. Blackwell Publishing Ltd, Oxford, pp.155-170.

Blessing, K., Sanders, D.S., Grant, J.J. (1998) Comparison of immunohistochemical staining of the novel antibody melan-A with S100 protein and HMB-45 in malignant melanoma and melanoma variants. *Histopathology* Vol.32(No.2): 139-146.

Blum, A., Jaworski, S., Metzler, G., Bauer, J. (2004) Lessons on dermoscopy: Dermoscopic pattern of hemosiderotic dermatofibroma. *Derm Surg* Vol.30(No.10): 1354.

Duggal ,R. & Srinivasan, R. (2010) Primary amelanotic melanoma of the cervix: case report with review of literature. *J Gynecol Oncol* Vol.21(No.3): 199-202.

Elmets, C.A. & Ceilley, R.I. (1980) Amelanotic melanoma as a pyogenic granuloma. *Cutis* Vol.25(No.2): 161–167.

Ferrari, A., Piccolo, D., Fargnoli, M.C., Biamonte, A.S., Peris, K. (2004) Cutaneous amelanotic melanoma metastasis and dermatofibromas showing a dotted vascular pattern. *Acta Derm Venereol* Vol.84(No.2): 164-165.

Gosselink, C.P., Sindone, J.L., Meadows, B.J., Mohammadi, A., Rosa, M. (2009) Amelanotic subungual melanoma: a case report. *J Foot Ankle Surg* Vol.48(No.2): 220-224.

Gualandri, L., Betti, R., Crosti, C. (2009) Clinical features of 36 cases of amelanotic melanomas and considerations about the relationship between histologic subtypes and diagnostic delay. *J Eur Acad Dermatol Venereol* Vol.23(No.3): 283-287.

Gupta, R.K. & Lallu, S. (1997) Cytodiagnosis of amelanotic metastatic malignant melanoma: an immunocytochemical study. *Diagn Cytopathol* Vol.16(No.3): 238-241.

Hoashi, T., Muller, J., Vieira, W.D., Rouzaud, F., Kikuchi, K., Tamaki, K., Hearing, V.J. (2006) The repeat domain of the melanosomal matrix protein PMEL17/GP100 is required for the formation of organellar fibers. *J Biol Chem* Vol.281(No.30): 21198-22208.

Hoashi, T., Watabe, H., Muller, J., Yamaguchi, Y., Vieira, W.D., Hearing, V.J. (2005) MART-1 is required for the function of the melanosomal matrix protein PMEL17/GP100 and the maturation of melanosomes. *J Biol Chem* Vol.280(No.14): 14006-14016.

Holder, J.E., Colloby, P.S., Fletcher, A., Camp, R.D. (1996) Amelanotic superficial spreading malignant melanoma mimicking Bowen's disease. *Br J Dermatol* Vol.134(No.3): 519-521.

Karimipour, D.J., Lowe, L., Su, L., Hamilton, T., Sondak, V., Johnson, T.M., Fullen, D. (2004) Standard immunostains for melanoma in sentinel lymph node specimens: which ones are most useful? *J Am Acad Dermatol* Vol.50(No.5) 759-764.

Kato, H., Inoue, Y., Ishihara, T., Kageshita, T., Ihn, H. (2010) Amelanotic malignant melanoma where primary lesion was discovered 5 years after metastasis in the lymph node. *J Dermatol* Vol.37(No.8): 730-734.

Kanoh, M., Amoh, Y., Tanabe, K., Maejima, H., Takasu, H., Katsuoka, K. (2010) Nestin is expressed in HMB-45 negative melanoma cells in dermal parts of nodular melanoma. *J Dermatol* Vol.37(No.6): 505-511.

Kawakami, Y., Eliyahu, S., Delgado, C.H., Robbins, P.F., Rivoltini, L., Topalian, S.L., Miki, T., Rosenberg, S.A. (1994) Cloning of the gene coding for a shared human melanoma antigen recognized by autologous T cells infiltrating into tumor. *Proc Natl Acad Sci U S A* Vol.91(No.9): 3515-3519.

Khaled, A., Hammami, H., Fazaa, B., Kourda, N., Kamoun, M.R., Ben Jilany, S., Zoghlami, A. (2009) Primary amelanotic anorectal melanoma: an uncommon neoplasia with poor prognosis. *Pathologica* Vol.101(No.3): 126-129.

Kushimoto, T., Basrur, V., Valencia ,J., Matsunaga, J., Vieira, W.D., Ferrans, V.J., Muller, J., Appella, E., Hearing, V.J. (2001) A model for melanosome biogenesis based on the purification and analysis of early melanosomes. *Proc Natl Acad Sci U S A* Vol.98(No.19): 10698-10703.

Martires, K.J., Capaldi, L., Pattee, S.F., Maloney, M.E., Bordeaux, J.S. (2010) Failed treatment of amelanotic lentigo maligna with imiquimod followed by pigment production. *Arch Dermatol* Vol.146(No.9): 1047-1048.

Matsuta, M., Segawa, I., Akasaka, T., Kon, S., Nara, T., Minato, S. (1990) A case of subungual amelanotic malignant melanoma: an electron microscopic study of aberrant melanosomes. *J Cutan Pathol* Vol.17(No.4): 246-250.

Menzies, S.W., Kreusch, J., Byth, K., Pizzichetta, M.A., Marghoob, A., Braun, R., Malvehy, J., Puig, S., Argenziano, G., Zalaudek, I., Rabinovitz, H.S., Oliviero, M., Cabo, H., Ahlgrimm-Siess, V., Avramidis, M., Guitera, P., Soyer, H.P., Ghigliotti, G., Tanaka, M., Perusquia, A.M., Pagnanelli, G., Bono, R., Thomas, L., Pellacani, G., Langford, D., Piccolo, D., Terstappen, K., Stanganelli, I., Llambrich, A., Johr, R. (2008) Dermoscopic evaluation of amelanotic and hypomelanotic melanoma. *Arch Dermatol* Vol.144(No.9): 1120-1127.

Notani, K., Shindoh, M., Yamazaki, Y., Nakamura, H., Watanabe, M., Kogoh, T., Ferguson, M.M., Fukuda, H. (2002) Amelanotic malignant melanomas of the oral mucosa. *Br J Oral Maxillofac Surg* Vol.40(No.3): 195-200.

Ohsie, S.J., Sarantopoulos, G.P., Cochran, A.J., Binder, S.W. (2008) Immunohistochemical characteristics of melanoma. *J Cutan Pathol* Vol.35(No.5): 433-444.

Oiso, N., Yoshida, M., Kawara, S., Kawada, A. (2010) Amelanotic vulvar melanoma with intratumor histological heterogeneity. *J Dermatol* Vol.37(No.6): 537-541.

Piccolo, D., Lozzi, G.P., Altamura, D., Fargnoli, M.C., Peris, K. (2010) Dermoscopic evolution of vascular pattern in two cases of amelanotic melanoma. *Acta Derm Venereol* Vol.90(No.1): 83-85.

Sashiyama, H., Tsujinaka, Y., Hamahata, Y., Tsutsumi, O., Hoshino, T., Minami, Y., Tsunoda, Y., Yano, M., Sato, Y. (2010) Primary amelanotic malignant melanoma of the colon. *Endoscopy* Vol.42 Suppl 2: E163-164.

Terada, T. (2009) Amelanotic malignant melanoma of the esophagus: report of two cases with immunohistochemical and molecular genetic study of KIT and PDGFRA. *World J Gastroenterol* Vol.215(No.21) 2679-2683.

Wain, E.M., Stefanato, C.M., Barlow, R.J. (2008) A clinicopathological surprise: amelanotic malignant melanoma. *Clin Exp Dermatol* Vol.33(No.3) 365-366.

Wang, S., Thamboo, T.P., Nga, M.E., Zin, T., Cheng, A., Tan, K.B. (2008) c-kit positive amelanotic melanoma of the oesophagus: a potential diagnostic pitfall. *Pathology* Vol.40(No.5): 527-530.

Yanagi, .T, Akiyama, M., Kasai, M., Yamakura, M., Nishio, M., Shimizu, H. (2005) Multiple skin metastases of amelanotic melanoma originating from the sinonasal mucosa. *Acta Derm Venereol* Vol.85(No.) 554-555.

Yasuoka, N., Ueda, M., Ohgami, Y., Hayashi, K., Ichihashi, M. (1999) Amelanotic acral lentiginous malignant melanoma. *Br J Dermatol* Vol.141(No.6): 370-372.

Zalaudek, I., Argenziano, G., Leinweber, B., Citarella, L., Hofmann-Wellenhof, R., Malvehy, J., Puig, S., Pizzichetta, M.A., Thomas, L., Soyer, H.P., Kerl, H. (2004) Dermoscopy of Bowen's disease. *Br J Dermatol* Vol.150(No.6): 1112-1116.

Zalaudek, I., Ferrara, G., Di Stefani, A., Argenziano, G. (2005) Dermoscopy for challenging melanoma. How to raise the "red flag" when melanoma clinically looks benign. *Br J Dermatol* Vol.153(No.1) 200–202.

Zubovits, J., Buzney, E., Yu, L., Duncan, L.M. (2004) HMB-45, S-100, NK1/C3, and MART-1 in metastatic melanoma. *Hum Pathol* Vol.35(No.2): 217-223.

18

The Interaction Between Melanoma and Psychiatric Disorder

Steve Kisely, David Lawrence, Gill Kelly, Joanne Pais and Elizabeth Crowe
Universities of Queensland and Western Australia
Australia

1. Introduction

This chapter explores the interaction between melanoma and psychiatric disorder, updating our work with another decade of population-based data. Although psychiatric and physical disorders, such as melanoma, frequently co-exist, the relationship between the two may be complex. Psychiatric complaints may be secondary to physical illness, may cause or exacerbate physical symptoms, or the two may merely occur by chance in the same individual. When psychiatric disorder is secondary to cancer, it can be due to cancer-related factors, cancer-treatment-related factors, psychiatric history factors and social factors.[1] Melanoma is no exception to this. This chapter examines some of these possible interactions.

2. Neuropsychiatric complications of interventions used to treat melanoma

One obvious association between melanoma and psychiatric disorders is that many of the medications used to treat melanoma have psychiatric complications. A significant proportion of patients diagnosed with any form of cancer experience psychiatric morbidity in association with diagnosis and treatment. Factors that influence or increase the risk of psychiatric co-morbidity can be categorised as cancer-related factors, cancer-treatment-related factors, psychiatric history factors and social factors.[1] When we say that an intervention is a cause of an adverse health outcome we mean that it is a contributory cause of that outcome in the sense that use of that intervention is one of a complex set of conditions that jointly produced it.[2] In order to infer that the intervention is a contributory cause we need evidence that: (1) medicine use and the health outcome co - vary; and (2) evidence that other explanations of the relationship are implausible, leaving medicine use as the most plausible explanation of the adverse health outcome.[2] However, it can often be difficult to attribute a particular psychiatric state to a specific cancer treatment/intervention. It is recognised that a range of cancer treatments can contribute to the development of psychiatric disorders in cancer patients. Disease modifying agents such as corticosteroids, chemotherapeutic agents (vincristine, vinblastine, asparaginase, intrathecal methotrexate, interferon, interleukin, amphotericin) and whole-brain radiation have all been associated with the development of depression, delirium or dementia. In addition, treatment of pain with high-dose opioids can be associated with acute confusional states (delirium), particularly in the elderly and terminally ill.[1]

There has been increasing concern about the psychiatric side effects of treatment with interferon (IFN), a therapy commonly used in the treatment of melanoma. Effects can occur shortly after beginning IFN therapy or later as a consequence of sustained treatment.[3] Neurologic and neuropsychiatric complications include headaches, visual changes, paresthesias, hyperkinesia, decreased attention and concentration, and impairments in visual scanning, verbal memory, executive function, and motor control. Psychiatric complications include depression, anxiety, mania, and suicidal ideation. More rarely, IFN may induce mixed affective states in patients with melanoma with both depressive and manic symptoms. Patients are at particular risk of developing hypomania or mania when IFN doses are changed or when IFN-induced depression is treated with antidepressants without concomitant mood stabilisers. The risk of mood fluctuation continues after treatment with IFN stops. Greenburg et al reported that 40% of interferon-treated melanoma patients reported depressed mood and 8% reported severe depression with functional impairment or suicidal ideation.[4] Adverse events following IFN treatment also include attempted and completed suicides.[3]

Neuropsychiatric effects of IFN resulting in depression and/or anxiety may be mistaken by clinicians as representing the flu-like syndrome of IFN treatment, or as a reaction to the trauma of the cancer diagnosis. It is important that clinicians are able to recognise the treatment related psychiatric side effects of IFN and other interventions used to treat melanoma.

3. The incidence and mortality of melanoma in people with psychiatric disorder

This chapter focuses on another interaction, the incidence and mortality of melanoma in people with psychiatric disorder. Studies of overall cancer incidence and mortality in psychiatric patients have had mixed results. Some authors have reported lower than expected cancer incidence or mortality in psychiatric patients, whilst others have found no association.[5-7] Still others have found an increased risk of incidence or mortality.[8, 9] Some of this discrepancy may be explained by differences between psychiatric diagnoses. Schizophrenia has particularly been associated with a reduced incidence of cancer, including melanoma.[10-15] The possible reasons for this are discussed in section 3.4. The use of different methodologies and cancer outcomes may also account for some of the conflicting results. For instance, some studies are restricted to patients in hospital.[16] The reporting of cohort age at study conclusion may be an additional critical confounder. Populations where patients are not followed up to an age when cancer incidence and mortality is maximal may underestimate cancer mortality and incidence, making SMRs complex to interpret. Finally, cancer mortality may not be an ideal marker of the risk of cancer as it is affected by both the susceptibility to developing the disorder, and subsequent survival rates.[17]

Our population-based studies from Western Australia and Nova Scotia addressed some of these issues by evaluating both the incidence and mortality associated with melanoma at the same time in the same population using a standard methodology.[18] The studies used the administrative databases of each jurisdiction, which have several advantages over community surveys or data derived from individual clinical settings[19], in that they provide accessible longitudinal data for an entire jurisdiction at relatively little cost. In both, rates were calculated using the inception cohort method.[20] The start of follow-up was taken as the date of each patient's first contact with mental health services. Patients were censored at the time of occurrence of the event under study, death, or the end of follow-up. The cohort was limited to people whose first contact with a clinician occurred in the study period, excluding people whose first contact occurred prior to the start of follow-up. This avoids the possibility of survivorship bias, which could otherwise occur if cancer risk changes with time since first contact with a clinician. After reviewing our previous work from Western Australia and Nova Scotia, we present another decade of Australian data to further explore these relationships through to 2007.

3.1 The psychiatric disorders of interest

The psychiatric disorders that form the focus of this chapter include all the mental and behavioural conditions covered in Chapter 5 of ICD9 (290 through 319 inclusive), or ICD10 chapter F. These capture organic psychiatric disorders such as dementia, alcohol and substance use disorders, psychosis, non-psychotic diagnoses including depression, anxiety, and somatoform conditions, and personality and adjustment disorders. Some of the studies also capture ICD external cause codes X60 – X84 (Intentional Self Harm) and non-Chapter 5 codes that cover health service use for mental health issues in the absence of a formal psychiatric diagnosis.

3.2 The Western Australia study 1982-1998

Within the WA Health Services Research Linked Database, we identified all psychiatric patients in Western Australia who had a diagnosis of cancer. The dataset contains information from several different core data sets. These were the Hospital Morbidity Data System (HMDS), the register of births, the register of deaths, Mental Health Information System, and the Cancer Registry. The Mental Health Information System (MHIS) is a register of patients who have had contact with state run community-based or outpatient mental health services in WA or who have been psychiatric inpatients of any public or private hospital in the state since 1966. Although the MHIS has been operating since 1966, the WA Cancer Register only commenced in 1982. Thus the linked cancer registrations covered the period 1982 to 1998. Diagnoses were coded according to ICD-8 until 1978 and according to ICD-9 from 1979 onwards. The last occurring psychiatric diagnosis across the episodes was then assigned as the principal diagnosis according to a hierarchy of diagnoses. If an earlier diagnosis was higher in the hierarchy than the last recorded diagnosis, then the earlier diagnosis was taken as the principal diagnosis. The hierarchy was as follows:

i. ICD-9 290, 293±296: dementia, organic psychotic conditions, schizophrenia and affective psychosis.
ii. ICD-9 291±292, 297±305, 313±315: alcohol and drug psychoses, paranoid states, other nonorganic psychoses, neurotic disorders, personality disorders, sexual deviations, alcohol and drug dependence, and childhood disorders.
iii. ICD-9 306±312, 317±319: adjustment reaction, reaction to stress, depressive disorders nec[1], conduct disorders nec, special syndromes nec and mental retardation.
iv. Other than chapter 5 (mental disorders) diagnoses.

Preference was given to diagnoses made in inpatient treatment units over diagnoses made in acute inpatient units or longer-term psychiatric residential units. Diagnoses made prior to 1979 were mapped from ICD-8 to ICD-9 using the nearest equivalent code. The purpose of these procedures was to allow more specific psychiatric diagnoses to take precedence over less specific diagnoses, and to favour an underlying condition rather than a non-specific

[1] Not elsewhere classified

symptom or event. Cancers were classified according to the ICD-9 classification of diseases at the three-digit level. This classification followed the same system used for classifying cancers by the WA Cancer Register.

Overall there were 672 melanoma patients, of whom 285 were male (Table 1). Males were significantly less likely to be diagnosed as having a melanoma while females had the same rate as that of the general population. There was little variation between psychiatric diagnoses although conclusions were limited by the small number of cases for some of the categories (Table 1). In no case was incidence higher than that of the general population (Table 1).

Proportional hazards regression analysis was used to examine the difference in case fatality between psychiatric patients with cancer and other cancer patients in the general population. After adjusting for demographic factors, there was a 103% higher case fatality following a diagnosis of melanoma in male psychiatric patients than in the general population (95% CI: 46% - 282%) and an 89% higher case fatality rate in females (95% CI: 43%-274%). This represented the highest case fatality rate ratios for any cancer site.

Psychiatric diagnosis	Male			Female		
	N	RR	95% CI		RR	95% CI
Dementia	12	0.67	(0.19 -2.45)	9	0.47	(0.02 – 14.5)
Alcohol/drug disorders	35	0.41	(0.18 -0.94)	12	0.46	(0.13 - 1.59)
Schizophrenia	22	0.76	(0.42 - 1.38)	20	0.93	(0.50 - 1.71)
Affective psychosis	19	0.70	(0.33 - 1.49)	43	1.06	(0.73 - 1.54)
Other psychoses	6	0.62	(0.15 -2.54)	12	0.49	(0.14 – 1.71)
Neurotic disorders	67	0.99	(0.76 - 1.30)	129	1.10	(0.91 - 1.33)
Personality disorders	20	1.29	(0.85 - 1.95)	15	1.26	(0.76 – 2.10)
Stress/Adjustment reaction	8	0.46	(0.09 - 2.37)	24	0.78	(0.45 - 1.38)
Depressive disorder	8	0.61	(0.19 - 1.93)	21	0.99	(0.57 - 1.70)
Other mental disorder	31	0.79	(0.48 - 1.30)	26	0.72	(0.38 - 1.34)
Attempted self-harm	14	0.68	(0.29 - 1.61)	26	1.14	(0.76 – 1.70)
Non-specific diagnosis	43	1.11	(0.84 - 1.46)	50	0.85	(0.60 - 1.21)
Total	285	0.75	(0.64 - 0.89)	387	0.92	(0.82 – 1.04)

Table 1. Cancer Site - Malignant Melanoma, by Principal Psychiatric Diagnosis. WA 1982 – 1998.

3.3 The Nova Scotian study

The West Australian administrative data do not include treatment for mental health disorders in private settings. Accordingly, studies from Australia, where both private health insurance and hospitals play a sizable role in providing medically necessary care, may not apply to jurisdictions such as Canada with universal health care provision. We therefore compared cancer incidence, first admission and mortality rates for people with psychiatric disorder in relation to the general population of one Canadian province, Nova Scotia. In addition, the Australian data were restricted to people in contact with specialist mental health services and did not include primary care where the majority of people with mental health problems are treated. Lastly Canadian data allowed for the study of patterns of melanoma in a less sunny environment.

Under the Canada Health Act, all Canadian residents are entitled to inpatient or outpatient care that is free at the point of delivery.[21] Patients receive treatment at publicly -funded facilities or are seen by private psychiatrists or general practitioners in the community who bill the Provincial health plan. However, the Provincial health plan does not cover visits to private psychologists or other mental health professionals in private practice. Importantly, there are no private psychiatric beds.[21]

We evaluated the association between mortality and psychiatric disorder for all patients of specialist services and primary care across Nova Scotia, using the province's linked administrative databases. The one-million residents have similar morbidity and mortality rates to the rest of Canada, although more live in rural areas than in other provinces. Halifax is the major metropolitan centre.

We evaluated the association between cancer mortality and psychiatric disorder for all patients of specialist services and primary care across Nova Scotia. We used the following Provincial administrative databases, held at the Population Health Research Unit (PHRU) of Dalhousie University, to identify anyone in contact with health services for psychiatric problems:[22]

- The Medical Services Insurance (MSI) database of all fee-for-service claims by physicians including patient demographics, date of service and diagnosis from the Clinical Modification of the 9th Revision of the International Classification of Diseases (ICD-9-CM). This includes family physicians and psychiatrists.
- The Canadian Institute for Health Information (CIHI) Discharge Abstract Database (DAD), which includes admissions, separation dates, diagnoses and procedures.
- Mental Health Outpatient Information System data (MHOIS), which records service contacts, demographics and diagnoses in the public sector. This includes contacts with all mental health clinicians, not just physicians.

This method was consistent with the definition used by the Public Health Agency of Canada (PHAC) for the surveillance of treated psychiatric disorder.[19, 23] As in Western Australia, we used an inception cohort. We included patients whose first psychiatric contact with primary or specialist services occurred between January 1, 1995 and December 31, 2001, and linked data using the provincial health card number as a unique identifier. Health card numbers are present in over 99% of records irrespective of database, and encrypted to ensure confidentiality.

We included everyone with ICD 9 codes of 290 through 319 inclusive, or their ICD-10 (chapter F) or DSM-IV equivalents. We also included non-specific mental disorders outside Chapter 5 of ICD-9 (formal mental disorders), such as injury of undetermined intention or psychosocial factors influencing health status, to ensure comparability with previous Australian work.[17] We did not include non-chapter 5 diagnoses of primary care patients, as they would not necessarily be psychiatric. We included contacts with primary or specialist services. We used a hierarchy of inpatient versus outpatient, and specialist versus primary care, reflecting both the increasing percentage of patients with severe mental illness and data reliability. It also allowed comparison with Australian data

We then transferred this data file to Cancer Care Nova Scotia who linked it to the Nova Scotia Cancer Registry (NSCR) to identify cancer incidence rates for the cohort. The NSCR has population-based incidence data that dates from 1964.[28] All malignant and in-situ tumours are reportable by law within the province. Other sources of data include Pathology Reports (1982 onwards) and death certificate information for all provincial deaths (from

1989 onwards). Registry operations meet the consensus on cancer registration standards outlined by both the Canadian Cancer Registry (CCR) and the North American Association of Central Cancer Registries (NAACCR).[18] The NSCR works collaboratively with Statistics Canada to ensure that Nova Scotia data is part of the national Canadian Cancer Registry. We classified cancers according to the ICD-9 classification of diseases at the three-digit level. This classification followed the same system used for classifying cancers by the NSCR. The cancer sites selected for analysis were the most frequent cancers in males and females.

We grouped disorders into dementia and other organic conditions (290-294), schizophrenia (295), other non-affective psychoses (297, 298.0, 298.1), alcohol/drug disorders (303-305), mood disorders (affective psychoses/depression-296, 298.2-298.9, 300.4, 311), neuroses (300 except 300.4), personality disorders (301), adjustment reactions (308-309), and other mental disorders (all remaining Chapter 5 diagnoses and those outside Chapter 5). Rates were again calculated using the inception cohort method.[20] The start of follow-up was taken as the date of each patient's first contact with a mental health clinician. Patients were censored at the time of occurrence of the event under study, death, or 31st December 2001. The cohort was limited to people whose first contact with a mental health clinician occurred in the study period, excluding people whose first contact occurred prior to the start of follow-up. We derived mortality rates from the Statistics Canada Vital Statistics Database. Person-years at risk were calculated separately for each outcome.

We calculated age- and sex-adjusted mortality, first admission and incidence rates for carcinoma by direct standardisation, using the average population distributions in Nova Scotia from 1995-2001 inclusive as the standard weights. We then calculated rate ratios (RRs) relative to the rate in the general NS population, using 95% confidence intervals to test for significance. Variance of the standardised rate ratios was calculated using expansion in Taylor series, using a logarithmic transformation of the ratio.[24] We assessed whether the rate ratios for mortality, first admission and incidence in psychiatric patients were significantly different from the general population of Nova Scotia as indicated by 95% confidence intervals that included a value of 1.0. We also assessed whether there were differences between mortality, first admission and incidence rate ratios. Unlike the Australian study, we were not able to investigate predictors of cancer incidence using Cox regression of NSRC records because of the nature of the data sharing agreement and therefore were unable to compare adjusted hazard ratios for incidence, first admission and mortality.

Table 2 presents the unadjusted rate ratios. Incidence rate ratios (RRs) were lower than might be expected given the mortality and first admission RRs, and no higher than that of the general population. By contrast the mortality rate was higher especially for men.

Gender	**Mortality rate**			**Cancer Incidence**		
	N	RR	95% CI	N	RR	95% CI
Males	17	2.18	(1.34-3.44)	151	1.05	(0.92-1.21)
Females	3	1.37	(0.64-2.92)	99	0.91	(0.73-1.07)
Total	20	2.00	(1.20 - 3.30)	250	0.98	(0.85-1.14)

Table 2. Comparing Cancer Incidence and Cancer Mortality rates: Nova Scotia, 1995 - 2001.

Melanoma was only one of a few cancers to show this pattern, the others being prostate, bladder and colorectal cancers. This pattern was especially noticeable in males (Figure 1).

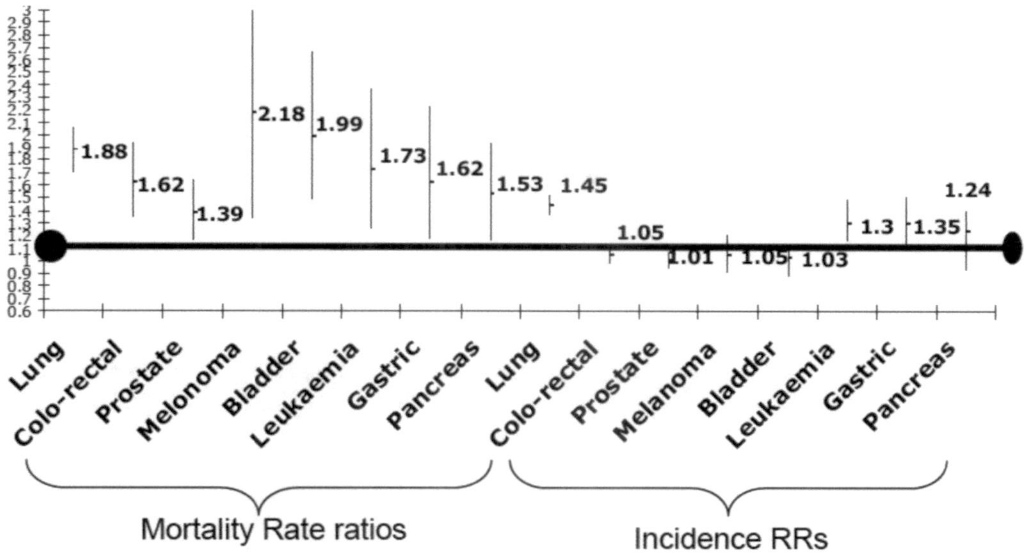

Fig. 1. Comparing cancer mortality & incidence in male Nova Scotian psychiatric patients

3.4 Implications of both studies

There is a common assumption that problems in self-care might explain the increased mortality from cancer, including melanoma, for patients with psychiatric disorder. If that were the sole explanation, incidence would consistently reflect the increased mortality rate. However, our work in both Canada and Australia suggests that psychiatric patients are no more likely to develop melanoma than the general population but still have increased mortality for the same condition. There may be a number of explanations for this increased case fatality rate. One might be that psychiatric patients present later, and with more advanced disease, than the general population. Another possibility is reduced access to general medical care. If doctors are less inclined to treat skin cancer in people with psychiatric disorder than in others, people with psychiatric disorder and skin cancer might be less likely to be admitted to hospital and therefore be selectively missed by researchers. This inequity would be of concern, and would confirm work from Ontario showing that other marginalised populations, such as those of low income, are less likely to receive specialist procedures such as adjuvant or palliative radiotherapy.[25]

Decreased screening for early lesions could also explain the increased mortality so that psychiatric patients only present when symptoms or signs become more obvious in later stages of the disease. In places without universal health care, ability to pay for care may be a factor. Even with universal health care, psychiatric patients may have problems in registering with a family physician, missed appointments, or difficulties in communication or scheduling appointments. Finally, psychiatric patients may have a worse prognosis even after adjusting for staging at presentation. Survival from cancer is associated with levels of depression, emotional expression and support. Some work suggests that individuals with depression prior to the diagnosis of the cancer have a worse survival rate than those with depression following diagnosis.[26] In the case of melanoma, several psychosocial variables measured at baseline are independently prognostic of survival. [26] The greatest protective effect was conferred by a belief that treatment would lead to cure or long-term survival and by marital status. [26] For those patients who were positive about the outcome of their treatment (i.e., who thought treatment would cure them or prolong their life long term), the risk of dying was reduced by 65%. Similarly, for patients who were married, the risk of dying was reduced by 50%. Two aspects of psychological adjustment were also protective. Patients who reported that their melanoma did not greatly affect their day-to-day life survived significantly longer than those who felt it was having a big impact on their lives, and those who exhibited greater levels of anger about their situation survived longer. Finally, quality of life scores were also significantly predictive of outcome. Further support for the importance of psychiatric factors in survival from melanoma comes from findings that structured group psychotherapy may help extend survival.

3.5 The special case of schizophrenia

In the case of schizophrenia, there is a suggestion that the incidence of skin cancer including melanoma is especially lower than the rest of the population. A Danish record linkage study investigated the incidence of cancer in a cohort of 9156 first admitted schizophrenic patients.[13] Reduced cancer incidence was particularly marked for genital cancers, and skin cancers, including malignant melanoma. The standardised incidence ratio for malignant melanoma was 0.14, although the study was limited by small numbers (1 case of melanoma). Goldacre and colleagues reported a similar finding in a cohort analysis of linked hospital and death records comparing cancer rates in people with schizophrenia with a reference cohort in the south of England[27]. They reported an adjusted rate ratio for melanoma of 0.2 (95% CI 0.02-0.74). A recent meta-analysis of cancer incidence rates in patients with schizophrenia combined 16 data collections from 15 studies. The pooled standardised incidence rate ratio of melanoma in patients with schizophrenia was significantly reduced (SIR 0.71 CI 0.57-0.87). A similar finding was reported for prostate cancer.[28]

Several biological hypotheses have been proposed to explain why people with schizophrenia might be protected against cancer in general, including a protective effect of excess dopamine, enhanced natural killer cell activity, an increase in the rate of apoptosis and modulation by antipsychotic drugs of the human cytochrome enzymes involved in mutagen activation and elimination[27].

There may be other reasons that are more specific to melanoma. One possibility is that people with schizophrenia may spend less time in the sun than the general population, and this may be compounded by issues such as weight gain (a common side effect of anti-psychotic medication) that may reduce both the desire and ability to engage in physical activity outdoors. Conversely if they do go out into the sun, people with schizophrenia might be less likely to take protective measures such as sunscreen or a hat. Against this explanation is that malignant melanoma is mainly related to childhood sun exposure,[29] and there is no evidence of reduced childhood sun exposure in individuals who subsequently develop schizophrenia.

In addition, sun exposure, perhaps through its role in vitamin D synthesis, may actually have a protective role in the development of schizophrenia. [30] McGrath has suggested that vitamin D deficiency in the neonate might be a risk factor for the subsequent development of schizophrenia. The same author also suggested that relative vitamin D deficiency might explain some of the epidemiological features of schizophrenia such as the excess of winter births, and the increased incidence of schizophrenia in dark-skinned migrants when they move to countries with more limited sunshine[31]. It is therefore possible that an inverse relationship between sun exposure and the development of schizophrenia could also partially explain why melanoma is seen less frequently in people with schizophrenia.

4. Our latest findings

We extended our work with another decade of data from Western Australia to further explore these relationships through to 2007. As before we used the linked administrative data from Western Australia from 1988 to 2007 employing the same databases. We also extended our study to the Australian State of Queensland, which has the highest rate of melanoma in Australia. On this occasion we investigated whether the pattern of psychiatric patients being no more likely to develop melanoma than the general population, but still having increased mortality for the same condition could be related to either:

1. delayed diagnosis or late presentation by comparing cancer staging at the time of diagnosis in psychiatric patients & the general population as determined by the presence of metastases; or
2. reduced access to specialised cancer therapy such as chemotherapy, radiotherapy and surgery once the diagnosis has been made.

If the former were true, it would indicate that specific action is required to ensure that clinicians and patients themselves consider the diagnosis of cancer in response to new symptoms, and that psychiatric patients are encouraged by their GP to attend, and are able to access appropriate routine cancer screening services. If the second were true it would indicate inequity of access to surgery, and adjuvant or palliative radio- and chemotherapy.

To investigate the first question, we calculated the proportion of patients with metastases at diagnosis, as melanoma staging is not collected in the cancer registry in WA. This was undertaken by extracting the behaviour code, which forms the end digit of the morphology code, a code that must be provided should a neoplasm ICD10 code be recorded (C00 - C96, D00 - D48). Behaviour code /6 refers to a malignant neoplasm that is stated or presumed to be secondary so a morphology code of M8720/6 refers to melanoma that is stated or presumed to be secondary. Also ICD10 code C80 is a malignant neoplasm of unknown primary origin; these have also been extracted to represent secondary cancers at diagnosis. In Queensland, the cancer registry does collect data on melanoma staging based on Clark's level, thickness and ulceration but it is impossible to determine when the cancer metastasised. Data on the time of metastasis were therefore extracted from hospital admissions using ICD10 codes C77 - C79, which are the particular ICD10 codes for a secondary cancer site. We also measured the proportion of patients developing metastases at 90 days and one year after presentation.

To investigate the second question, we collected basic information on cancer treatment, including chemotherapy (yes/no), radiotherapy (yes/no) and surgery (yes/no). For surgery we also collected information on time to surgery from diagnosis. For palliative care we assessed the proportion of cases that had at least one course of palliative radiotherapy (PRT) in the last 2 years of life. This measure has been used elsewhere as a proxy for access to radiotherapy services.[32] For surgery we collected information on time to surgery from diagnosis. We used the method of Valery, Coory et al in their studies of cancer services in Indigenous Queenslanders to compare access to chemotherapy, radiotherapy and surgery.[23]

4.1 Aims

The aims were to investigate the following:

1. To compare the incidence and mortality of melanoma in psychiatric patients and the general population of Western Australia and Queensland from 1988 to 2007 (2002 to 2007 in the case of Queensland) and to determine whether there are significant

differences between types of psychiatric illness (e.g. schizophrenia, affective disorder) in incidence, and mortality rates.

2. To determine whether psychiatric patients present at a more advanced stage of melanoma at diagnosis than the general population as determined by the presence of metastases and whether there is a difference in cancer stage at presentation between male and female psychiatric patients.
3. To determine whether psychiatric patients have a poorer prognosis after controlling for cancer stage at presentation and whether there is a difference in prognosis between males and females.
4. To determine whether psychiatric patients diagnosed with cancer access surgical services equally in comparison with the general population diagnosed with cancer, and whether there is a difference in access by gender.
5. To determine whether psychiatric patients diagnosed with cancer access adjuvant or palliative chemotherapies & radiotherapies equally in comparison with the general population , and whether there is a difference by gender

4.2 The hypotheses

The hypotheses were that:

1. Psychiatric patients would be more likely to present with more advanced cancer, as determined by the presence of metastases.
2. Psychiatric patients would also be less likely to receive the appropriate specialist surgical procedures, adjuvant or palliative chemotherapies & radiotherapies than the general population, even after adjusting for socio-demographic and clinical features (including the presence of metastases).
3. These effects would be more marked for patients with severe mental illnesses in terms of either diagnoses (e.g. schizophrenia) or of having ever required admission to a psychiatric unit, and more marked in men than women.

4.3 Study design

This was a population-based record-linkage analysis from the two Australian states (Western Australia and Queensland), using a historical cohort to calculate rate ratios. In the case of the Western Australian data we also calculated rate ratios using the inception cohort method. We could not do the same for the Queensland data as these did not extend far enough to identify an inception cohort. It is important to do both. Inception cohort studies that study incident psychiatric cases over a period of time are less subject to survivorship bias given that the majority of excess deaths due to physical causes occur in the first seven years after psychiatric diagnosis.[17] However as they are based on incident cases, there may be fewer subjects than a study based on prevalence, and so a greater chance of insufficient statistical power. This is particularly relevant for less common outcomes such as mortality in individual psychiatric diagnoses that are less common such as schizophrenia. Using an inception cohort also allowed comparison with our previous studies from Western Australia and Canada. Historical cohorts are based on prevalent psychiatric cases and so yield larger numbers. They are therefore more appropriate for rarer outcomes. In this case, use of an historical cohort allowed the addition of Queensland data, so further increasing statistical power. On the other hand, historical cohorts may underestimate overall mortality risk because of survivorship bias.

4.4 Data sources

The project used linked datasets provided by the data linkage centres of Queensland and Western Australia. Both form part of Australia's Population Health Research Network (PHRN) (Figure 2). PHRN is a national network of Australia's extensive health data that provides linkage across data sets in all States and Territories for population health research (Figure 2). Subject anonymity was preserved by a rigorous privacy protocol, as it was not possible to obtain informed consent given we were using large population datasets. In each case, the relevant data custodian provided demographic data, but no other information, to data linkage centres within the Health Department of each jurisdiction. Within the linkage centre, probabilistic and deterministic matching were used to link within and between the datasets based on identifying information (ID), including name, date of birth, aliases, sex, and Indigenous status. Each person was assigned a unique project ID that was returned to the data custodians. The data custodian attached the relevant clinical or service information to the unique project ID, but no identifying information. These anonymised data extracts were then released to the researchers.

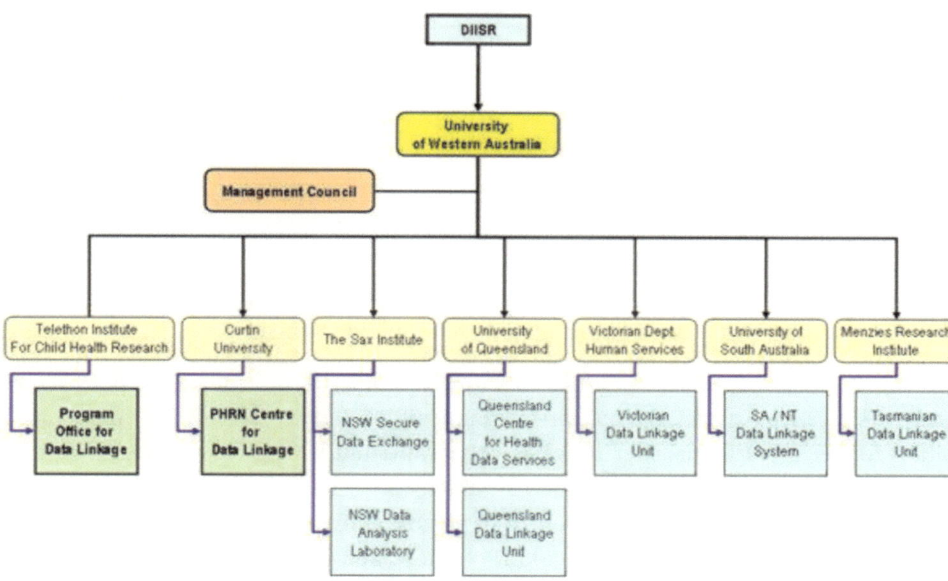

Fig. 2. Australia's Population Health Research Network.

4.4.1 Western Australia

We identified users of mental health services in WA with cancer registrations and death records, using the WA Health Services Research Linked Database. In this database, individual patient records have been linked by means of probabilistic matching, using the Automatch software package,[33] as there are no unique identification numbers in use on the core data sets. Name, residential address, date of birth and sex are the principal fields used in the probabilistic matching.[20] The probabilistic matching technique is based on estimating the probability that any two records represent the same person (or event), while allowing for the possibility of errors or changes in the identifying information used for matching.[20] The dataset contains information from several different core data sets. As before, we used the following: Hospital Morbidity Data System (HMDS), the register of births, the register of deaths, Mental Health Information System, and the Cancer Registry (Figure 3). The Mental Health Information System is a register of patients who have had contact with state run community-based or outpatient mental health services in WA or who have been psychiatric inpatients of any public or private hospital in the state.

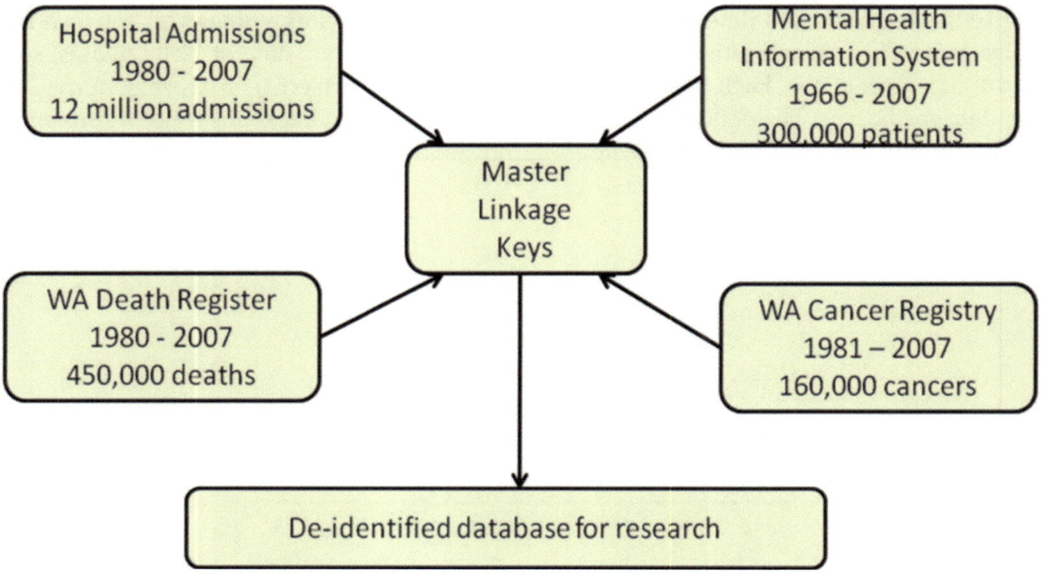

Fig. 3. Schema of the WA Health Services Research Linked Database

Within the WA Health Services Research Linked Database, we identified all psychiatric patients in Western Australia who had a diagnosis of cancer. We used the same case definition for psychiatric disorder that has been validated by the Public Health Agency of Canada (PHAC) for use in administrative databases.[23] This is any contact with a health service with an ICD-9 diagnosis of 290-319 or ICD10 equivalent. As stated previously, we used both the historical and inception cohort method. For the latter, we restricted the study cohort to those patients whose first contact with mental health services occurred between 1988 and December 2007. The start of follow-up was the date of each patient's first contact with mental health services.

Patients were censored at the occurrence of the event under study, death, or 31st December 2007. We compared the outcomes of this cohort to the general population through the calculation of age-, sex-standardised rates, which were then adjusted for confounders using multivariate analyses (see section 4.6 on statistical methods). Outcomes were mortality, metastases and access to surgery or radiotherapy. Data linkage of all administrative data, including epidemiological databases, was carried out by the Data Linkage Branch at the WA Department of Health which houses the Western Australian Health Linked Database.

4.4.2 Queensland

We used a similar methodology in Queensland. We extracted data from the following datasets: the Queensland Hospital Admitted Patients' Data Collection (QHAPDC), the Client Event Services Application (CESA - now called CIMHA, community integrated mental health application), Queensland Cancer Registry (including death data), BreastScreen QLD and the Australian Bureau of Statistics Estimated Resident Population (Table 3). As in Western Australia, we identified all psychiatric patients in Queensland with the diagnosis of cancer using the Public Health Agency of Canada (PHAC) case definition of psychiatric disorder. In this case, the Link King software package was used to link individual patient records probabilistically and deterministically.

Data source	Data obtained
Queensland Hospital Admitted Patients' Data Collection	In-patients receiving treatment in a designated psychiatric unit in a public hospital or public psychiatric hospital in QLD; all cancer admissions in public & private hospitals and all co morbidity data in the twelve months prior to the cancer diagnosis (Charlson Deyo)
Client Event Services Application (CESA)	Clients receiving treatment in a public-sector community mental health service
Queensland Cancer Registry	All QLD cancer registrations, with details of diagnosis including date, ICD-10 site code, morphology code. Data on people who die of cancer or cancer patients who die of other diseases linked to mortality files of the Registrar of Births, Deaths & Marriages & linked to hospital & pathology data.
BreastScreen QLD	All voluntary screening records for patients subsequently diagnosed with breast cancer
Australian Bureau of Statistics	Estimated resident population for all of Queensland

Table 3. Queensland data sources

4.5 Data quality

The WA Health Services Research Linked Database is unique in Australia and one of only a small number of comprehensive record linkage systems in the world.[20] These include the Oxford Record Linkage Study, the Scottish Record Linkage System, the Rochester Epidemiology Project, the Manitoba Population Health Information System, the Nova Scotian linkable database system and the Scandinavian case registers. Probabilistic matching of records is based on estimating the probability that any two records represent the same person (or event), while allowing for the possibility of errors or changes in the identifying information used for matching. The WA Data Linkage System uses a chain of links method to map the linkage of records. Each individual source record from each of the component data sets is assigned a unique record number. Separate individuals are then identified by assigning a number to identify the chain, called the root number. This root number is the record number of the first record in the chain for each person. A master linkage file records pointers specifying the root number for each individual source record in the system, enabling chains of records for each individual to be created.

The master linkage file is date stamped and records the history of all updates to the system, so the state of the linkage can be reconstructed as it existed on any previous date.[20] The construction of the WA Linked Database and its ongoing maintenance are performed by an extramural unit of the Centre for Health Services Research located within the Health Information Centre. Access to identifying information is restricted to the staff of the extra-mural unit. Once the data have been linked, a second de-identified copy of the WA Linked Database is created. The de-identified version does not contain names, addresses (except for postcode), dates of birth (except for month and year of birth), individual hospital identifiers or individual doctor identifiers. Most research is conducted from this second de-identified copy of the database. The system allows for the protection of the confidentiality of individual patients and the information contained in the administrative health records, while still allowing population-based health services research to be performed.

The WA Health Services Research Linked Database currently contains in excess of 12 million records, and occupies over 12 Gb of storage space. By far the largest component of the database is the Hospital Morbidity Data System (HMDS) which contains over 7 million records. The register of births contains around 400,000 entries, while the register of deaths contains approximately 450,000 entries. The MHIS contains details for just over 300,000 patients of mental health services (Figure 3). As the WA Data Linkage System brings together separate records for each person, it is possible to examine the consistency of recording fixed personal characteristics such as sex, aboriginality, and date of birth. For each of these characteristics, the entire set of records for each patient have been examined to check that the field was recorded the same in all core data records regardless of their source. Overall, sex was consistently recorded across all records for 98.5% of the study population, aboriginality was consistently recorded for 97.3% of the study population and date of birth was consistently recorded (to an exact date) for 83.3% of the study population

Data linkage in Queensland has not progressed as far as that in Western Australia since the state has only recently begun developing linkage infrastructure whereas WA began this process in 1995. There are a large number of databases available but currently linkages exist only within the Queensland Hospital Admitted Patient Data Collection (QHAPDC) for years 2003/04-2008/09 and between QHAPDC and the Registrar General's (RG) Mortality data. RG mortality data is available from 1996 onward and contains approximately 360,000 records. RG birth data (over 64,000 records in 2010) is also available but the exact dates that are available for research are yet to be determined and this collection hasn't yet been linked with other databases. QHAPDC data collection began in January 1993 and on average there are about 1.8 million episodes of care added to the QHAPDC database each year. Episodes of care for admitted mental health patients are also captured within this database and a mental health module was added in July 1996. Non-admitted mental health patients that are seen by community mental health facilities are included in the Consumer Integrated Mental Health Application (CIMHA) database which, over a five year period (2006 - 2010), contained over 280,000 consumer (patient) records.

There is also less information on the quality of the Queensland data as these datasets have only recently been used for research. Some published information is available on the quality of variables such as Indigenous status, which can be defined either through place of residence or through the recording of Indigenous status in datasets such as the Queensland Hospital Admitted Patient Data Collection (QHAPDC). Indigenous status is correctly identified in about 89% of cases with variation by definition used.[34]

4.6 Statistical methods

We identified cancer type, cancer stage at diagnosis by cancer type, principle psychiatric diagnosis, and time from psychiatric contact with service until cancer incidence. We initially calculated the age- and sex-standardised mortality rate, cancer incidence and proportion with metastases at diagnosis for all cancers for anyone meeting the PHAC case definition of psychiatric disorder. We used the method of Lawrence et al. to group cases in terms of severity of psychiatric diagnosis.[20] We also calculated separate age- and sex-standardised ratios for cases who had ever had inpatient psychiatric treatment as opposed to those who had only had outpatient treatment, as a marker of psychiatric disease severity. Finally we calculated rates of surgery, and adjuvant or palliative radio- and chemotherapy in the same way.

The average population distribution in Western Australia over the period 1988-2007 was used as a standard weight. In all cases we used direct standardisation. Rates were calculated overall, and by principal psychiatric diagnosis. Relative risks for mortality, 1st admissions, incidence, and cancer stage for different cancer types were calculated in groups of patients in the study cohort relative to the rate in the WA population. Denominators were taken from estimated resident population counts. We compared relative risks by psychiatric diagnosis, cancer type, diagnostic case complexity and treatment setting (ever admitted as an in-patient versus outpatient or community care).

The relative importance of factors that were identified on univariate analysis as being associated with the particular outcome under study (e.g. presence of metastases, mortality) were further analysed using the Cox proportional hazards model. This methodology requires the identification of a terminal event that marks either survivors or non-survivors. Consequently, there are two basic requirements for a survival analysis design- time of origin into the study and the meaning of failure. In our study, the former was entry into the study, and the failure was defined as mortality. One advantage of survival analysis is that it allows an examination of data from all participants who entered the study over the sampling timeframe (until the end of the study) without imposing arbitrary cut-off dates on the data. Participants who were still alive at the end of the study were treated as censored observations (i.e. an observation for which the event does not occur). Cox's model allowed us to quantify the weight of or significance of variables that increased or decreased the risk of admission. Using the statistical technique of "backward elimination," we eliminated non-significant variables from each group of variables sequentially in order to retain the relative risk of each significant variable. For longitudinal items (e.g. mortality), we included the presence of metastases, as well as all other relevant socio-demographic & clinical variables. Survival analysis is more appropriate than logistic regression for studying time to event data (e.g. time to mortality following cancer diagnosis) while logistic regression is useful in developing an initial model.

4.7 Preliminary results

We present initial results from the Western Australian arm of the study, as Queensland data are as yet unavailable. Because the results are confined to Western Australia, we have given greater prominence to the inception, as opposed to historical cohort although we present the results of both. For all persons in WA between 1988 - 2007, malignant melanoma represented approximately 10% of all diagnosed cancers in people with a psychiatric disorder (n 618 / 6586).

4.7.1 Baseline characteristics

During this period there were 618 psychiatric patients in the inception cohort who had a diagnosis of malignant melanoma, 285 of whom were male (Table 4). There were 14,059 non psychiatric patients with melanoma. Both males and females were significantly less likely to be diagnosed as having a melanoma than the general population. There was little variation between psychiatric diagnoses although conclusions were limited by the small number of cases for some of the categories. The only disorders associated with increased incidence were Other Psychoses and Other Mental Disorders (both male and female) as well as Attempted Self Harm (females). Melanoma incidence in patients with schizophrenia was no higher than that of the general population, although the 95% confidence intervals were wide, reflecting the small number (24) of patients with schizophrenia who developed melanoma (Table 4). Some diagnoses were actually associated with increased melanoma risk: attempted self harm in females and other psychoses and other mental disorder in both males and females. There was no clear pattern with the other diagnoses, again possibly because of small numbers and wide confidence intervals.

Psychiatric diagnosis	Male			Female		
	N	RR	95% CI	N	RR	95% CI
Dementia	37	0.87	(0.63 - 1.19)	52	0.90	(0.80 - 1.02)
Alcohol/drug disorders	20	0.79	(0.51 - 1.21)	7	1.10	(0.78 - 1.54)
Schizophrenia	12	0.90	(0.68 - 1.19)	12	1.21	(0.86 - 1.71)
Affective psychosis	39	1.03	(0.79 - 1.35)	40	0.86	(0.63 - 1.19)
Other psychoses	28	1.33	(1.05 - 1.69)	18	2.12	(1.71 - 2.63)
Neurotic disorders	17	0.72	(0.43 - 1.19)	42	0.93	(0.66 - 1.29)
Personality disorders	6	1.47	(0.93 - 2.32)	5	1.30	(0.91 - 1.86)
Stress/Adjustment reaction	37	0.83	(0.55 - 1.25)	48	0.86	(0.56 - 1.32)
Depressive disorder	40	0.89	(0.63 - 1.25)	62	1.12	(0.90 - 1.39)
Other mental disorder	28	1.35	(1.01 - 1.80)	13	1.44	(1.12 - 1.86)
Attempted self-harm	5	1.38	(0.95 - 2.02)	5	2.24	(1.62 - 3.11)
Non-specific diagnosis	16	1.05	(0.73 - 1.51)	29	1.14	(0.91 - 1.43)
Total	285	0.72	(0.61 - 0.86)	333	0.84	(0.73 - 0.96)

Table 4. Cancer Site - Malignant Melanoma, by principal psychiatric diagnosis. WA, 1988 – 2007 (inception cohort).

In both psychiatric patients and the general population, melanoma incidence rate increased with age. The rate was higher in males than in females, except in psychiatric patients between the ages of 35-55 years. The peak incidence for both the general population and psychiatric patients was between 75 – 85 years of age (Figure 4).

In the case of the historical cohort, there were 1,166 psychiatric patients who had a diagnosis of malignant melanoma, 526 of whom were male (Table 5). On average, incidence rates using the historical cohort method were slightly lower than those calculated using the inception cohort approach. As in the inception cohort, males and females were significantly less likely to be diagnosed as having a melanoma. There was little variation between psychiatric diagnoses although conclusions were again limited by the small number of cases for some of the categories. As before, rates increased with age and the rate was higher in males than in females, except between the ages of 35-55 years (data not shown).

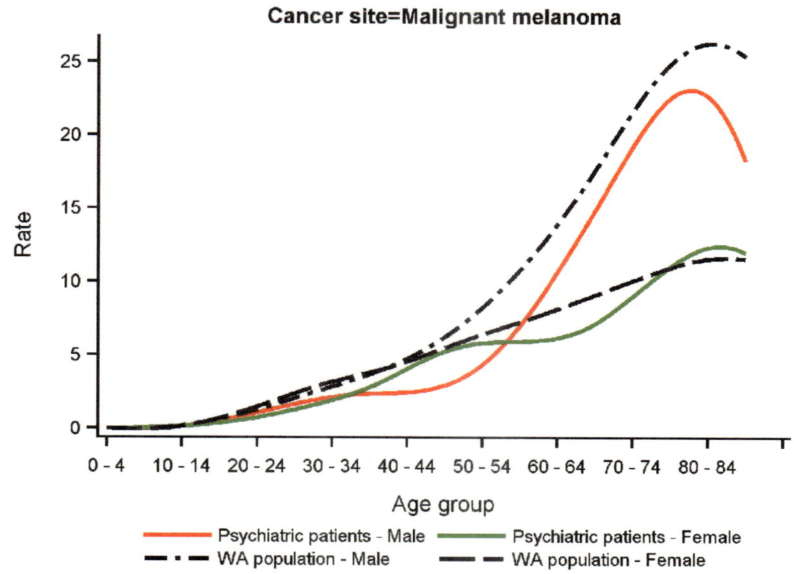

Fig. 4. Age-specific melanoma incidence rates, psychiatric patients versus WA population (inception cohort).

With greater numbers (n=57), melanoma incidence in people with schizophrenia was significantly lower in both males (0.51 - 95% CI 0.29 - 0.92) and females (0.68 - 95% CI 0.46 - 0.99). Again with more subjects and narrower confidence intervals, melanoma incidence was also lower in dementia and affective psychoses in both sexes. They were lowest in males with alcohol and drug disorders. The only situation where incidence was higher than that of the general population was for females who attempted self harm (Table 5).

Psychiatric diagnosis	Male			Female		
	N	RR	95% CI	N	RR	95% CI
Dementia	59	0.69	0.51 - 0.93	67	0.79	0.71 - 0.88
Alcohol/drug disorders	36	0.49	0.29 - 0.82	16	0.78	0.52 - 1.18
Schizophrenia	33	0.51	0.29 – 0.92	24	0.68	0.46 – 0.99
Affective psychosis	67	0.71	0.51 – 0.99	88	0.68	0.50 – 0.93
Other psychoses	44	0.81	0.58 – 1.15	29	1.08	0.70 – 1.67
Neurotic disorders	48	0.76	0.54 – 1.06	83	0.78	0.58 – 1.04
Personality disorders	19	0.98	0.67 – 1.44	15	0.91	0.60 – 1.38
Stress/Adjustment reaction	53	0.61	0.39 – 0.98	84	0.69	0.46 – 1.03
Depressive disorder	68	0.68	0.48 – 0.95	135	0.90	0.74 – 1.09
Other mental disorder	44	1.06	0.77 – 1.48	24	1.16	0.86 – 1.55
Attempted self-harm	6	1.13	0.86 – 1.48	11	1.61	1.17 – 2.20
Non-specific diagnosis	49	0.86	0.64 – 1.16	64	1.02	0.79 – 1.30
Total	526	0.60	0.52 – 0.70	640	0.71	0.64 – 0.80

Table 5. Cancer Site - Malignant Malignant Melanoma, by principal psychiatric diagnosis. WA, 1988 – 2007 (historical cohort).

4.7.2 Presence of metastases at baseline or follow-up

50 inception cohort patients with primary melanoma had metastasised at time of original diagnosis as determined from the tumour behaviour code (8.1%) This was not significantly different from that of the general population (9.9% - p = 0.107).
Ninety days later, 3 patients had developed metastases. Again there was no difference between psychiatric patients and the general population (0.5% and 0.6% p=0.771). By one year, 7 patients had developed metastases. As before, there was no difference between psychiatric patients and the general population (1.2% and 1.6% respectively P=0.332).
For the historical cohort, 86 (7.4%) patients with an assigned primary melanoma had metastasised at time of original diagnosis as determined from the tumour behaviour code. This was slightly yet significantly different from the general population 9.9% p=0.002. Ninety days later, 7 patients had developed metastases. Again there was no difference between psychiatric patients and the general population (0.6% and 0.6% respectively p=0.720). By one year, 12 patients had developed metastases. As before, there was no difference between psychiatric patients and the general population (1.1% and 1.6% respectively p=0.157).

4.7.3 Receipt of chemotherapy or radiotherapy and time to surgery

We then investigated differences between psychiatric patients and the general population with regards access to surgery and receipt of chemotherapy and radiotherapy. 0.7% (n=4) of psychiatric patients received chemotherapy for their melanoma within 90 days of diagnosis compared with 1% of melanoma patients with no contact with MHS. This difference was not statistically significant (p=0.216, Table 6). A similar proportion of psychiatric patients and people from the general population received radiotherapy (p=0.196 Table 6).

Procedure	Cohort	
	Inception	No contact with MHS
Started chemotherapy within 90 days of cancer diagnosis	0.7%	1.0%
Received radiotherapy	1.4%	2.1%

Table 6. Receipt of chemotherapy and radiotherapy.

We found similar results for the historical cohort (data not shown).
Finally, we investigated time to surgical removal of tumour. In the inception cohort 126 psychiatric patients with malignant melanoma received surgical intervention within 90 days of cancer diagnosis. There was no significant difference between psychiatric patients and the general population in time to surgery (Figure 5) (p=0.473). Again, we found similar results for the historical cohort (data not shown).

4.7.4 Mortality in psychiatric patients with melanoma

Using the inception cohort approach, 149 psychiatric patients with malignant melanoma died during the follow-up period. Of these deaths, 58 were coded as primary cause of death being malignant melanoma (Table 7). Of the 2,840 deaths during the follow-up period among malignant melanoma patients who had not had any prior contact with mental health services, 1,558 deaths were classified as malignant melanoma being the primary cause (Table 7).

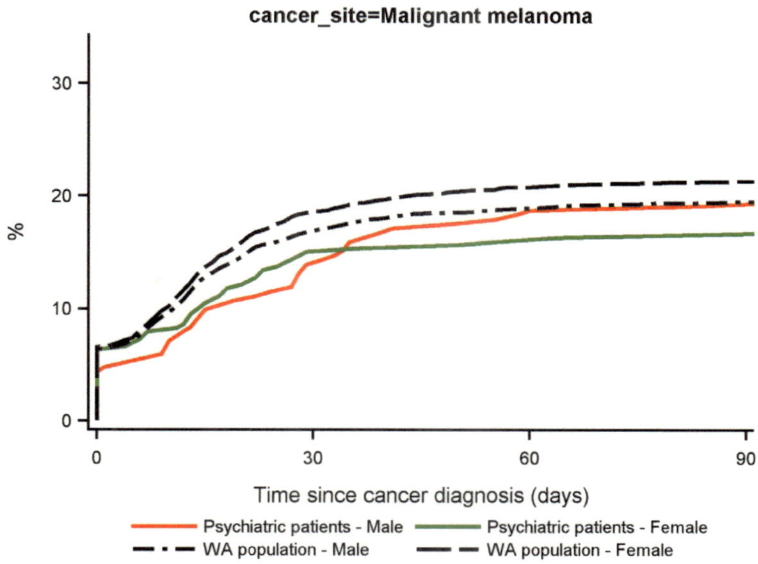

Fig. 5. % of patients who accessed surgery up to 90 days after diagnosis of their melanoma, WA, 1988 - 2007.

	Inception cohort		**Historical cohort**	
	Psychiatric case	Non Psychiatric case	Psychiatric case	Non Psychiatric case
All cause mortality	149	2840	263	2840
All cause hazard ratio	1.81 (1.53 - 2.14)		1.67 (1.47 - 1.90)	
Cancer specific mortality	58	1558	118	1558
Cancer specific hazard ratio	1.34 (1.03 - 1.74)		1.32 (1.10 - 1.60)	
Total patients with melanoma	618	14059	1166	14059

Table 7. Mortality in Psychiatric Patients with Melanoma WA, 1988 - 2007.

We compared the mortality rates between melanoma patients with and without a history of contact with mental health services using proportional hazards regression. This model allowed us to adjust for differences in the age and sex make-up of the two different cohorts. After adjusting for age, sex and socio-economic status (based on area of residence), psychiatric patients had a higher risk of all cause- and melanoma-specific mortality (Table 7). The difference between these two rates indicates that melanoma patients with a history of contact with mental health services were more likely to die as a direct result of melanoma, and also more likely to die from other causes. After malignant melanoma itself, the most common cause of death among melanoma patients with a history of contact with mental health services was coronary heart disease. In common with our findings on cancer incidence, all-cause and cancer specific mortally were lower in the historical than in the inception cohort. However both were significantly greater than those of the general population.

5. Discussion

There is literature on the adverse affect of depression on survival from melanoma. There is also literature on the incidence of melanoma in people with schizophrenia, and whether this is lower than that of the general population.[35, 36] Lastly, there is limited literature comparing incidence and mortality in patients of specialist psychiatric services.[17] To our knowledge, these studies conducted in WA and QLD are the first to investigate melanoma incidence and mortality rates in people with psychiatric disorder that include outpatient data, where the vast majority of people receive treatment. Our findings therefore give a fuller picture of the relationship between psychiatric disorder and melanoma. Another strength is the use of both inception and historical cohort data, exploiting the advantages of each. Historical cohorts may have greater statistical power because of increased numbers, but may underestimate mortality risk because of survivorship bias. Our findings of lower incidence and mortality rates in the historical as opposed to inception cohort would be consistent with this pattern. Inception cohorts may be more sensitive to the increased mortality risk faced by patients but be underpowered to detect rarer outcomes. Again, this was suggested by our study where analysis of subgroups, such as schizophrenia only yielded significant results in our historical cohort.

Our latest findings confirm our previous work on melanoma from Western Australia and Canada. With a further 10 years of data we found a continued pattern of an incidence that was lower, or no higher, than that of the general population alongside a mortality that was higher. This pattern is not unique to melanoma and has been identified for other cancers such as lung, colorectal, breast and prostate cancers even after adjusting for factors such as smoking.[28] Studying melanoma has particular advantages as this site may be less affected by potential medication or lifestyle confounders such as diet or alcohol and substance use. Studies of cancers, such as colorectal and lung, can only control for known lifestyle confounders and, even then, it is not possible to adjust for all of these.[28] By contrast, malignant melanoma is mainly related to childhood sun exposure,[29] and there is no evidence of reduced childhood sun exposure in individuals who subsequently develop psychiatric disorder.[28] As such, this cancer may be less subject to confounding by concurrent factors of lifestyle.

As regards schizophrenia, our historical cohort findings are consistent with a large meta-analysis by Catts et al that reported significantly reduced standardised incidence ratios (SIRs) for malignant melanoma of 0.71 for patients with schizophrenia (CI 0.57–0.87; P = 0.002).[28] The absence of any significant reduction in our inception cohort may be partly explained by the low numbers (n=24). Our historical cohort results also suggest that this effect extends to other psychiatric diagnoses, which tends to militate against biological hypotheses of why people with schizophrenia might be protected against cancer in general. Biological explanations include a protective effect of excess dopamine, enhanced natural killer cell activity, increased apoptosis, or modulation by antipsychotic drugs of cytochrome enzymes involved in mutagen activation and elimination, as well as the hypothesis of relative vitamin D deficiency.[27]

If biological explanations may be less applicable to the pattern we observed for melanoma for people with all types of psychiatric disorder, other hypotheses merit consideration. One is that cancer is undiagnosed in people with psychiatric disorder. Reduced cancer incidence rates in psychiatric disorder in general, and schizophrenia in particular, could be due to lower detection rates related to poorer self-care and substandard preventive health care.[28] However, it has been argued that while medical comorbidity in general is under-recognized, this does not seem to apply to cancer in general.[28] For instance, post-mortem data collected between 1966 and 1980 in Denmark, where the autopsy rates were in the order of 30–50% in both patients with schizophrenia and the general population, indicated that the post-mortem diagnosis of previously unrecognized cancer was rare. It is unclear whether these findings would apply to melanoma because unlike cancers such as lung or colorectal cancer, there may be few obvious early symptoms.[28]

Another explanation is that people with psychiatric disorder receive poorer care. Work from Ontario shows that other marginalised populations, such as those of low income, are less likely to receive specialist procedures such as adjuvant or palliative radiotherapy, even under universal health care.[32] We have also shown that psychiatric patients are less likely to receive appropriate specialised procedures for cardiovascular disease in both Australia and Canada.[17, 37] In the case of the former, one explanation might be that many of the procedures are carried out in the private health system for which people with many psychiatric disorders would be unable to find insurance. This would not apply to Canada, where the private health sector has no role in the provision of medically necessary procedures.

It is possible that physicians are reluctant to offer some procedures because of the ensuing psychological stress, concerns about capacity or compliance with postoperative care, or the presence of contra-indications such as smoking. In addition, psychiatric patients may be more at risk of developing complications following medical or surgical interventions[38] or to have poorer outcomes post-operatively.[39]

So what do our latest results suggest about the role of under-diagnosis, delayed diagnosis or inequity in treatment? Our project could not address the first explanation as this would require a detailed investigation of death register or post-mortem records to ascertain the presence of melanoma at death that had not been previously treated. Our study does not particularly shed light on the other two explanations. Psychiatric patients in the historical cohort were significantly more likely to have metastases at time of original diagnosis ($p=0.002$). Otherwise, psychiatric patients were no more likely to present with metastases, or develop them 90 days or 1 year afterwards, than the general population. Neither were they less likely to receive specialised procedures such as radio- or chemotherapy.

These findings would be consistent with work on cancer in general showing there is little evidence of delayed detection in people with psychiatric disorder such as schizophrenia.[28] However, as discussed in the following paragraph, this study may have been under-powered to detect any difference in the presence of metastases, or of treatment access.

5.1 Study limitations

We used routinely collected administrative data to maximise coverage across the state, keep within budget and maximise statistical power. However reliance on secondary data meant that we were unable to collect information on quality of life. The WA cancer register does not contain information on staging other than the presence or absence of metastases. Administrative data may also be subject to recording bias, especially for diagnosis. Most data concerning the validity of our case–definition of treated psychiatric disorder are for overall morbidity rather than specific diagnoses. We have therefore emphasised overall psychiatric morbidity, not sub-categories, to minimise possible bias. We were unable to study the effects of lifestyle such as use of sunscreen and sun exposure. However, this would not explain our finding of an increased risk of mortality in the presence of an incidence that was no higher than that of the general population. We were unable to separately study the relationship between specific psychiatric disorder and melanoma because of small numbers. In a similar vein, this study may have been under-powered to detect any difference in the presence of metastases, or of treatment access. Our results so far have been confined to Western Australia. The addition of Queensland data covering a population that is more than double that of Western Australia may address study power. In addition, the Queensland Cancer Registry has the advantage over Western Australia of collecting staging data on melanoma. Lastly, we were only able to capture data on access to surgery as well as admissions for radio- or chemotherapy, and so cannot comment on access to other interventions for melanoma.

6. Conclusions

This chapter has illustrated some of the complex interactions between melanoma and psychiatric disorder. It extends our previous work with another decade of Australian data to further explore these relationships through to 2007. These findings provide further evidence of a melanoma incidence in psychiatric patients that was lower or no higher than that of the general population alongside a mortality that was higher. Furthermore, this pattern extends to a broad range of psychiatric disorders and not just schizophrenia, where the low incidence of melanoma was first described. Although we were unable to show any clear reason in terms of delays in presentation as shown by metastases, or of access to treatment, the availability of just West Australian data may have meant the study was underpowered. The addition of Queensland data may rectify this. More research is certainly needed on why psychiatric patients with melanoma are more likely to die of the condition, but no more likely to develop it in the first place. This has implications for both primary and secondary care, including access to appropriate treatment for psychiatric patients with melanoma, as well as of awareness of the psychiatric symptoms of treatments for melanoma.

7. Acknowledgements

Funding for this study came from the Griffith Institute for Health and Medical Research and the Cancer Council of Queensland.

8. References

[1] Breitbart W. Identifying patients at risk for, and treatment of major psychiatric complications of cancer. *Support Care Cancer*. 1995;3:45-60.

[2] Hall W, Kisely S, Wilson F. *Report of the Psychiatric Drug Safety Expert Advisory Panel*. Canberra: Therapeutic Goods Administration, Australian Government Department of Health and Ageing; 2009.

[3] Trask PC, Esper P, Riba M, et al. Psychiatric side effects of interferon therapy: prevalence, proposed mechanisms, and future directions. *J Clin Oncol*. 2000;18:2316-26.

[4] Greenberg DB, Jonasch E, Gadd MA, et al. Adjuvant therapy of melanoma with interferon-alpha-2b is associated with mania and bipolar syndromes. *Cancer*. 2000;89:356-62.

[5] Black DW, Winokur G. Cancer mortality in psychiatric patients: the Iowa Record-linkage Study. *Int J Psychiatry Med.* 1986;16:189-97.
[6] Casadebaig F, Quemada N. Mortality in psychiatric inpatients. *Acta Psychiatr Scand.* 1989;79:257-64.
[7] Saku M, Tokudome S, Ikeda M, et al. Mortality in psychiatric patients, with a specific focus on cancer mortality associated with schizophrenia. *Int J Epidemiol.* 1995;24:366-72.
[8] Lichtermann D, Ekelund J, Pukkala E, et al. Incidence of cancer among persons with schizophrenia and their relatives. *Arch Gen Psychiatry.* 2001;58:573-8.
[9] Brown S, Inskip H, Barraclough B. Causes of the excess mortality of schizophrenia. *Br J Psychiatry.* 2000;177:212-7.
[10] Barak Y, Achiron A, Mandel M, et al. Reduced cancer incidence among patients with schizophrenia. *Cancer.* 2005;104:2817-21.
[11] Cohen M, Dembling B, Schorling J. The association between schizophrenia and cancer: a population-based mortality study. *Schizophr Res.* 2002;57:139-46.
[12] Dalton SO, Mellemkjaer L, Thomassen L, et al. Risk for cancer in a cohort of patients hospitalized for schizophrenia in Denmark, 1969-1993. *Schizophr Res.* 2005;75:315-24.
[13] Mortensen PB. The occurrence of cancer in first admitted schizophrenic patients. *Schizophr Res.* 1994;12:185-94.
[14] Grinshpoon A, Barchana M, Ponizovsky A, et al. Cancer in schizophrenia: is the risk higher or lower? *Schizophr Res.* 2005;73:333-41.
[15] Gulbinat W, Dupont A, Jablensky A, et al. Cancer incidence of schizophrenic patients. Results of record linkage studies in three countries. *Br J Psychiatry Suppl.* 1992:75-83.
[16] Hippisley-Cox J, Vinogradova Y, Coupland C, et al. Risk of malignancy in patients with schizophrenia or bipolar disorder: nested case-control study. *Arch Gen Psychiatry.* 2007;64:1368-76.
[17] Lawrence D, Holman CD, Jablensky AV, et al. Excess cancer mortality in Western Australian psychiatric patients due to higher case fatality rates. *Acta Psychiatr Scand.* 2000;101:382-8.
[18] Kisely S, Sadek J, MacKenzie A, et al. Excess cancer mortality in psychiatric patients. *Can J Psychiatry.* 2008;53:753-61.
[19] Kisely S, Lin E, Lesage A, et al. Use of administrative data for the surveillance of mental disorders in 5 provinces. *Can J Psychiatry.* 2009;54:571-5.
[20] Lawrence D, Jablensky AV, Holman CD. *Preventable physical illness in people with mental illness.* Perth: University of Western Australia; 2001.
[21] Kisely S, Smith M, Lawrence D, et al. Mortality in individuals who have had psychiatric treatment: population-based study in Nova Scotia. *Br J Psychiatry.* 2005;187:552-8.
[22] Population Health Research Unit. Research Data Repository. Halifax: Dalhousie University; 2007; Available from: http://metadata.phru.dal.ca/.
[23] Gilbert C, Jones W, Schopflocher D, et al. *Use of provincial administrative data for surveillance of mental disorders: feasibility study.* Ottawa: Surveillance Division, Centre for Chronic Disease Prevention and Control, Public Health Agency of Canada; 2007.
[24] Rothman KJ. *Modern Epidemiology.* Boston, MA: Little, Brown and Company; 1986.

[25] Paszat LF, Mackillop WJ, Groome PA, et al. Radiotherapy for breast cancer in Ontario: rate variation associated with region, age and income. *Clin Invest Med.* 1998;21:125-34.
[26] Butow PN, Coates AS, Dunn SM. Psychosocial predictors of survival in metastatic melanoma. *J Clin Oncol.* 1999;17:2256-63.
[27] Goldacre MJ, Kurina LM, Wotton CJ, et al. Schizophrenia and cancer: an epidemiological study. *Br J Psychiatry.* 2005;187:334-8.
[28] Catts VS, Catts SV, O'Toole BI, et al. Cancer incidence in patients with schizophrenia and their first-degree relatives - a meta-analysis. *Acta Psychiatr Scand.* 2008;117:323-36.
[29] Marks R. Epidemiology of melanoma. *Clin Exp Dermatol.* 2000;25:459-63.
[30] Kellett J, James WH, Moskovitz RA. Seasonality in Schizophrenia. *Lancet.* 1978;311:664.
[31] McGrath J. Hypothesis: is low prenatal vitamin D a risk-modifying factor for schizophrenia? *Schizophr Res.* 1999;40:173-7.
[32] Huang J, Zhou S, Groome P, et al. Factors affecting the use of palliative radiotherapy in Ontario. *J Clin Oncol.* 2001;19:137-44.
[33] Jaro M. *Automatch Generalized Record Linkage System. User's Manual.* Burtonsville, MD: Matchware Technologies Inc; 1996.
[34] Kennedy B, Howell S, Breckell C. *Indigenous identification in administrative data collections and the implications for reporting Indigenous health status.* Brisbane: Queensland Health, Health Statistics Centre; 2009.
[35] Levav I, Lipshitz I, Novikov I, et al. Cancer risk among parents and siblings of patients with schizophrenia. *Br J Psychiatry.* 2007;190:156-61.
[36] Osborn DP, Levy G, Nazareth I, et al. Relative risk of cardiovascular and cancer mortality in people with severe mental illness from the United Kingdom's General Practice Rsearch Database. *Arch Gen Psychiatry.* 2007;64:242-9.
[37] Kisely S, Smith M, Lawrence D, et al. Inequitable access for mentally ill patients to some medically necessary procedures. *CMAJ.* 2007;176:779-84.
[38] Daumit GL, Pronovost PJ, Anthony CB, et al. Adverse events during medical and surgical hospitalizations for persons with schizophrenia. *Arch Gen Psychiatry.* 2006;63:267-72.
[39] Mallik S, Krumholz HM, Lin ZQ, et al. Patients with depressive symptoms have lower health status benefits after coronary artery bypass surgery. *Circulation.* 2005;111:271-7.